State of the Art in Idiopathic Pulmonary Fibrosis

State of the Art in Idiopathic Pulmonary Fibrosis

Editors

Malgorzata Wygrecka
Elie El Agha

MDPI • Basel • Beijing • Wuhan • Barcelona • Belgrade • Manchester • Tokyo • Cluj • Tianjin

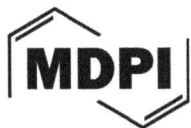

Editors

Malgorzata Wygrecka
Department of Internal Medicine
Justus-Liebig University Giessen
Giessen
Germany

Elie El Agha
Department of Internal Medicine
Justus-Liebig University Giessen
Giessen
Germany

Editorial Office
MDPI
St. Alban-Anlage 66
4052 Basel, Switzerland

This is a reprint of articles from the Special Issue published online in the open access journal *Cells* (ISSN 2073-4409) (available at: www.mdpi.com/journal/cells/special_issues/Cells_Idiopathic_Pulmonary_Fibrosis).

For citation purposes, cite each article independently as indicated on the article page online and as indicated below:

LastName, A.A.; LastName, B.B.; LastName, C.C. Article Title. *Journal Name* **Year**, *Volume Number*, Page Range.

ISBN 978-3-0365-6385-5 (Hbk)
ISBN 978-3-0365-6384-8 (PDF)

© 2023 by the authors. Articles in this book are Open Access and distributed under the Creative Commons Attribution (CC BY) license, which allows users to download, copy and build upon published articles, as long as the author and publisher are properly credited, which ensures maximum dissemination and a wider impact of our publications.

The book as a whole is distributed by MDPI under the terms and conditions of the Creative Commons license CC BY-NC-ND.

Contents

Preface to "State of the Art in Idiopathic Pulmonary Fibrosis" vii

Elie El Agha and Malgorzata Wygrecka
State of the Art in Idiopathic Pulmonary Fibrosis
Reprinted from: *Cells* **2022**, *11*, 2487, doi:10.3390/cells11162487 1

Roxana Maria Wasnick, Irina Shalashova, Jochen Wilhelm, Ali Khadim, Nicolai Schmidt and Holger Hackstein et al.
Differential LysoTracker Uptake Defines Two Populations of Distal Epithelial Cells in Idiopathic Pulmonary Fibrosis
Reprinted from: *Cells* **2022**, *11*, 235, doi:10.3390/cells11020235 7

Yu-Qing Lv, Ge-Fu Cai, Ping-Ping Zeng, Qhaweni Dhlamini, Le-Fu Chen and Jun-Jie Chen et al.
FGF10 Therapeutic Administration Promotes Mobilization of Injury-Activated Alveolar Progenitors in a Mouse Fibrosis Model
Reprinted from: *Cells* **2022**, *11*, 2396, doi:10.3390/cells11152396 29

Ana Ivonne Vazquez-Armendariz, Margarida Maria Barroso, Elie El Agha and Susanne Herold
3D In Vitro Models: Novel Insights into Idiopathic Pulmonary Fibrosis Pathophysiology and Drug Screening
Reprinted from: *Cells* **2022**, *11*, 1526, doi:10.3390/cells11091526 47

Ashesh Chakraborty, Michal Mastalerz, Meshal Ansari, Herbert B. Schiller and Claudia A. Staab-Weijnitz
Emerging Roles of Airway Epithelial Cells in Idiopathic Pulmonary Fibrosis
Reprinted from: *Cells* **2022**, *11*, 1050, doi:10.3390/cells11061050 59

Fabian Schramm, Liliana Schaefer and Malgorzata Wygrecka
EGFR Signaling in Lung Fibrosis
Reprinted from: *Cells* **2022**, *11*, 986, doi:10.3390/cells11060986 87

Stefan Preisendörfer, Yoshihiro Ishikawa, Elisabeth Hennen, Stephan Winklmeier, Jonas C. Schupp and Larissa Knüppel et al.
FK506-Binding Protein 11 Is a Novel Plasma Cell-Specific Antibody Folding Catalyst with Increased Expression in Idiopathic Pulmonary Fibrosis
Reprinted from: *Cells* **2022**, *11*, 1341, doi:10.3390/cells11081341 103

Vahid Kheirollahi, Ali Khadim, Georgios Kiliaris, Martina Korfei, Margarida Maria Barroso and Ioannis Alexopoulos et al.
Transcriptional Profiling of Insulin-like Growth Factor Signaling Components in Embryonic Lung Development and Idiopathic Pulmonary Fibrosis
Reprinted from: *Cells* **2022**, *11*, 1973, doi:10.3390/cells11121973 125

Kazutaka Takehara, Yasuhiko Koga, Yoshimasa Hachisu, Mitsuyoshi Utsugi, Yuri Sawada and Yasuyuki Saito et al.
Differential Discontinuation Profiles between Pirfenidone and Nintedanib in Patients with Idiopathic Pulmonary Fibrosis
Reprinted from: *Cells* **2022**, *11*, 143, doi:10.3390/cells11010143 139

Martina Korfei, Poornima Mahavadi and Andreas Guenther
Targeting Histone Deacetylases in Idiopathic Pulmonary Fibrosis: A Future Therapeutic Option
Reprinted from: *Cells* **2022**, *11*, 1626, doi:10.3390/cells11101626 . . . . **151**

Peter Braubach, Christopher Werlein, Stijn E. Verleden, Isabell Maerzke, Jens Gottlieb and Gregor Warnecke et al.
Pulmonary Fibroelastotic Remodelling Revisited
Reprinted from: *Cells* **2021**, *10*, 1362, doi:10.3390/cells10061362 . . . . **197**

Preface to "State of the Art in Idiopathic Pulmonary Fibrosis"

Idiopathic pulmonary fibrosis (IPF) is a lethal disease of unknown etiology, elusive pathogenesis, and very limited therapeutic options. The onset and progression of IPF are influenced by multiple environmental and intrinsic factors such as exposure to harmful substances, aging, and genetic predisposition; however, the magnitude of the contribution of these factors to IPF and the chronological order of downstream pathogenic events remain uncertain. The main hallmarks of IPF are the abnormal activation of lung epithelial cells and the accumulation of fibroblasts/myofibroblasts, along with the excessive deposition of extracellular matrix proteins. The aforementioned processes eventually lead to irreversible alveolar scarring, organ malfunction, and death. Moreover, the incidence and prevalence of IPF are increasing at an alarming rate with the aging population. Recent technological advances and interdisciplinary approaches have unmasked the involvement of a broad spectrum of molecular and cellular mediators in the pathogenesis of IPF. Molecules as diverse as lipids, RNAs, and peptides, along with a plethora of inflammatory, epithelial, and mesenchymal cell subpopulations, have turned out to drive maladaptive remodeling in the lung. The multifactorial nature of IPF and the lack of robust translational models represent an enormous challenge for the development of successful therapeutic approaches. Thanks to the excellent content provided by the contributing authors, we hope that this reprint will provide a platform for conceptual and technological innovation in the field of IPF and that it will shed light on new therapeutic strategies that may become part of future treatment options.

Malgorzata Wygrecka and Elie El Agha
Editors

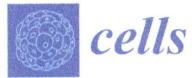

Editorial

State of the Art in Idiopathic Pulmonary Fibrosis

Elie El Agha [1,2,3,4,*] and Malgorzata Wygrecka [1,3,4,*]

1. Department of Medicine II, Internal Medicine, Pulmonary and Critical Care, Universities of Giessen and Marburg Lung Center (UGMLC), Justus-Liebig University Giessen, German Center for Lung Research (DZL), 35392 Giessen, Germany
2. Department of Medicine V, Internal Medicine, Infectious Diseases and Infection Control, Universities of Giessen and Marburg Lung Center (UGMLC), Justus-Liebig University Giessen, German Center for Lung Research (DZL), 35392 Giessen, Germany
3. Cardio-Pulmonary Institute (CPI), Justus-Liebig University Giessen, 35392 Giessen, Germany
4. Institute for Lung Health (ILH), Justus-Liebig University Giessen, 35392 Giessen, Germany
* Correspondence: elie.el-agha@innere.med.uni-giessen.de (E.E.A.); malgorzata.wygrecka@innere.med.uni-giessen.de (M.W.)

Citation: El Agha, E.; Wygrecka, M. State of the Art in Idiopathic Pulmonary Fibrosis. *Cells* 2022, 11, 2487. https://doi.org/10.3390/cells11162487

Received: 3 August 2022
Accepted: 9 August 2022
Published: 11 August 2022

Publisher's Note: MDPI stays neutral with regard to jurisdictional claims in published maps and institutional affiliations.

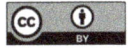

Copyright: © 2022 by the authors. Licensee MDPI, Basel, Switzerland. This article is an open access article distributed under the terms and conditions of the Creative Commons Attribution (CC BY) license (https://creativecommons.org/licenses/by/4.0/).

Idiopathic pulmonary fibrosis (IPF) is a form of usual interstitial pneumonia (UIP), though its origin is unknown. IPF remains one of the most aggressive and lethal forms of interstitial lung diseases. Extensive basic and clinical research during the past decade has uncovered critical aspects related to the pathophysiological events that lead to the formation of fibrotic scars in the lungs of IPF patients. Our current understanding of IPF pathogenesis includes repetitive/chronic injury to alveolar epithelial type 2 cells (AEC2) that triggers an aberrant wound healing response associated with the activation of fibroblasts and the infiltration of immune cells. This leads to the excessive accumulation of myofibroblasts that deposit extracellular matrix (ECM) proteins, particularly collagen and fibronectin. All aforementioned processes culminate in detrimental scarring of the lung tissue, loss of AEC2 and AEC1, and respiratory failure [1].

In this Special Issue, Wasnick et al. describe two subsets of AEC2 in both healthy and fibrotic lungs [2]. Using the lysosomal dye, LysoTracker, to stain lamellar bodies in AEC2, the authors demonstrate that *bona fide* AEC2 (Lyso^{high}) is the predominant AEC2 subset in the healthy lung, and that this population is largely replaced by an intermediate AEC state (Lyso^{low}) in bleomycin-induced pulmonary fibrosis and in human IPF. Lyso^{low} cells express, in addition to typical AEC2 markers, markers of basal cells, thus highlighting epithelial cell plasticity as a source of cellular heterogeneity in IPF [3–7]. Lyso^{low} cells are also reminiscent of the tdTomato-low (tdTom)^{low} cells, identified using the AEC2 lineage-tracing mouse line (*Sftpc*$^{Cre-ERT2}$; *tdTomato*^{flox}) [8–10]. Such tdTom^{low} cells have been shown to expand during compensatory lung growth following pneumonectomy and were therefore dubbed injury-activated alveolar progenitors (IAAPs) [8,9]. In this Special Issue, Lv et al. show that upon bleomycin injury in mice, IAAPs are amplified alongside a loss of mature AT2 cells [11]. They also show that the intratracheal instillation of recombinant fibroblast growth factor 10 (rFGF10) is both preventive and therapeutic against bleomycin-induced pulmonary fibrosis. These findings accord with previous data that utilized a transgenic approach to overexpress *Fgf10* [12]. Importantly, Lv et al. also demonstrate that therapeutic rFGF10 treatment further boosts IAAP expansion [11]. In the future, it will be worth comparing the colony-forming efficiency of human AT2 subsets and their mode of interaction with mesenchymal niche cells using organotypic co-culture models. In this context, Vazquez-Armendariz et al. provide a comprehensive review on various three-dimensional (3D) models that can be used to study cell–cell interactions [13]. These 3D models include hydrogels, precision-cut lung slices (PCLSs), lung organoids, and lung-on-chip devices. These approaches can be particularly useful in analyzing intermediate cell states that persist during fibrosis, and in evaluating molecular signaling pathways which drive lung tissue scarring. The ultimate goal of such approaches is to improve our understanding of the events that mediate the onset, progression, and resolution of lung fibrosis, and to identify novel therapeutic targets via high-throughput drug screening.

Despite the fact that IPF is considered as a "distal" lung disease, with a central role of AEC2 malfunction during its pathogenesis, Chakraborty et al. highlight recent developments that point towards the involvement of airway epithelial cells in IPF pathobiology [14]. The contribution of airway epithelial cells to the development of IPF is supported by multiple lines of evidence, including the cellular composition and morphological alterations of IPF airways, strong associations between the *MUC5B* promoter *rs35705950* polymorphism and the risk of IPF, and the bronchiolization of distal airspaces in IPF lungs. The contribution of airway epithelial cells to IPF pathogenesis is also addressed by Schramm et al., who discuss the role of the ErbB receptor–ligand system in lung fibrosis [15]. Intriguingly, the deregulation of the ErbB receptor-ligand axis is mainly observed in the regions of alveolar bronchiolization. This underlies the pivotal role of ErbB receptors in the reprogramming of airway epithelial cells, and thereby honeycomb cyst formation and IPF progression. The authors of this comprehensive review emphasize the dual role of ErbB receptors and their ligands in lung fibrosis and indicate the need to elaborately characterize the dynamics and causal flows in the ErbB signaling networks in acute versus chronic lung injury [15].

The cellular heterogeneity of IPF is further discussed by Preisendörfer et al., who stress the potential role of B cells in IPF pathobiology [16]. The pathological relevance of B-cell accumulation in the lungs of IPF patients is supported by the presence of circulating autoantibodies and the increased concentration of B-lymphocyte stimulator factor (BLyS) in IPF plasma. The authors build upon these findings and show increased levels of FK506-binding protein 11 (FKBP11), an antibody-folding catalyst, in IPF lungs. Mechanistically, they demonstrate that FKBP11 expression is elevated following the differentiation of B cells into antibody-secreting plasma cells and upon the induction of ER stress in A549 cells. The latter may lead to higher susceptibility of A549 cells to ER stress-induced cell death. Although the authors failed to demonstrate the importance of FKBP11 for antibody production in the loss-of-function approaches, these results provide further evidence for the role of auto-immunogenicity in IPF pathogenesis [16].

IPF is also associated with a set of metabolic disorders and targeting cellular metabolism, particularly in mesenchymal cells, represents an exciting therapeutic avenue [17–21]. Kheirollahi et al. provide a systematic gene expression analysis of insulin-like growth factor (IGF) signaling components during embryonic murine lung development, as well as bleomycin-induced pulmonary fibrosis in mice and human IPF [22]. The authors demonstrate significant upregulation of IGF1 and several IGF binding proteins (IGFBPs) in parallel with marked downregulation of IGF1 receptor (IGF1R) in lung fibrosis. They also address the impact of matrix stiffness on the fibroblast response to IGF1 treatment and the interconversion to either lipofibroblasts or myofibroblasts [22]. The lipofibroblast–myofibroblast interconversion was recently shown to be involved in the development and resolution of experimental lung fibrosis [21,23,24].

One of the factors that contribute to the incurable nature of IPF is the fact that patients are already in advanced disease stages at the time of diagnosis. As such, treatment mainly focuses on treating the symptoms and slowing down disease progression rather than treating early events that initiate downstream pathological signaling cascades. Accordingly, efforts that seek to find alternative therapeutic agents against IPF are still ongoing.

Current treatment modalities for IPF patients rely on two approved drugs: pirfenidone, which is believed to act as a transforming growth factor beta 1 and hedgehog signaling inhibitor [25], and nintedanib, which is a small molecule inhibitor of multiple receptor tyrosine kinases (RTKs). Although these two medications slightly prolong survival of IPF patients, they do not halt disease progression. Moreover, they possess a marked side-effect profile, which may lead to the discontinuation of antifibrotic therapy. In this Special Issue, Takehara et al. [26] retrospectively analyzed the discontinuation rates of pirfenidone and nintedanib in a cohort of 261 patients in Japan, 77 of which were excluded because either the antifibrotic agent was switched or the observation period was less than a year. Analysis of the remaining patient data showed that the discontinuation rate was around half within one year of treatment. Over the entire treatment period, the discontinuation rates were similar for the two drugs; however, discontinuation due to adverse events was higher for nintedanib, with diarrhea and liver dysfunction being the more common reasons for cessation. Discontinuation due to disease progression or hospital transfer was higher for pirfenidone than nintedanib. The authors associated the adverse effects of nintedanib with a lower body mass index (BMI) and recommended a reduced starting dose and closer attention paid to adverse events at the initiation of nintedanib treatment to improve tolerability, achieve longer treatment, and improve prognosis [26].

Korfei et al. contribute to the Special Issue with a comprehensive review on the current knowledge regarding IPF pathophysiology, the associated cellular and molecular mechanisms, clinical management, as well as novel therapeutic targets and therapies in development [27]. Importantly, the authors draw lessons about histone deacetylases (HDACs) from the cancer field and highlight the imbalance between increased HDAC activity in fibroblasts and bronchiolar basal cells, and decreased HDAC activity in AEC2 in IPF. Such an imbalance leads to fibroblast proliferation, ECM deposition and bronchiolar basal cell hyperproliferation from one side, and AEC2 endoplasmic reticulum (ER) stress, senescence, and apoptosis from the other side. All these processes ultimately culminate in fibrosis development and progression. Accordingly, the authors propose targeting HDACs as a novel therapeutic option for IPF [27].

Braubach et al. go beyond IPF and provide a broad characterization of fibroelastotic remodeling (FER), its anatomic distribution, and clinical association [28]. FER is observed in pleuroparenchymal fibroelastosis (PPFE), which can either be of idiopathic origin or linked to autoimmune disorders. All PPFE manifestations share a rather poor prognosis and a similar histological feature of the fibrous obliteration of alveolar airspaces. The authors stress the need of histological characterization of FER and its clear demarcation from other interstitial lung diseases, as this may provide the basis for studies addressing molecular mechanisms underlying PPFE development [28].

In conclusion, we present a collection of articles in this Special Issue that touch on all aspects of IPF, from the molecular mechanisms driving disease development and progression, to translational models enabling high-throughput drug screening, finishing on clinical studies evaluating adverse effect profiles of drugs approved for IPF treatment. Despite immense improvements in understanding the molecular basis of IPF, further research is urgently needed to pursue innovative translational studies in order to learn more about the enormous repertoire of molecular tricks that lung cells use to adapt to stress conditions and fight against damaging agents.

Author Contributions: E.E.A. and M.W. drafted and edited the manuscript. All authors have read and agreed to the published version of the manuscript.

Funding: E.E.A. acknowledges financial support from the Institute for Lung Health (ILH) and the German Research Foundation (DFG; KFO309 P7, SFB CRC 1213 268555672 project A04 and EL 931/4-1). M.W. acknowledges financial support from the DZL (82 DZL 005A1) and the Else Kröner-Fresenius Foundation (2014_A179).

Acknowledgments: E.E.A. acknowledges the excellence cluster Cardio-Pulmonary Institute (CPI, EXC 2026, Project ID: 390649896) and the German Center for Lung Research (DZL).

Conflicts of Interest: The authors declare no conflict of interest.

References

1. Günther, A.; Korfei, M.; Mahavadi, P.; von der Beck, D.; Ruppert, C.; Markart, P. Unravelling the Progressive Pathophysiology of Idiopathic Pulmonary Fibrosis. *Eur. Respir. Rev.* **2012**, *21*, 152–160. [CrossRef]
2. Wasnick, R.M.; Shalashova, I.; Wilhelm, J.; Khadim, A.; Schmidt, N.; Hackstein, H.; Hecker, A.; Hoetzenecker, K.; Seeger, W.; Bellusci, S.; et al. Differential LysoTracker Uptake Defines Two Populations of Distal Epithelial Cells in Idiopathic Pulmonary Fibrosis. *Cells* **2022**, *11*, 235. [CrossRef]

3. Strunz, M.; Simon, L.M.; Ansari, M.; Kathiriya, J.J.; Angelidis, I.; Mayr, C.H.; Tsidiridis, G.; Lange, M.; Mattner, L.F.; Yee, M.; et al. Alveolar Regeneration through a Krt8+ Transitional Stem Cell State That Persists in Human Lung Fibrosis. *Nat. Commun.* **2020**, *11*, 3559. [CrossRef]
4. Adams, T.S.; Schupp, J.C.; Poli, S.; Ayaub, E.A.; Neumark, N.; Ahangari, F.; Chu, S.G.; Raby, B.A.; DeIuliis, G.; Januszyk, M.; et al. Single-Cell RNA-Seq Reveals Ectopic and Aberrant Lung-Resident Cell Populations in Idiopathic Pulmonary Fibrosis. *Sci. Adv.* **2020**, *6*, eaba1983. [CrossRef]
5. Habermann, A.C.; Gutierrez, A.J.; Bui, L.T.; Yahn, S.L.; Winters, N.I.; Calvi, C.L.; Peter, L.; Chung, M.-I.; Taylor, C.J.; Jetter, C.; et al. Single-Cell RNA Sequencing Reveals Profibrotic Roles of Distinct Epithelial and Mesenchymal Lineages in Pulmonary Fibrosis. *Sci. Adv.* **2020**, *6*, eaba1972. [CrossRef]
6. Reyfman, P.A.; Walter, J.M.; Joshi, N.; Anekalla, K.R.; McQuattie-Pimentel, A.C.; Chiu, S.; Fernandez, R.; Akbarpour, M.; Chen, C.I.; Ren, Z.; et al. Single-Cell Transcriptomic Analysis of Human Lung Provides Insights into the Pathobiology of Pulmonary Fibrosis. *Am. J. Respir. Crit. Care Med.* **2019**, *199*, 1517–1536. [CrossRef]
7. Xu, Y.; Mizuno, T.; Sridharan, A.; Du, Y.; Guo, M.; Tang, J.; Wikenheiser-Brokamp, K.A.; Perl, A.-K.T.; Funari, V.A.; Gokey, J.J.; et al. Single-Cell RNA Sequencing Identifies Diverse Roles of Epithelial Cells in Idiopathic Pulmonary Fibrosis. *JCI Insight* **2016**, *1*, e90558. [CrossRef]
8. Ahmadvand, N.; Khosravi, F.; Lingampally, A.; Wasnick, R.; Vazquez-Armendariz, I.; Carraro, G.; Heiner, M.; Rivetti, S.; Lv, Y.; Wilhelm, J.; et al. Identification of a Novel Subset of Alveolar Type 2 Cells Enriched in PD-L1 and Expanded Following Pneumonectomy. *Eur. Respir. J.* **2021**, *58*, 2004168. [CrossRef]
9. Ahmadvand, N.; Lingampally, A.; Khosravi, F.; Vazquez-Armendariz, A.I.; Rivetti, S.; Jones, M.R.; Wilhelm, J.; Herold, S.; Barreto, G.; Koepke, J.; et al. Fgfr2b Signaling Is Essential for the Maintenance of the Alveolar Epithelial Type 2 Lineage during Lung Homeostasis in Mice. *Cell. Mol. Life Sci.* **2022**, *79*, 302. [CrossRef]
10. Ahmadvand, N.; Carraro, G.; Jones, M.R.; Shalashova, I.; Noori, A.; Wilhelm, J.; Baal, N.; Khosravi, F.; Chen, C.; Zhang, J.-S.; et al. Cell-Surface Programmed Death Ligand-1 Expression Identifies a Sub-Population of Distal Epithelial Cells Enriched in Idiopathic Pulmonary Fibrosis. *Cells* **2022**, *11*, 1593. [CrossRef]
11. Lv, Y.-Q.; Cai, G.-F.; Zeng, P.-P.; Dhlamini, Q.; Chen, L.-F.; Chen, J.-J.; Lyu, H.-D.; Mossahebi-Mohammadi, M.; Ahmadvand, N.; Bellusci, S.; et al. FGF10 Therapeutic Administration Promotes Mobilization of Injury-Activated Alveolar Progenitors in a Mouse Fibrosis Model. *Cells* **2022**, *11*, 2396. [CrossRef]
12. Gupte, V.V.; Ramasamy, S.K.; Reddy, R.; Lee, J.; Weinreb, P.H.; Violette, S.M.; Guenther, A.; Warburton, D.; Driscoll, B.; Minoo, P.; et al. Overexpression of Fibroblast Growth Factor-10 during Both Inflammatory and Fibrotic Phases Attenuates Bleomycin-Induced Pulmonary Fibrosis in Mice. *Am. J. Respir. Crit. Care Med.* **2009**, *180*, 424–436. [CrossRef]
13. Vazquez-Armendariz, A.I.; Barroso, M.M.; El Agha, E.; Herold, S. 3D In Vitro Models: Novel Insights into Idiopathic Pulmonary Fibrosis Pathophysiology and Drug Screening. *Cells* **2022**, *11*, 1526. [CrossRef]
14. Chakraborty, A.; Mastalerz, M.; Ansari, M.; Schiller, H.B.; Staab-Weijnitz, C.A. Emerging Roles of Airway Epithelial Cells in Idiopathic Pulmonary Fibrosis. *Cells* **2022**, *11*, 1050. [CrossRef]
15. Schramm, F.; Schaefer, L.; Wygrecka, M. EGFR Signaling in Lung Fibrosis. *Cells* **2022**, *11*, 986. [CrossRef]
16. Preisendörfer, S.; Ishikawa, Y.; Hennen, E.; Winklmeier, S.; Schupp, J.C.; Knüppel, L.; Fernandez, I.E.; Binzenhöfer, L.; Flatley, A.; Juan-Guardela, B.M.; et al. FK506-Binding Protein 11 Is a Novel Plasma Cell-Specific Antibody Folding Catalyst with Increased Expression in Idiopathic Pulmonary Fibrosis. *Cells* **2022**, *11*, 1341. [CrossRef]
17. Zhao, Y.D.; Yin, L.; Archer, S.; Lu, C.; Zhao, G.; Yao, Y.; Wu, L.; Hsin, M.; Waddell, T.K.; Keshavjee, S.; et al. Metabolic Heterogeneity of Idiopathic Pulmonary Fibrosis: A Metabolomic Study. *BMJ Open Respir. Res.* **2017**, *4*, e000183. [CrossRef]
18. Yan, F.; Wen, Z.; Wang, R.; Luo, W.; Du, Y.; Wang, W.; Chen, X. Identification of the Lipid Biomarkers from Plasma in Idiopathic Pulmonary Fibrosis by Lipidomics. *BMC Pulm. Med.* **2017**, *17*, 174. [CrossRef]
19. Sato, N.; Takasaka, N.; Yoshida, M.; Tsubouchi, K.; Minagawa, S.; Araya, J.; Saito, N.; Fujita, Y.; Kurita, Y.; Kobayashi, K.; et al. Metformin Attenuates Lung Fibrosis Development via NOX4 Suppression. *Respir. Res.* **2016**, *17*, 107. [CrossRef]
20. Rangarajan, S.; Bone, N.B.; Zmijewska, A.A.; Jiang, S.; Park, D.W.; Bernard, K.; Locy, M.L.; Ravi, S.; Deshane, J.; Mannon, R.B.; et al. Metformin Reverses Established Lung Fibrosis in a Bleomycin Model. *Nat. Med.* **2018**, *24*, 1121–1127. [CrossRef]
21. Kheirollahi, V.; Wasnick, R.M.; Biasin, V.; Vazquez-Armendariz, A.I.; Chu, X.; Moiseenko, A.; Weiss, A.; Wilhelm, J.; Zhang, J.-S.; Kwapiszewska, G.; et al. Metformin Induces Lipogenic Differentiation in Myofibroblasts to Reverse Lung Fibrosis. *Nat. Commun.* **2019**, *10*, 2987. [CrossRef]
22. Kheirollahi, V.; Khadim, A.; Kiliaris, G.; Korfei, M.; Barroso, M.M.; Alexopoulos, I.; Vazquez-Armendariz, A.I.; Wygrecka, M.; Ruppert, C.; Guenther, A.; et al. Transcriptional Profiling of Insulin-like Growth Factor Signaling Components in Embryonic Lung Development and Idiopathic Pulmonary Fibrosis. *Cells* **2022**, *11*, 1973. [CrossRef]
23. El Agha, E.; Moiseenko, A.; Kheirollahi, V.; De Langhe, S.; Crnkovic, S.; Kwapiszewska, G.; Szibor, M.; Kosanovic, D.; Schwind, F.; Schermuly, R.T.; et al. Two-Way Conversion between Lipogenic and Myogenic Fibroblastic Phenotypes Marks the Progression and Resolution of Lung Fibrosis. *Cell Stem Cell* **2017**, *20*, 261–273. [CrossRef]
24. El Agha, E.; Kramann, R.; Schneider, R.K.; Li, X.; Seeger, W.; Humphreys, B.D.; Bellusci, S. Mesenchymal Stem Cells in Fibrotic Disease. *Cell Stem Cell* **2017**, *21*, 166–177. [CrossRef]

25. Didiasova, M.; Singh, R.; Wilhelm, J.; Kwapiszewska, G.; Wujak, L.; Zakrzewicz, D.; Schaefer, L.; Markart, P.; Seeger, W.; Lauth, M.; et al. Pirfenidone Exerts Antifibrotic Effects through Inhibition of GLI Transcription Factors. *FASEB J.* **2017**, *31*, 1916–1928. [CrossRef]
26. Takehara, K.; Koga, Y.; Hachisu, Y.; Utsugi, M.; Sawada, Y.; Saito, Y.; Yoshimi, S.; Yatomi, M.; Shin, Y.; Wakamatsu, I.; et al. Differential Discontinuation Profiles between Pirfenidone and Nintedanib in Patients with Idiopathic Pulmonary Fibrosis. *Cells* **2022**, *11*, 143. [CrossRef]
27. Korfei, M.; Mahavadi, P.; Guenther, A. Targeting Histone Deacetylases in Idiopathic Pulmonary Fibrosis: A Future Therapeutic Option. *Cells* **2022**, *11*, 1626. [CrossRef]
28. Braubach, P.; Werlein, C.; Verleden, S.E.; Maerzke, I.; Gottlieb, J.; Warnecke, G.; Dettmer, S.; Laenger, F.; Jonigk, D. Pulmonary Fibroelastotic Remodelling Revisited. *Cells* **2021**, *10*, 1362. [CrossRef]

Article

Differential LysoTracker Uptake Defines Two Populations of Distal Epithelial Cells in Idiopathic Pulmonary Fibrosis

Roxana Maria Wasnick [1,*], Irina Shalashova [1], Jochen Wilhelm [1,2,3,4], Ali Khadim [1,4], Nicolai Schmidt [1], Holger Hackstein [5], Andreas Hecker [6], Konrad Hoetzenecker [7], Werner Seeger [1,2,3,4], Saverio Bellusci [1,2,4], Elie El Agha [1,4], Clemens Ruppert [1,2,8] and Andreas Guenther [1,2,4,6,8,9]

1. Universities of Giessen and Marburg Lung Center (UGMLC), The German Center for Lung Research (DZL), 35392 Giessen, Germany; irn.bry@yandex.ru (I.S.); jochen.wilhelm@innere.med.uni-giessen.de (J.W.); Ali.Khadim@innere.med.uni-giessen.de (A.K.); nschmidt97@hotmail.de (N.S.); Werner.Seeger@innere.med.uni-giessen.de (W.S.); saverio.bellusci@innere.med.uni-giessen.de (S.B.); Elie.El-Agha@innere.med.uni-giessen.de (E.E.A.); Clemens.Ruppert@innere.med.uni-giessen.de (C.R.); Andreas.Guenther@innere.med.uni-giessen.de (A.G.)
2. Excellence Cluster Cardiopulmonary Institute (CPI), 35392 Giessen, Germany
3. Max-Planck-Institute for Heart and Lung Research, 61231 Bad Nauheim, Germany
4. Institute for Lung Health (ILH), 35392 Giessen, Germany
5. Department of Clinical Immunology and Transfusion Medicine, 35392 Giessen, Germany; Holger.Hackstein@uk-erlangen.de
6. Department of General and Thoracic Surgery, University Hospital Giessen, 35392 Giessen, Germany; Andreas.Hecker@chiru.med.uni-giessen.de
7. Department of Thoracic Surgery, Medical University of Vienna, 1090 Vienna, Austria; konrad.hoetzenecker@meduniwien.ac.at
8. European IPF Registry/UGLMC Giessen Biobank, 35392 Giessen, Germany
9. Lung Clinic Waldhof-Elgershausen, 35753 Greifenstein, Germany
* Correspondence: roxana.wasnick@cellergon.de

Abstract: Idiopathic pulmonary fibrosis (IPF) is a progressive and fatal degenerative lung disease of unknown etiology. Although in its final stages it implicates, in a reactive manner, all lung cell types, the initial damage involves the alveolar epithelial compartment, in particular the alveolar epithelial type 2 cells (AEC2s). AEC2s serve dual progenitor and surfactant secreting functions, both of which are deeply impacted in IPF. Thus, we hypothesize that the size of the surfactant processing compartment, as measured by LysoTracker incorporation, allows the identification of different epithelial states in the IPF lung. Flow cytometry analysis of epithelial LysoTracker incorporation delineates two populations (Lyso^{high} and Lyso^{low}) of AEC2s that behave in a compensatory manner during bleomycin injury and in the donor/IPF lung. Employing flow cytometry and transcriptomic analysis of cells isolated from donor and IPF lungs, we demonstrate that the Lyso^{high} population expresses all classical AEC2 markers and is drastically diminished in IPF. The Lyso^{low} population, which is increased in proportion in IPF, co-expressed AEC2 and basal cell markers, resembling the phenotype of the previously identified intermediate AEC2 population in the IPF lung. In that regard, we provide an in-depth flow-cytometry characterization of LysoTracker uptake, HTII-280, proSP-C, mature SP-B, NGFR, KRT5, and CD24 expression in human lung epithelial cells. Combining functional analysis with extracellular and intracellular marker expression and transcriptomic analysis, we advance the current understanding of epithelial cell behavior and fate in lung fibrosis.

Keywords: IPF; alveolar epithelial cells; intermediate epithelial cells; transitional states; LysoTracker; flow cytometry; lung transcriptomic profile; CK5; NGFR; CD24

1. Introduction

The human lung is a highly complex organ designed specifically for gas exchange. In idiopathic pulmonary fibrosis (IPF), chronic epithelial injury leads to excessive deposition of rigid extra-cellular matrix and a progressive decrease in lung compliance and gas-exchange surface, causing inevitable and fatal lung failure within 2–5 years after diagnosis [1–3]. Although new therapies significantly increased the duration and quality of life of IPF patients, a therapeutic regimen that can arrest or, even better, reverse disease progression remains to be discovered [4]. Partly responsible for this situation is our limited understanding of the cellular states and processes that each of the more than 40 cell types in the lung undergoes, in an active (causative) or reactive manner in homeostatic and injury contexts [5,6]. A number of recent studies clearly identified the chronic injury of the alveolar type 2 epithelial cells (AEC2s) as the initial site of injury in the IPF lung [7–9]. AEC2s are facultative progenitors in the distal lung, which, in a differentiated state, serve the vital function of surfactant production and secretion, but can also act as progenitors for other AEC2s and AEC1s in homeostatic and injury-repair situations [10,11].

Pulmonary surfactant is a phospholipoprotein mixture secreted exclusively by AEC2s which reduces the alveolar surface tension necessary for alveoli reopening during the respiratory cycle. The protein component is represented by the surfactant proteins (SP) A, B, C and D, with two of them, SP-B and SP-C, holding tension-active properties. Following the processing from the pro- forms (proSP-B and proSP-C) to the mature forms (mSP-B and mSP-C), they are secreted in their mature forms specifically by AEC2s [12–14]. The processing and assembly of pulmonary surfactant proteins take place in the lamellar bodies of AEC2s, specialized organelles characterized by very low pH [15].

In IPF, repeated alveolar injury results in the recruitment of the AEC2 progenitors necessary for the repair process [11,16–18]. In this process, the differentiated function of bona fide AEC2s, defined as AEC2s which synthesize, process, and secrete alveolar surfactant, is impaired and leads to increased alveolar surface tension and increased alveolar collapse, which propagates the injury even further, thus creating a self-propagating cycle of injury and repair [19–22]. The acute AEC1/2 injury creates a microenvironment where other reactive cell types, such as alveolar macrophages and fibroblasts, are quickly activated and recruited to cover the basement membrane and prevent fluid leakage into the airspace [23]. However, as the AEC2 progenitor pool is exhausted by injury or by extensive proliferation, the long-term repair after or during the chronic and repeated injury relies on the recruitment of other local epithelial progenitors, several of which have already been identified in the mouse lung [17,24–26]. In humans, the profound histological changes found in the distal IPF lung are consistent with the expansion of a cytokeratin 5 (CK) progenitor, but its origin and differentiating trajectory remain to be determined [27]. Recent landmark papers described the transcriptomic signatures of disease-free (donor) and IPF epithelial cells at single-cell level, leading to the identification of transcriptomic signatures for many known epithelial cell types in the lung and the identification of novel ones (ionocytes and CK17+/CK5- aberrant AEC2s) [16,28–32]. However, it is unclear how these transcriptomic signatures translate into the stable or transitional cellular states and processes responsible for the disease phenotype [33]. The repair process in IPF is ultimately ineffective, underlying the disease progression that leads to organ failure. Thus, the ability to correlate scNGS data with protein expression and functional behavior would greatly increase our understanding of these epithelial fates and states and turn this into a therapeutically actionable process for the benefit of IPF patients.

Here, we ask if the aberrant or intermediate transcriptional programs recently identified in IPF [29,31] result in functional transitional states that can be identified by the low/intermediate ability to process and secrete surfactant proteins (SP). To that end, we analyze the size of the surfactant processing compartment in dissociated human donor and IPF lung epithelial cells, thus defining two functional alveolar epithelial states present in both donor and IPF lung. Based on known intracellular cell surface proteins and LysoTracker incorporation, coupled with transcriptomic analysis, we show that the LysoTracker^{high} population consists of bona fide AEC2s and is drastically diminished in IPF. A second population of LysoTracker^{low} cells, which uniformly expresses and processes surfactant proteins but bears the transcriptional footprint of a CK5-derived (basal) population, is increased in IPF.

2. Materials and Methods

2.1. Animal Studies

Animal studies were performed in accordance with the Helsinki convention for the use and care of animals and were approved by the local authorities at Regierungspräsidium Giessen V54-19 c 2015 (1) GI 20/10 Nr. 109/2011 (Bleomycin) or V54-19 c 20 15 h 02 GI 20/10 Nr. A53/2012 (untreated controls).

2.2. Patient Material

The study protocol was approved by the Ethics Committee of the Justus-Liebig-University School of Medicine (No. 31/93, 29/01, and No. 111/08: European IPF Registry), and informed consent was obtained in written form from each subject. Explanted lungs ($n = 31$ for sporadic IPF, IPF_{LTX}; $n = 6$ for COPD) or non-utilized donor lungs or lobes fulfilling transplantation criteria ($n = 27$; human donors) were obtained from the Dept. of Thoracic Surgery in Giessen, Germany and Vienna, Austria and provided by the UGMLC Giessen Biobank, a member of the DZL platform Biobanking. All IPF diagnoses were made according to the American Thoracic Society (ATS)/European Respiratory Society (ERS) consensus criteria [34], and a usual interstitial pneumonia (UIP) pattern was proven in all IPF patients.

2.3. Bleomycin Model of Lung Fibrosis

C57BL/6N mice (Charles River Laboratories, Sulzfeld, Germany) between 10 and 16 weeks old were used. Mice were intubated and bleomycin (Hexal, 2.5U/Kg body weight in 0.9% saline) was aerosolized using a microsprayer (Penncentury). At each time point, saline-treated and/or untreated mice were used as controls. Mice were weighed every day and sacrificed 3, 7, 14, 21 and 28 days later for cell dissociation and flow cytometry analysis.

2.4. Lung Tissue Dissociation

For both mouse and human lung, standard dispase-based dissociation protocols were used, as previously described [22,35,36] and detailed in the Supplemental Materials.

2.5. Flow Cytometry Analysis and Cell Sorting

Standard [37], previously published methods [22,35,36] were used for sample preparation and intracellular and extracellular staining in preparation for flow cytometry and fluorescence-activated cell sorting. Detailed methods and reagents, including all antibodies, are described in the Supplemental Materials. Single color controls were used to compensate for spectral overlap. Fluorescence-minus-one (FMO) controls were used whenever possible for positive/negative population gating. In the case of indirect intracellular staining, no primary control samples, consisting of the FMO control in the particular channel to which only the secondary antibody was added, were used for data interpretation and quantification. Data were acquired on a BD FACSCanto II (BD Biosciences) using BD FACSDiva software (BD Biosciences). Data were further analyzed using FlowJo vX software (FlowJo, LLC).

2.6. Immunofluorescence Analysis

The staining procedures were based on standard, previously published techniques and the reagents are listed in the Supplemental Materials and Supplemental Tables S1 and S2. However, given that both the mature SP-B and proSP-B antibodies were raised in the same species (rabbit), the standard protocol was modified, as follows. Following standard deparaffinization and blocking (see Supplemental Materials), slides were incubated with a mature SP-B antibody at a very low concentration (1:2000, 10 times lower than for traditional mature SP-B staining) and the fluorescent signal was amplified using the Alexa Fluor™ 555 Tyramide SuperBoost™ Kit, goat anti-rabbit IgG (Thermo Scientific, Waltham, MA, USA). This resulted in the covalent attachment of Alexa Fluor 555 Tyramide at the base of the antigen, which allowed the consequent stripping of the rabbit anti-mature SP-B antibody using the standard citrate-based antigen retrieval solution, as described in the Supplemental Materials. Samples were re-blocked with 5% BSA in PBS solution and incubated with the rabbit anti-proSP-B antibody, followed by an Alexa Fluor 488-labeled donkey anti-rabbit secondary antibody. Appropriate controls demostrating the lack of cross-reactivity were used to ascertain the specificity of the two signals (see Supplemental Materials). The stained amsples were imaged on a wide-field fluorescence microscope (Axio Observer.Z1 fluorescence microscope, Carl Zeiss MicroImaging, Jena, Germany) and a confocal microscope (TCS SP5, Leica Microsystems) and the images were processed and quantified using the Fiji package of ImageJ image analysis software ((https://imagej.net, version 20.0-rc-65/1.51w, accessed on 31 January 2018).

2.7. Microarray Analysis

Purified total RNA was amplified using the Ovation PicoSL WTA System V2 kit (NuGEN Technologies, Bemmel, The Netherlands). For each sample, 2 µg of amplified cDNA was Cy3-labeled using the SureTag DNA labeling kit (Agilent, Waldbronn, Germany). Hybridization to 8 × 60K 60mer oligonucleotide spotted microarray slides (Human Whole Genome, SurePrint G3 Human GE v3 8 × 60K Microarray; Agilent Technologies, design ID 072363) and the subsequent washing and drying of the slides was performed following the Agilent hybridization protocol in Agilent hybridization chambers with the following modifications: 2 µg of the labeled cDNA were hybridized for 22 h at 65 °C. The cDNA was not fragmented before hybridization. The dried slides were scanned at a 2 µm/pixel resolution using the InnoScan is900 (Innopsys, Carbonne, France). Image analysis was performed with Mapix 8.2.5 software, and calculated values for all spots were saved as GenePix result files. Stored data were evaluated using the R software (www.r-project.org, version R3.6.3 GUI1.70 ElCapitan, accessed on 29 February 2020) and the limma package [38] from BioConductor [39]. Log_2 mean spot signals were taken for further analysis. Data were background corrected using the NormExp procedure on the negative control spots and were quantile-normalized [38,40] before averaging. Log_2 signals of replicate spots were averaged, and, from several different probes addressing the same gene, only the probe with the highest average signal was used. Genes were ranked for differential expression using a moderated t-statistic [38]. Pathway analyses were performed using gene set tests on the ranks of the t-values [38,41]. Pathways were taken from the KEGG database (http://www.genome.jp/kegg/pathway.html, accessed on 11 October 2021).

Heatmaps are generated from the normalized log_2 spot intensities (I) and show the gene-wise z-values (where $z_j = (I_j - mean(I))/SD(I)$ for $j = 1\ldots n$).

2.8. Data Analysis

2.8.1. Flow Cytometry Data Analysis

The frequency of parent and mean fluorescence intensity (MFI) data were exported from FlowJo v.10 and analyzed using MicrosoftExcel, R software (www.r-project.org, version R3.6.3 GUI1.70 ElCapitan, accessed on 29 February 2020) or GraphPad Prism (GraphPad Software). For the bleomycin experiments, the percentages of $Lyso^{high}$ and $Lyso^{low}$ cell populations in control vs. treated samples were first log-transformed and Student's T-test was used to determine the statistical significance of their differences at each time point. To evaluate the dynamic of the $Lyso^{high}$ and $Lyso^{low}$ populations over time (Figure 1C), we related the proportion of each $Lyso^{high}$ or $Lyso^{low}$ population in each group (bleomycin or saline) to the total LysoTracker-incorporating population in the control animals at each time point, as follows: each point on the line represents the % change log10 of the respective $Lyso^{high}$ or $Lyso^{low}$ at DayX, calculated as $log10(Lyso^{high\ or\ low})$ $DayX_{bleo\ or\ control}/log10(Lyso^{high}DayX + Lyso^{low}DayX)_{control}$. To determine the relative difference between the $Lyso^{high}$ and $Lyso^{low}$ populations in each epithelial group at each time point (Figure 1D), we analyzed the log odds ratio of these two populations using the R statistical analysis software. A log odds ratio of 0 means that the two populations are similar, and, therefore, the probability that an epithelial cell is a $Lyso^{high}$ cell is equal to that of it being a $Lyso^{low}$ cell. Positive log odds ratios indicate that the two populations are different, and, therefore, the probability of a cell belonging to one population is larger than the probability of it belonging to the other one. Flow cytometry data collected from human samples were analyzed in a similar manner. Student's t-tests or two-way ANOVAs were used, as appropriate (stated in the figure legend), to test the null hypotheses that the log-transformed MFI of the percentage of parent values were different in each comparison.

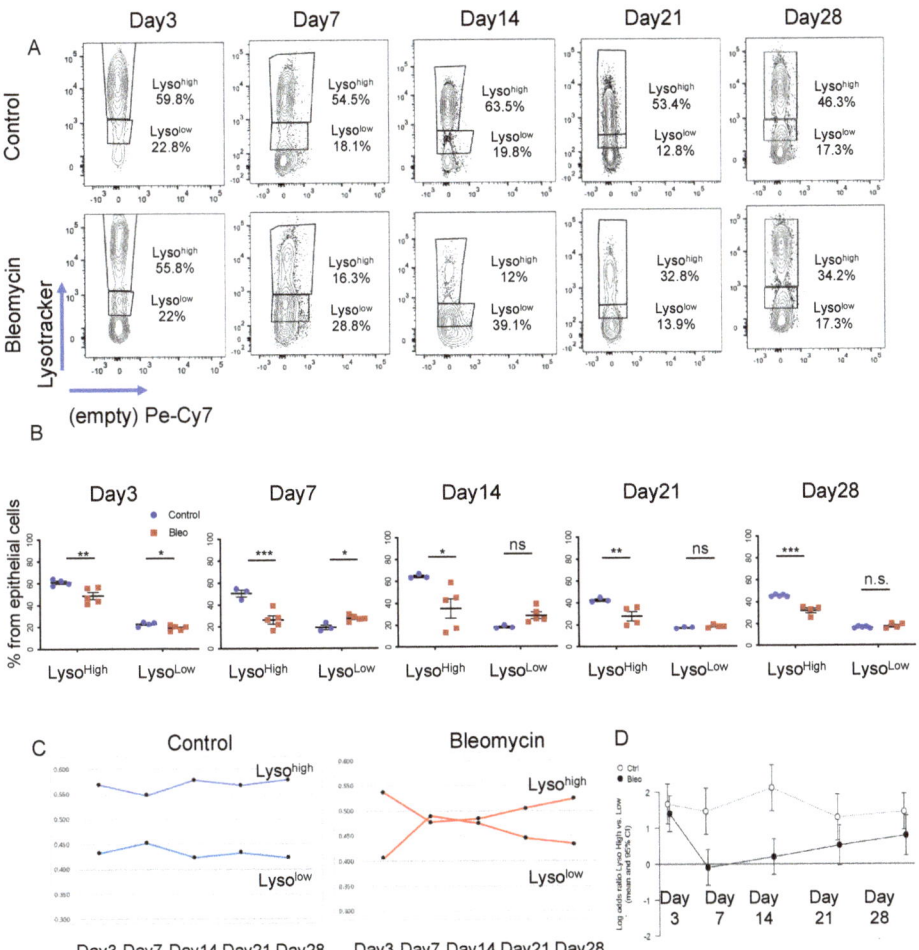

Figure 1. Characterization of AEC2s in a bleomycin model of lung fibrosis. (**A–D**) Bleomycin or saline were intratracheally instilled into the lungs of C57B6 mice, which were analyzed after 3 (control $n = 4$, bleomycin $n = 5$), 7 (control $n = 3$, bleomycin $n = 5$), 14 (control $n = 3$, bleomycin $n = 5$), 21 (control $n = 3$, bleomycin $n = 4$) and 28 (control $n = 4$, bleomycin $n = 4$) days. The flow cytometry analysis of the AEC2s in the epithelial compartment, defined as DAPI$^-$ CD45$^-$ CD31$^-$ PDP$^-$ EpCAM$^+$. (**A**) Representative panels of LysoTracker uptake (Lyso^{high} and Lyso^{low}) as a percentage of the parent epithelial compartment of bleomycin-treated mice. (**B**) Statistical analysis of the Lyso^{high} and Lyso^{low} populations at each time point. Data are presented as the means ± SEM. * $p < 0.05$, ** $p < 0.01$, *** $p < 0.001$, n.s. = not significant by ANOVA. (**C**) Time-course analysis of the Lyso^{high} and Lyso^{low} populations in control mice (left panel) and bleomycin-treated mice (right panel). (**D**) Analysis of the log odds ratio of the Lyso^{high} vs. Lyso^{low} population (log Lyso^{high}/Lyso^{low}) during the time course of bleomycin recovery. Data are presented as the means and 95% confidence intervals.

2.8.2. Immunoflurescence Quantification and Analysis

Fluorescence intensity was analyzed using the Fiji/Image J (https://imagej.net, version 20.0-rc-65/1.51w, accessed on 31 January 2018) image analysis software and fluorescence intensity data was exported and statistically analyzed and plotted using Microsoft Excel.

3. Results

3.1. LysoTracker Incorporation Delineates Two Populations of Epithelial Cells in Bleomycin-Induced Injury

To determine the dynamic behavior of AEC2s during bleomycin injury, C57BL6 mice were treated with bleomycin (2.5U/kg) and analyzed 3, 7, 14, 21, and 28 days post-administration. Saline or untreated mice (generally termed controls) were used as controls at each time point. Mice were sacrificed and their lungs were dissociated into a single-cell suspension whose cellular composition was analyzed by flow cytometry at each time point. To identify AEC2s, dead cells (PI^+ or $DAPI^+$) and AEC1 cells (podoplanin-$PDPN^+$) were first excluded, and the epithelial compartment was further identified by EpCAM expression within the $CD45^-$ (non-hematopoietic) and $CD31^-$ (non-endothelial) population (full gating path is in Supplemental Figure S1A). The proportion of the $DAPI^-$ $CD45^-$ $CD31^-$ $PDPN^-$ $EpCAM^+$ population (the epithelial cell compartment from here on) was slightly decreased in bleomycin-treated mice starting on day 14 and reached statistical significance on day 28 (Supplemental Figure S1B). To identify AEC2s within the epithelial compartment, we took advantage of their specific ability to uptake LysoTracker dyes [12,42]. The dynamic of LysoTracker uptake was analyzed during the bleomycin recovery time course, revealing three distinct populations: a $LysoTracker^{neg}$ ($Lyso^{neg}$), a $LysoTracker^{low}$ ($Lyso^{low}$) and a $LysoTracker^{high}$ ($Lyso^{high}$) population (Figure 1A). At all time-points analyzed, the $Lyso^{high}$ population was decreased in number, with the greatest decrease registered at days 7 and 14, when AEC2 injury was maximal [43,44]. This was paralleled by a proportional increase in the $Lyso^{low}$ population that reached a maximum increase at the same time points (Figure 1B). The time-course analysis of the population dynamic showed that $Lyso^{high}$ and $Lyso^{low}$ populations behaved complementary to each other, with a maximum relative change at day 7 and a partial recovery by days 21 and 28. The paired analysis of the log odds ratio of the $Lyso^{high}$ and $Lyso^{low}$ populations (log $Lyso^{high}/Lyso^{low}$) further supported our conclusion that the difference between the two populations was maximal in control samples and early time points but decreased significantly at days 7 and 14 (log value of zero) (Figure 1D). Of note, LysoTracker uptake was not completely recovered at day 28, suggesting long-lasting alterations in cellular phenotype (Figure 1B–D).

3.2. LysoTracker Uptake in Human Lung Epithelium

Next, we asked if the behavior of these populations is similar in the distal human donor and IPF lung. To that end, subpleural tissue from six donor and six end-stage IPF explanted lungs were dissociated into single-cell suspensions and analyzed by flow cytometry. The gating strategy was similar to that of the mouse lung, where the epithelium was identified as live $CD45^-$ $CD31^-$ $EpCAM^+$ cells (Supplemental Figure S2A). Fluorescence-minus-one (FMO) samples were used for appropriate gating (Supplemental Figure S2B). There was no statistically different proportion of epithelial cells between the groups (Supplemental Figure S2D). Similar to the mouse data, the proportion of IPF $Lyso^{high}$ cells was dramatically decreased compared to donors, from an average of 50.3% in donors to 10.1% in IPF. The $Lyso^{low}$ population behaved in a complementary fashion, increasing from an average of 15.2% in donors to 37.1% in IPF patients (Figure 2A,B). Individual panels from each patient are shown in Supplemental Figure S2C.

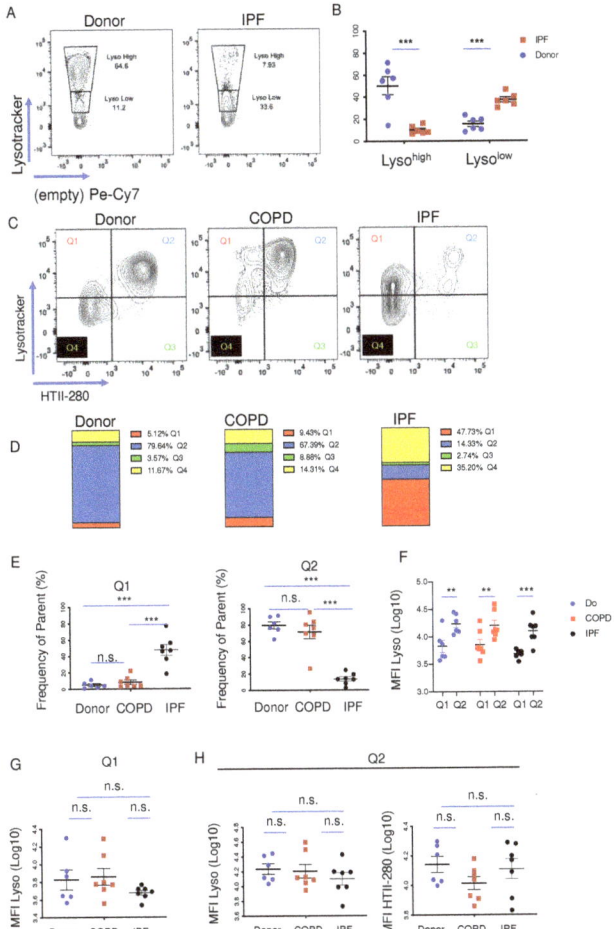

Figure 2. LysoTracker uptake in the epithelial compartment of the human lung. (**A**) Representative panels of flow cytometry analysis of the LysoTracker uptake (Lyso^{high} and Lyso^{low}) in the epithelial compartment (DAPI$^-$ CD45$^-$ CD31$^-$ EpCAM$^+$) of human donor ($n = 6$) and IPF ($n = 6$) lungs. (**B**) Quantification of the Lyso^{high} and Lyso^{low} populations in donor and IPF samples in (**A**). (**C**) Representative panels of LysoTracker uptake (y-axis) as a function of HTII-280 reactivity (x-axis) in the epithelial compartment of donor ($n = 6$), COPD ($n = 7$) and IPF ($n = 7$) lungs. Quadrant gating identifies four different populations as follows: Q1 (Lyso^{pos}/HTII-280^{neg}), Q2 (Lyso^{pos}/HTII-280^{pos}), Q3 (Lyso^{neg}/HTII-280^{pos}) and Q4 (Lyso^{neg}/HTII-280^{neg}). (**D**) Quantification of the data shown in (**C**) showing the relative contribution of the Q1 to Q4 populations to the epithelial compartment of donor, COPD and IPF lungs. (**E**) Quantification of Q1 (left diagram) and Q2 (right diagram) as the frequency of the parent (DAPI$^-$ CD45$^-$ CD31$^-$ EpCAM$^+$) population. (**F**) Comparison of the LysoTracker uptake in the LysoTracker-positive populations, Q1 and Q2, in donor, COPD and IPF patients, as measured by the MFI of the respective populations. (**G**) Comparison of the LysoTracker uptake in the Q1 population in donor, COPD and IPF patients, as measured by the MFI of the respective populations. (**H**) Comparison of the LysoTracker uptake (left panel) and HTII280 reactivity (right panel) in the Q2 population in donor, COPD and IPF patients, as measured by the MFI of the respective populations. Data are presented as the means ± SEM of the percentage of cells from the parent population. Statistical analysis was performed on log(10) values. ** $p < 0.01$, *** $p < 0.001$, n.s. = not significant by ANOVA.

To further understand the identity of the Lyso^{high}- and Lyso^{low}-incorporating cells, we analyzed the expression of HTII-280, a well-known AEC2 marker, as a function of LysoTracker incorporation [45]. In addition to donor ($n = 6$) and IPF ($n = 7$) samples, COPD samples ($n = 7$) were added as non-IPF related controls. Quadrant gating of LysoTracker versus HTII-280 expression in the epithelial cell population, as in Figure 2A, led to the identification of four populations: Q1 (Lyso^{pos}/HTII-280^{neg}), Q2 (Lyso^{pos}/HTII-280^{pos}), Q3 (Lyso^{neg}/HTII-280^{pos}), and Q4 (Lyso^{neg}/HTII-280^{neg}) (Figure 2C). In donor and COPD samples, the largest proportion of epithelial cells comprised bona fide AEC2s (Q2: 79.64% Donor and 67.39% COPD), which were Lyso^{pos}/HTII-280^{pos}. In contrast, in the IPF samples, the proportion of Q2 cells was markedly reduced to an average of 14.33%, consistent with the well-established chronic injury of AEC2s characteristic of IPF. This decrease in Q2 was paralleled by a marked increase in Q1, which represents the Lyso^{pos}/HTII-280^{neg} cells, from 5.12% in donor samples and 9.43% in COPD samples to 47.73% in IPF (Figure 2D,E). Populations Q3 and Q4 were not significantly altered in all comparisons, with the exception of a slight but statistically increase in Q4 in the comparison of COPD and IFP samples (Supplemental Figure S2E). The analysis was very consistent from patient to patient, with some variability noted in the Q4 (Lyso^{neg}/HTII-280^{pos}) population, as shown in Supplemental Figure S2F.

At a first glance, the gating strategy suggests that the Q2 population consists mostly of Lyso^{high} cells, while the Lyso^{low} cells belong to Q1. Thus, we compared the mean fluorescence intensity (MFI) of the LysoTracker-incorporating populations Q1 and Q2, which showed a constant and statistically significant increase in LysoTracker incorporation in Q2 compared to Q1, demonstrating that Q2 comprises mostly Lyso^{high} cells and Q1 comprises mostly Lyso^{low} cells. This difference was maintained in all three groups, regardless of their disease status (Figure 2F), suggesting that these two parameters define two distinct cellular states and, in this regard, functionally homogeneous populations (Figure 2G,H). Taken together, our data suggest the existence of two distinct epithelial populations with distinct LysoTracker uptake characteristics that vary in an inversely correlated manner, suggestive of compensatory behavior in IPF patients compared to donors. Moreover, the Lyso^{high} population is marked by the well-established HTII-280 antibody, confirming its bona fide AEC2 identity.

3.3. Surfactant Protein Expression Defines Two Populations of AEC2s in Donor and IPF Lung

Surfactant protein production, processing and secretion is the most defining characteristic of AEC2s. Thus, we asked what the pattern of proSPC expression is in relation to HTII-280. To that end, following the usual cell surface staining (CD45, CD31, EpCAM, and HTII-280), the same six donor and six IPF single-cell preparations used in the previous analysis were fixed, permeabilized, and stained intracellularly with a proSP-C specific antibody. Because the LysoTracker signal is lost during the fixation process, we relied on HTII-280 reactivity for the identification of the bona fide AEC2s (DAPI^{neg} CD45^{neg} CD31^{neg} EpCAM^{pos} HTII-280^{pos}). Analysis of HTII-280 vs. proSPC expression in these samples resulted in four populations: Q1 (proSP-C^{pos}/HTII-280^{neg}), Q2 (proSP-C^{pos}/HTII-280^{pos}), Q3 (proSP-C^{neg}/HTII-280^{pos}) and Q4 (proSP-C^{neg}/HTII-280^{neg}) (Figure 3A and Supplemental Figure S3A,B). Similar to the Lyso/HTII-280 analysis (Figure 2), donor bona fide AEC2s (Q2, proSP-C^{pos}/HTII-280^{pos}) were the highest represented population (Q2 = 66.7%) and their proportion was markedly decreased to 6.75% in IPF samples (Figure 3B). Moreover, a population that was HTII-280^{neg} but expressed lower levels of proSP-C than Q2 was present in both patient groups, and it was markedly increased in IPF (donor Q1 = 17.31% vs. IPF Q1 = 33.84%, Figure 3B,C). Confirming previously known data, analysis of the amount of proSP-C expressed, as measured by the proSP-C MFI of each population, showed that in IPF the bona fide AEC2s (Q2) expressed significantly less proSP-C compared to donors. However, the Q1 (proSP-C^{pos}/HTII-280^{neg}) population, which was increased proportionally in IPF patients, did not differ in the amount of proSP-C expressed (Figure 3B–D). This suggests that, while in IPF the number and SP-producing function of AEC2s is decreased, the potentially compensatory proSP-C^{low} HTII-280^{neg} (Q1) population expresses lower levels of proSP-C. Additionally, there was a statistically significant increase in the proSP-C^{neg} HTII-280^{neg} (Q4) population, which suggested the increased presence of non-AEC2 cells in the distal IPF lung (Figure 3D). The Q3 population, representing proSP-C^{neg} HTII-280^{pos} cells was negligible and did not vary significantly with the disease state (Supplemental Figure S3C).

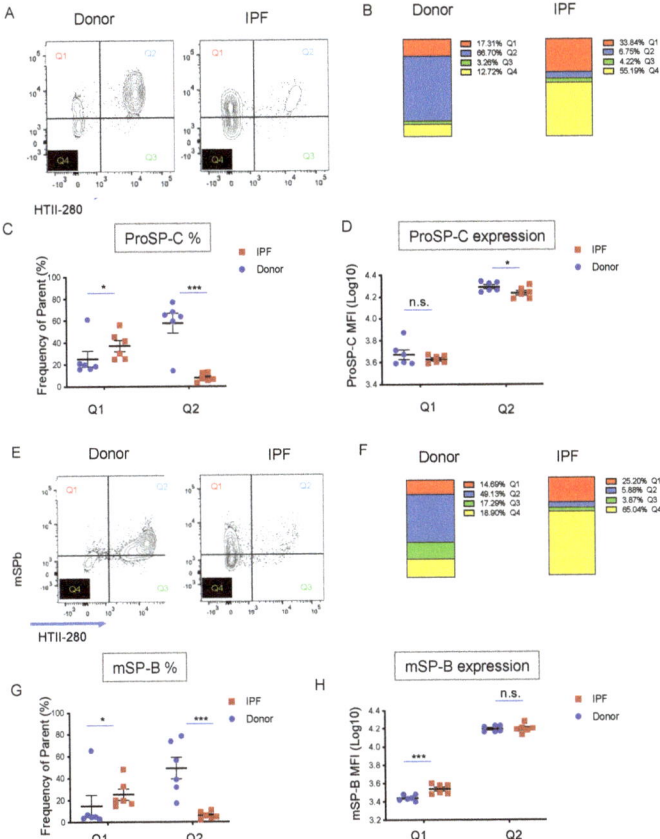

Figure 3. Surfactant protein expression in the epithelial compartment of donor and IPF lung. (**A**) Representative flow cytometry panels of proSP-C and HTII-280 expression in the epithelial compartment (DAPI$^-$ CD45$^-$ CD31$^-$ EpCAM$^+$) of donor ($n = 6$) and IPF ($n = 6$) lung preparations. (**B**) Average contribution of the Q1–Q4 populations to the epithelial compartment of the samples shown in (**A**), showing the change in epithelial composition in IPF lung compared to donors. Left column: donors; right column: IPF. (**C**) Quantification of the population frequency of Q1 and Q2 in donor (blue dot) and IPF (red square) lung samples shown in (**A**). (**D**) Quantification of the MFI as a measure of proSP-C expression level (log10 MFI) in the Q1 and Q2 populations of the samples shown in (**A**). (**E**) Representative flow cytometry panels of mSP-B and HTII-280 expression in the epithelial compartment (DAPI$^-$ CD45$^-$ CD31$^-$ EpCAM$^+$) of donor ($n = 6$) and IPF ($n = 6$) lung preparations. (**F**) Average contribution of the Q1–Q4 populations to the epithelial compartment of the samples shown in (**E**). Left column: donors; right column: IPF. (**G**) Quantification of the population frequency of Q1 and Q2 in donor and IPF lung samples in (**E**). (**H**) Quantification of the MFI as a measure of mSP-B expression level in the Q2 population of the samples in (**E**). Data are presented as the means ± SEM of the log10 (MFI) values. * $p < 0.05$, *** $p < 0.001$, ns = not significant by Student t-test.

Although characteristic for the alveolar epithelium, expression of proSP-C and proSP-B has been previously noted in the non-alveolar compartment of the human lung. However, only AEC2s have the unique ability to process and secrete the mature forms (mSP-C and mSP-B). Thus, we analyzed the expression of mature SP-B (mSP-B) by intracellular staining of the same donor ($n = 6$) and IPF ($n = 6$) samples as in the previous analyses in conjunction with the usual cell surface markers. Similar to the proSP-C data, mSP-B was expressed in the majority of the bona fide AEC2s (Q2: HTII-280^{pos} mSP-B^{pos}) in both donor and IPF, and their proportion was drastically reduced in IPF (Figure 3E,F and Supplemental Figure S3D). However, the IPF Q1 (HTII-280^{neg} mSP-B^{pos}) population expressed higher levels of mSP-B than donor Q1, suggesting an upregulation of the surfactant processing ability in this population in disease conditions. Of note, the expression level of mSP-B in Q1 of IPF remained below that of Q2 (HTII-280^{pos} mSP-B^{pos}), suggesting a distinct functional state of this population (Figure 3E–H). Similar to the proSP-C data, there was no significant change in the proportion of the Q3 (HTII-280^{pos} mSP-B^{neg}) population but there was a significant increase in Q4 (HTII-280^{neg} mSP-B^{neg}) cells.

Throughout our analysis, we noticed very consistent similarities among the LysoTracker, proSP-C and mSP-B expression pattern in relation to HTII-280: the Q1 and Q2 populations behaved similarly in all samples in each analysis. The co-staining of LysoTracker with intracellular markers is technically not feasible because of the loss of LysoTracker fluorescence during the fixation/permeabilization process necessary for intracellular staining. However, comparative and concomitant analysis of the Q1–Q4 profile with the three markers in the same donor ($n = 6$) and IPF ($n = 6$) patient samples showed that the proportion of cells belonging to Q1–4 in each population was very similar in the three parallel analyses (Figure 4A). This suggested, in a correlative manner, that the Q1 population represents a Lyso^{low}, proSP-C^{low}, mSP-B^{low} population of AEC2-like cells while the Q2 population represents the Lyso^{high}, proSP-C^{high}, mSP-C^{high} population of bona fide AEC2s. To confirm the existence of mSP-B expressing cells outside of the LysoTracker-incorporating compartment, donor and IPF peripheral lung tissue sections were co-stained for mSP-B and ABCA3, a protein specifically expressed in the lamellar bodies of mature AEC2s. Indeed, in the donor lung, mSP-B was present in almost all ABCA3-expressing AEC2s, while in IPF extensive epithelial areas (identified morphologically) were characterized by mSP-B expression in the absence of ABCA3 (Figure 4B). The expression of LysoTracker and proSP-C was very consistent within each patient group (Do vs. IPF and Supplemental Figure S4). However, the intensity of the mSP-B staining was highly variable within the same patient group, suggesting the existence of a variable mSP-B processing capacity (Figure 4A and Supplemental Figure S4A). To confirm that the variable processing ability of AEC2 cells was not an artefact of the cell isolation procedure, donor ($n = 4$) and IPF ($n = 4$) paraffin-embedded tissue sections were co-stained for proSP-B and mSP-B, and the fluorescence intensity of each was quantified. A linear regression analysis showed that the processing ability of each sample, represented by the regression's slope, was variable within each group, but an overall flattening of the slope was noted between IPF and donor samples. Moreover, the two values yielded were positively correlated in most donor samples (positive R^2 values), but this correlation was lost in three out of the four IPF samples ($R^2 = 0$, Figure 4C,D). When analyzing the spatial distribution of the two signals, we noticed that in donors they were tightly co-expressed (Figure 4D upper panels), but in IPF there was a heterogeneous distribution of the areas of mature and proSP-B co-localization (particularly in non-affected areas, Figure 4D panels in rows 2 and 4) and areas where the mSP-B was low or absent in cells that expressed the pro forms (Figure 4D—panels in row 3). Together, these data show that while it is variable in donor samples, mSP-B processing ability is decreased in IPF.

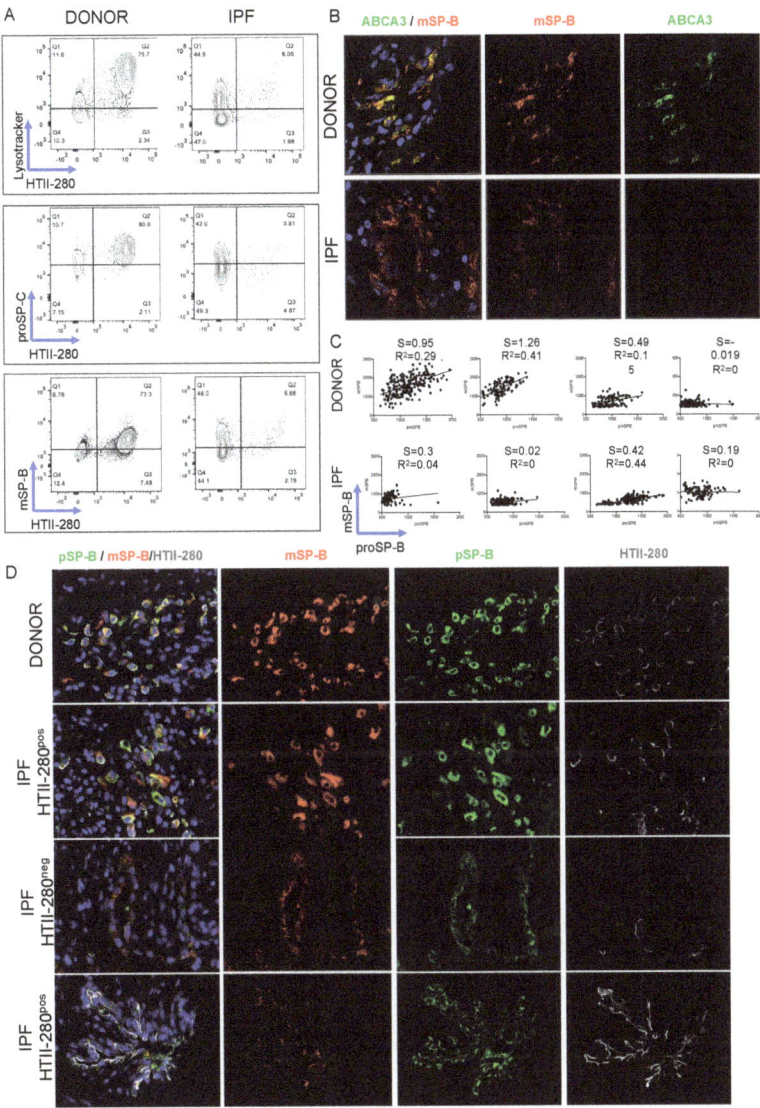

Figure 4. Comparative expression of LysoTracker, proSP-C and mSP-B expression in donor and IPF lung. (**A**) Six donor and six IPF lung preparations were co-stained in parallel with HTII-280, LysoTracker, proSP-C and mSP-B. Representative flow cytometry panels of LysoTracker (upper), proSP-C (middle) and mSP-B (lower) vs. HTII-280 expression in the epithelial compartment of one donor (left column) and one IPF (right column) lung. (**B**) Representative immunofluorescence images of mature (red) and ABCA3 (green) in donor and IPF paraffin-embedded lung tissues. (**C**) Quantification of the fluorescence intensity of the mature SP-B and proSP-B immunofluorescence signals in four donor (upper row) and four IPF (lower row) patients, showing the slope (s) of the linear regression and the correlation index (R^2) for each patient. (**D**) Representative immunofluorescence images of the mature (red) and proSP-B (green) in donor and IPF tissues shown in (**C**).

3.4. Transcriptional Characterization of the IPF Lyso^{low} Population

Given the recent single-cell NGS data that identified the existence of transitional AEC2 states with distinct transcriptomic signatures in normal and IPF lungs [28–31,46], we asked if the Lyso^{low} population in IPF, which has an intermediate expression profile in terms of LysoTracker and surfactant protein expression, resembled any of the previously mentioned intermediate populations. Thus, we used microarray analysis to compare the transcriptomic profile of eight FACS-sorted donor Lyso^{pos} AEC2s, composed, in the majority, of Lyso^{high} cells (see Figure 2A), and Lyso^{pos} cells from six IPF lungs, consisting, in the majority, of Lyso^{low} cells (Figures 2A and 5A). Principal component analysis of the data showed the lack of variance between the two groups (Supplemental Figure S5A), suggesting great similarities between the two populations. However, in this analysis, 612 genes were upregulated (LFC > 2) and 1382 genes were downregulated (LFC < −2) in IPF Lyso^{pos} compared to donor Lyso^{pos} AEC2s. Interestingly, the first 50 upregulated genes in the Lyso^{pos} population of IPF patients included several genes known to be upregulated in IPF while several surfactant-related genes were noted in the 50 most downregulated genes (Figure 5B and Supplemental Figure S5B). Validating our data, KEGG analysis identified metabolic pathways and pathways related to protein synthesis/processing and oxidative phosphorylation as being the most significantly downregulated pathways in IPF (Figure 5C). To determine the phenotype of the Lyso^{pos} IPF population, we superimposed the transcriptomic signatures of several relevant cell types from two recent publications onto our differentially expressed gene expression data [29,31]. First, we defined the signatures of all relevant cell types in each data set using the first 30 most differentially expressed genes for each cell type: AEC2, signaling AEC2, basal, differentiating and proliferating basal, AEC1, ciliated and club cells (Travaglini et al.), and AEC2, AEC1, basal, aberrant basal, ciliated and club (Adams et al.). These signatures were then superimposed onto our Donor/IPF LysoTracker comparison, showing an overall downregulation of the AEC2 signature in the IPF Lyso^{pos} population. However, a closer look at the surfactant compartment genes revealed the significant downregulation of several surfactant synthesis and processing genes (*NAPSA, ABCA3, LAMP3, LPCAT1*), while the surfactant protein genes *SFTPB* and *SFTPC* were not significantly regulated (*SFTPC* LFC = −0.25, LOG(p) = 0.24 and *SFTPB* LFC = −0.30, LOG(p) = 0.50). This suggested that the two populations, which homogeneously express proSP-B and proSP-C mRNA (Figure 5D) and protein (Figure 3), differ in the expression of the processing machinery that would normally commit them to a bona fide AEC2 fate. In addition, two fundamental regulators of AEC2 fate had opposite patterns of expression: IPF Lyso^{pos} cells expressed markedly decreased levels of *ETV5* (LFC =−3.42, LOG(p) = 2.32), but *SOX9* (LFC = 3.25, LOG(p) = 8.93) was one of the top overexpressed genes in our data set (Figure 5D and Supplemental Figure S5C,D). Further analysis showed the upregulation of basal, differentiating basal and aberrant basal transcriptomic signatures in IPF, suggesting the presence of cells belonging to the basal cell lineage. Ciliated, club and AEC1 signatures did not unequivocally superimpose with any of the up or downregulated transcriptomic profiles (Figure 5E and Supplemental Figure S5C,D). Taken together, this data demonstrates that the Lyso^{pos} population in IPF most likely represents a heterogeneous population of basal-derived cells with the common property of surfactant protein B and C expression but lacking a mature surfactant processing compartment necessary to compensate for the surfactant defects known to occur in IPF.

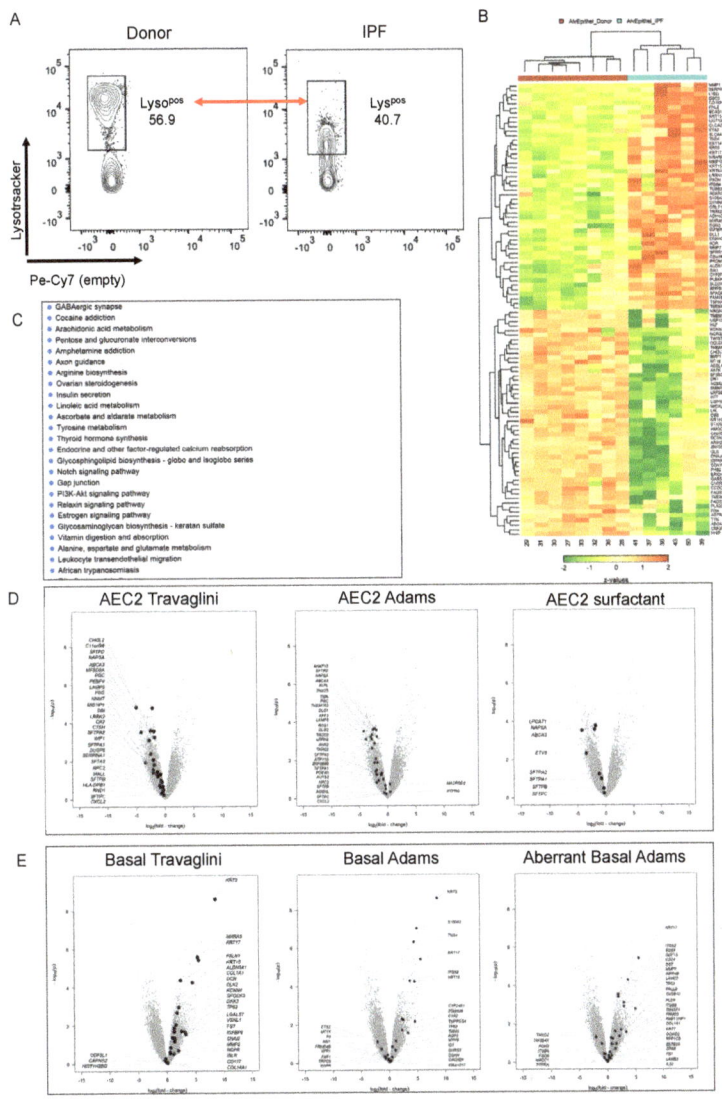

Figure 5. Transcriptomic profiling of the Lyso^{pos} population in IPF. Donor Lyso^{pos} ($n = 8$) and IPF Lyso^{pos} ($n = 6$) epithelial cells were isolated by flow cytometry and their transcriptomic profiles were determined by microarray analysis. (**A**) Flow cytometry panels showing the sorting strategy for the two populations. (**B**) Heat map of the first upregulated and downregulated genes in IPF Lyso^{pos} vs. donor Lyso^{pos}. (**C**) KEGG pathway analysis showing the first 20 most differential regulated pathways. (**D**) The transcriptomic signatures of AEC2 that were identified by Travaglini et al. and Adams et al. were superimposed on the vulcano plots depicting the upregulated and downregulated genes in IPF Lyso^{pos} compared to donor Lyso^{pos} (left and middle plots). The right plot shows the distribution of surfactant production and processing genes. (**E**) The transcriptomic signatures of various populations of donor and IPF basal cells that were identified by Travaglini et al. and Adams et al. were superimposed on the vulcano plots depicting the upregulated and downregulated genes in IPF Lyso^{pos} compared to donor Lyso^{pos}.

3.5. Basal Cell Marker Expression in Donor and IPF Lung

Our data, in consensus with the existing literature, suggested an increase in basal and aberrant basaloid cells in the distal lung epithelium of IPF patients, which have, in the past, been identified by their intracellular expression of cytokeratin 5 (CK5, the protein product of *KRT5* mRNA) or cell surface expression of NGFR [47,48]. First, we determined by flow cytometry the expression of the CK5 protein in the epithelial compartment of six donor and six IPF lungs. Of note, CK5 expression as a function of HTII-280 demonstrated that HTII-280^{pos} cells did not express CK5 in donor or IPF lung, and the CK5 upregulation was strictly limited to the HTII-280^{neg} compartment (Figure 6A and Supplemental Figure S6A). Indeed, the number of CK5^{pos} cells was greatly increased in the epithelial compartment of IPF lung (average Q3 = 37.86%) compared to donor lung (average Q3 = 12.15% Figure 6A,B and Supplemental Figure S6B). We also determined, in a similar manner, the cell surface expression of NGFR in six donor and six IPF lung cell preparations (Figure 6C,D and Supplemental Figure S6C,D). While the number of NGFR^{pos} cells also increased significantly in proportion in IPF compared to donor epithelial cells (average 20.1% IPF vs. 3% donor), their proportion was much lower than that of CK5^{pos} cells in both groups (donor and IPF), suggesting the existence of a population of CK5^{pos} cells that do not express NGFR. Of note, in our transcriptomic analysis, NGFR showed levels of expression in both AEC2 populations below the threshold above which a gene was considered to be expressed (Figure 6B and Supplemental Figure S6B). We next asked if the expression of the two markers defines distinctly localized populations of epithelial cells in either donor and/or IPF lung. Thus, we analyzed by immunofluorescence staining the pattern of expression of CK5 and NGFR together with the AEC2 marker ABCA3 in six donor and six IPF lung samples. Representative confocal images (Figure 6E) show that, in both donor and IPF lungs, ABCA3-expressing AEC2s expressed neither CK5 nor NGFR, confirming the flow cytometry data in Figure 6A,C. Additionally, in donor's lung, extensive areas of basal cells were labeled with either CK5 alone or co-expressed with NGFR (CK5^{pos} NGFR^{pos} cells) in a clonal fashion. In the IPF lung, CK5^{pos} NGFR^{pos} cells were found in either normal-appearing basal cells in the conducting airways or in the simple or pseudo-stratified epithelium lining epithelial cysts in distal fibrotic areas. CK5^{pos} NGFR^{neg} cells were present, predominantly as highly metaplastic areas in the fibrotic distal lung (Figure 6D). Together, these data demonstrate that NGFR expression can differentiate two populations of CK5^{pos} basal cells with different behavior in IPF.

3.6. CD24 Upregulation in IPF

CD24 was identified as a cell surface marker highly expressed by aberrant basaloid cells [31] and in the KRT5-/KRT17+ intermediate cells [32] (Figure 7A and Supplemental Figure S7A). In our transcriptomic analysis, CD24 was also markedly increased in IPF Lyso^{low} cells (LFC = 2.92, LOG(p) = 3.1). To determine which epithelial cells express CD24, we stained four donor and three IPF lung cell preparations with the usual cell surface markers in combination with a CD24 antibody, and its expression was analyzed in the epithelial compartment as a function of LysoTracker uptake. In donor epithelial cells, the proportion of CD24^{pos} cells was very small (average 1.4% in Lyso^{high} and 3.41% in Lyso^{low} population), but its expression was markedly increased in both IPF Lyso^{high} and Lyso^{low} populations (average 15.2% and 28.5% respectively, Figure 7B–D; individual patient data in Supplemental Figure S7B,C). Given the basal/AEC2 profile of the Lyso^{low} CD24^{pos} population suggested by our transcriptomic data, our cell surface expression analysis allows us to speculate that the CD24^{pos} Lyso^{low} cells might represent a sub-population of an IPF-specific intermediate cell type.

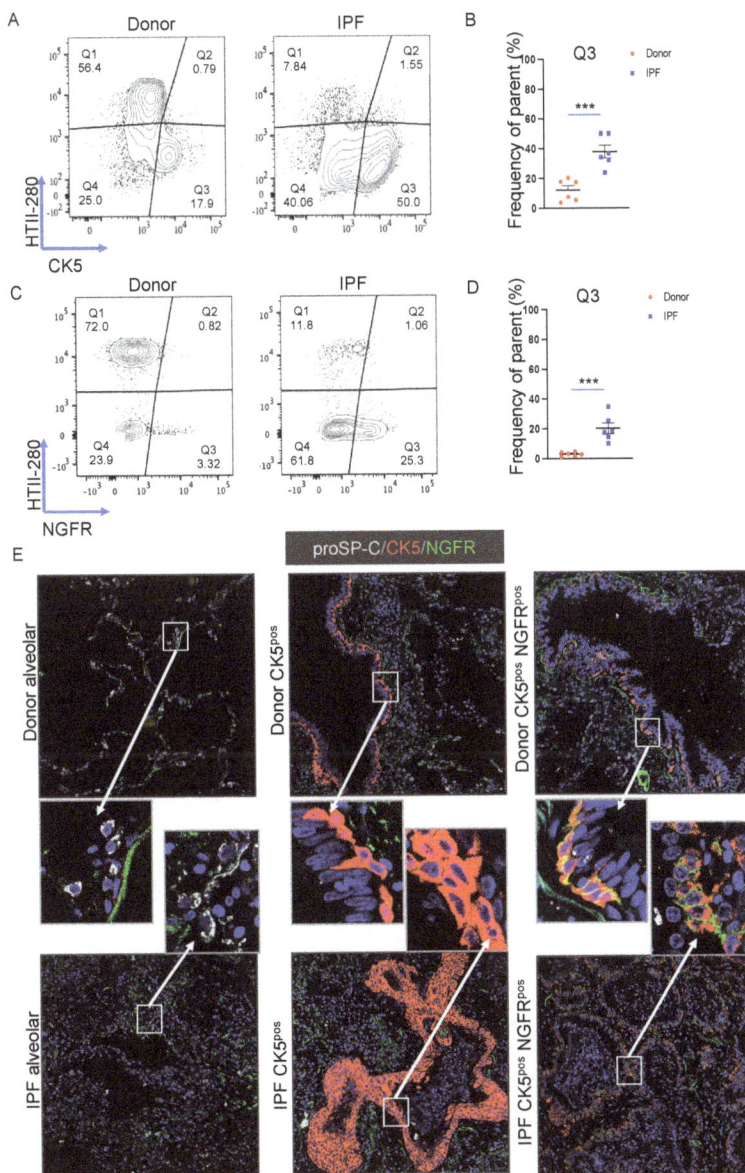

Figure 6. CK5 and NGFR expression in donor and IPF epithelial cells. (**A**) Representative flow cytometry panels of CK5 vs. HTII-280 expression in the epithelial cell compartment of donor ($n = 6$, left) and IPF ($n = 6$, right) lungs. (**B**) Quantification of the CK5^{pos} HTII-280^{neg} (Q3) population shown in (**A**). (**C**) Representative flow cytometry panels of NGFR vs. HTII-280 expression in the epithelial cell compartment of donor ($n = 6$, left) and IPF ($n = 6$, right) lungs. (**D**) Quantification of the NGFR^{pos} HTII-280^{neg} (Q3) population shown in (**C**). Data are presented as the means ± SEM of the percentage of cells from the parent population. Statistical analysis was performed on log(10) values. *** $p < 0.001$, n.s. = not significant by ANOVA. (**E**) Representative confocal images of proSP-C (white signal), CK5 (red signal) and NGFR (green signal) in different locations of donor (upper images) and IPF (lower images) lung.

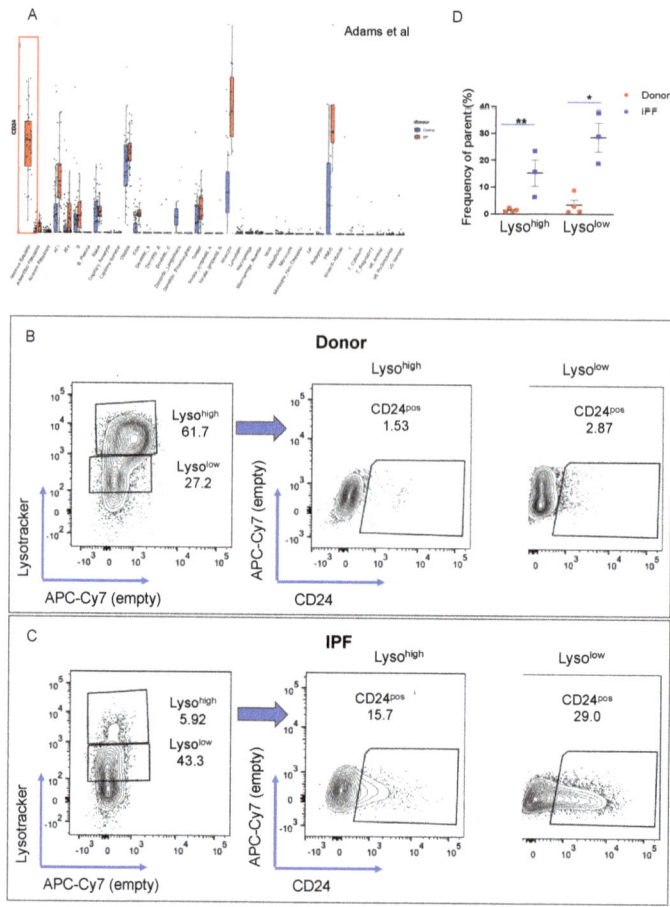

Figure 7. CD24 expression in donor and IPF lung. (**A**) Differential expression of CD24 in donor and IPF scNGS data published by Adams et al. (**B**), (**C**) Flow cytometry analysis of donor (n = 4) (**B**) and IPF (n = 3) (**C**) samples of LysoTracker incorporation in the epithelial cell compartment (left panel). Right panels show the expression of CD24 in the Lyso^{high} and Lyso^{low} populations shown in the panels on the left. (**D**) Quantification of the data in (**B**,**C**) showing the difference between donor and IPF Lyso^{high} and Lyso^{low} populations. Average donor Lyso^{high} CD24^{pos} 1.4%, donor Lyso^{low} CD24^{pos} 0.34%; IPF Lyso^{high} CD24^{pos} 15.2% and IPF Lyso^{low} CD24^{pos} 28.53%. Data are presented as the means ± SEM of the percentage of cells from the parent population. Statistical analysis was performed on log(10) values. * $p < 0.05$, ** $p < 0.01$, n.s. = not significant by ANOVA.

4. Discussion

Here we provide an in-depth phenotypical analysis of human alveolar epithelial cells isolated from donor and end-stage IPF explanted lungs. In doing so, we identify two populations that differ markedly in their ability to process and secrete surfactant, the defining differentiated function of AEC2s. During bleomycin-induced lung fibrosis, the two populations vary in complementary directions, suggestive of correlative behavior. Comparing the transcriptome of the IPF and donor Lyso^{pos} populations in human lung, we determine that the IPF Lyso^{pos} population co-expresses markers of basal and AEC2 lineages. We further confirm by flow cytometry and immunofluorescence analysis the

CK5^{pos} cell expansion in IPF and show that CK5 and NGFR expression define two distinct basal cell populations with differential behavior in IPF.

CD24 is a widely expressed glycophospholipid (GPI)-anchored cell surface protein localized to lipid rafts with a versatile signaling ability through cis- and trans-association with various transmembrane receptors [49]. Its epithelial expression was recently identified as the core of the ligand-receptor interactome in the development of human lung adenocarcinoma [50]. Interestingly, in ovarian and breast cancer, CD24 functions as a checkpoint inhibitory molecule, mediating macrophage-phagocytosis evasion through its interaction with Siglec 10 [51]. In IPF, its expression is specifically increased in aberrant epithelial cells, ionocytes, and pulmonary neuroendocrine cells [30–32]. Our data confirm the increased cell-surface expression of CD24 in the intermediate Lyso^{low} population in IPF, thus offering a potential cell surface marker to sub-type, together with LysoTracker incorporation, various populations of epithelial cells in donor and IPF lung. A possible correlation between CD24 expression and the well-documented increase in lung adenocarcinoma development in IPF patients is intriguing and remains to be addressed experimentally [50].

The emergence of single-cell transcriptomics led to the in-depth profiling of already known populations of cells and the identification of other novel populations in the mouse and human lung [27,29–32,52]. Recent landmark papers led to the identification of epithelial populations with an intermediate transcriptomic signature in the IPF lung. First, a population of cells with an "intermediate phenotype" that resembled the transcriptomic profiles of both AEC2s and basal cells was identified by Xu et al. [28]. Recently, a similar population of cells specific for IPF called aberrant basal cells was described by Reyfman et al. and by Adams et al. [30,31].

Similarly, we find that the Lyso^{pos} population in IPF expresses several markers defining these intermediate populations. Characteristic markers, such as KRT5, 15 and 17, ITGA2, Sox4, Sox9, and CD24, are expressed at high levels, together with the AEC2 genes SFTPB and C. Genes involved in surfactant protein processing and secretion are also expressed in the IPF Lyso^{pos} population, although they do not reach the level of expression of the donor AEC2s, which correlates well with the low and intermediate levels of LysoTracker incorporation in this population. Interestingly, two genes defining the AEC2 cell fate, *ETV5* and *SOX9*, are also expressed in the IPF Lyso^{pos} population, but while *SOX9* is expressed at levels exceeding that of bona fide AEC2s, *ETV5* expression is much lower, suggesting that they regulate different aspects of the IPF alveolar epithelial fate. Indeed, *SOX9* is crucial for mouse and human distal lung epithelium specification [53–56], while *ETV5*, acting downstream of *SOX9* [56–59] and FGF signaling [60,61], is crucial for AEC2 fate maintenance and is downregulated in transitional states, such as the AEC2 to AEC1 transition [61]. Interestingly, a recent paper identified a population with similar characteristics in the mouse lung [62]. Lineage tracing of alveolar epithelial cells using the SFTPCcreER/Rosa26^{TdTomato} double transgenic mice revealed a TdTomato^{low} population of cells which express low levels of the AEC2 markers proSP-C, *etv5* and *Fgfr2b* that has progenitor cell properties. This suggests that a similar population with intermediate AEC2 characteristics and progenitor properties exists in the mouse lung, which is supported by our data showing the maximum expansion of the Lyso^{low} population at the peak of epithelial proliferation (day 14) following bleomycin injury.

There are multiple circumstances that require the transition through an intermediate fate. First, it has been shown that multiple progenitors can participate in the repair of the alveolar epithelium [63]. It is, thus, conceivable that they converge on a common intermediate state on their way to becoming fully differentiated AEC2s. Second, aberrant progenitors, that in a normal state do not participate in alveolar repair, can be recruited when the local progenitor pool is exhausted, as is the case in the IPF lung, converging towards the same intermediate fate. Third, AEC2 divergent intermediate fates could also emerge, such as (1) AEC2s differentiating into AEC1s [43], (2) AEC2s de-differentiating in order to assume a progenitor function [22] or (3) AEC2s that temporarily limit their differentiated function to allow recovery from injury. Thus, although the Lyso^{low} population appears homogeneous from a phenotypic perspective, as seen by the surfactant protein expression and LysoTracker incorporation, one cannot exclude that it might represent a lineage-diverse population. Based on our data, we propose that the Lyso^{low} population represents a stable cellular state on the way to or from a mature AEC2, rather than a particular cell type. Our population level transcriptomic analysis does not allow us to draw conclusions about the lineage composition or transcriptomic heterogeneity of the Lyso^{low} population, but flow cytometry analysis offers a modality of isolating cells in this intermediate state for further analysis.

In conclusion, we show that LysoTracker incorporation defines two cellular states in donor and IPF distal epithelial lung, with the Lyso^{high} state representing bona fide AEC2s and the Lyso^{low} state characterizing an intermediate cell population displaying both basal and AEC2 characteristics.

Supplementary Materials: The following supporting information can be downloaded at: https://www.mdpi.com/article/10.3390/cells11020235/s1, Figure S1: Characterization of lung cells in bleomycin model of lung fibrosis and human IPF lung (A) Representative panels showing the gating strategy of dissociated mouse lung: cell-debris discriminated based on size and granularity ("cells" gate); elimination of PDP+ and PI+ cells ("live PDP-" gate); identification of epithelial cells (EpCAM+ CD45- CD31-); doublet exclusion in the epithelial population ("single-cell" gate). (B) Flow cytometry panels of Lysotracker incorporation in a control mouse lung (left) and the corresponding fluorescence minus one (FMO) gating control. (C) Statistical analysis of the epithelial compartment (PI- CD45- CD31- PDP- EpCAM+); Figure S2: Lysotracker uptake in the epithelial compartment of the human lung. (A) Representative panels showing the gating strategy of dissociated human lung: cell-debris discriminated based on size and granularity ("cells" gate); elimination of DAPI+ cells ("live" gate); identification of epithelial cells (EpCAM+ CD45- CD31-); doublet exclusion in the epithelial population ("single-cell" gate). (B) Flow cytometry panels of Lysotracker incorporation in a control human lung (left) and the corresponding fluorescence minus one (FMO) gating control. Statistical analysis of the proportion of epithelial cells (DAPI- CD45- CD31- EpCAM+) in donor and IPF samples. Data are presented as the mean ± SEM. * $p < 0.05$, ** $p < 0.01$, *** $p < 0.001$, ns = not significant by Student t-test. (C) Individual panels of Lysotracker incorporation in the epithelial compartment of each donor and IPF patient. (D) Gating controls for the Lysotracker / HTII-280 analysis. First two panels correspond to the respective FMO controls for Lysotracker and HTII-280, the third panel shows the background of the secondary antibody used to detect HTII-280. (E) Statistical analysis of the proportion of Q3 and Q4 populations in donor, COPD and IPF patients. Data are presented as the mean ± SEM of Log10 (MFI). Statistical analysis was performed on Log(10) values. ** $p < 0.01$, n.s. = not significant by ANOVA. (F) Individual panels of Lysotracker/HTII-280 distribution in the epithelial compartment of each donor, COPD and IPF patient; Figure S3: Surfactant protein expression in the epithelial compartment of donor and IPF lung. (A) Staining controls used to define the gating of the proSP-C and mSP-B vs HTII-280 analysis. First panel shows the "no primary" FMO control which is shared by the proSP-C and mSP-B, second panel shows the "no primary" FMO control for HTII-280. (B) Quantification of the population frequency of Q3 and Q4 in proSP-C stained donor and IPF lung samples shown in Figure 3A. (C) Quantification of the population frequency of Q3 and Q4 in mSP-B stained donor and IPF lung samples shown in Figure 3E. (D) Analysis of mSP-B expression (histogram) in the bona-fide AEC2s defined as HTII-280pos cells in donor and IPF epithelial cells (same data set as Figure 3E–H). Upper panels show the gating strategy of the HTII-280pos population (donor and IPF). Lower left, the overlay histogram of mSP-B expression in the HTII-280pos population in donor (blue) and IPF (red) is shown. Lower right shows the quantification of the % of mSP-B cells within the HTII-280pos population in donor (blue) and IPF (red) patients; Figure S4: Individual flow cytometry panels of Lysotracker, proSP-C and mSP-B vs HTII-280 expression in the epithelial compartment (DAPI- CD45- CD31- EpCAM+) of all donor (left column, n = 6) and IPF (right column, n = 6) lung preparations shown in Figure 4; Figure S5: Transcriptomic profiling of the Lysopos population in IPF. (A) PCA analysis of the IPF Lysopos (blue triangles) and Donor Lysopos(orange circles). (B) List of the 20 most up-regulated (left)and down-regulated (right) genes in IPF Lysopos vs donor Lysopos population. (C), (D) The transcriptomic signatures of AEC2 identified by Travaglini et al. and Adams et al. were superimposed on the vulcano plots depiction of the up and downregulated genes in IPF Lysopos compared to donor

Lysopos. (C)Transcriptomic signatures of different epithelial cell populations in donor lung identified by Travaglini et al. transposed onto our Do/IPF data. (D) Transcriptomic signatures of different epithelial cell populations in IPF lung identified by Adams et al. transposed onto our Do/IPF data; Figure S6. CK5 and NGFR expression in donor and IPF epithelial cells. (A) FMO gating control for CK5. (B) CK5 HTII-280 flow cytometry plots for individual donor and IPF patients shown in Figure 6. (C) No primary HTII-280 and NGFR FMO controls. (D) NGFR HTII-280 flow cytometry plots for individual donor and IPF patients shown in Figure 6; Figure S7: CD24 expression in donor and IPF lung. (A) Differential expression of CD24 in donor and IPF scNGS data published by Habermann et al. (B), (C)Individual flow cytometry panels of n = 4 donor (B) and n = 3 IPF (C) of Lysotracker incorporation in the epithelial cell compartment (left panel) shown in Figure 7. Table S1: Important materials; Table S2: Antibodies used in experiments.

Author Contributions: Conceptualization, R.M.W. and A.G.; Data curation, J.W.; Formal analysis, R.M.W., I.S., J.W., A.K., N.S. and E.E.A.; Investigation, R.M.W., I.S., J.W. and E.E.A.; Methodology, J.W., A.K., N.S. and H.H.; Project administration, W.S.; Resources, H.H., A.H., K.H., W.S., C.R. and A.G.; Supervision, A.G.; Writing—original draft, R.M.W.; Writing—review and editing, R.M.W., S.B., E.E.A., C.R. and A.G. All authors have read and agreed to the published version of the manuscript.

Funding: This study was supported, in part, by the RARE-ILD consortium (European Joint Program on Rare Diseases, EJP-RD), the Lung Fibrosis Stipend of the Lung Clinic Waldhof Elgershausen, the Clinical Research Group (KFO309 Project 7 284237345) and the Institute for Lung Health (ILH).

Institutional Review Board Statement: The study was conducted according to the guidelines of the Declaration of Helsinki and was approved by the Ethics Committee of the Justus-Liebig-University School of Medicine (No. 31/93, 29/01, and No. 111/08: European IPF Registry), and informed consent was obtained in written form from each subject. Animal studies were performed in accordance with the Helsinki convention for the use and care of animals and were approved by the local authorities at Regierungspräsidium Giessen V54-19 c 2015 (1) GI 20/10 Nr. 109/2011 (Bleomycin) or V54-19 c 20 15 h 02 GI 20/10 Nr. A53/2012 (untreated controls).

Informed Consent Statement: Informed consent was obtained from all subjects involved in the study prior to biospecimen collection.

Data Availability Statement: Transcriptomic data is publicly available at the following location: https://www.ncbi.nlm.nih.gov/geo/query/acc.cgi?acc=GSE185691.

Acknowledgments: The authors would like to acknowledge the technical assistance of Simone Becker and Gabriele Dahlem. We would like to thank Gabriela Michel and Neli Baal from the Zentrum für Transfusionsmedizin und Hämotherapie, Institut für Klinische Immunologie (UKGM Giessen) for their priceless assistance with flow cytometry. We also acknowledge the extremely valuable contributions of the Multiscale Imaging Platform and the Genomic and Bioinformatics Platform of the Institute for Lung Health (ILH-Giessen). We would also like to thank Walter Klepetko and the surgical team for collecting the patient material, Ludger Fink for the pathological assessment and the patients themselves without whom this work would not have been possible.

Conflicts of Interest: The authors declare no conflict of interest.

References

1. Günther, A.; Korfei, M.; Mahavadi, P.; von der Beck, D.; Ruppert, C.; Markart, P. Unravelling the progressive pathophysiology of idiopathic pulmonary fibrosis. *Eur. Respir. Rev.* **2012**, *21*, 152–160. [CrossRef]
2. Raghu, G.; Remy-Jardin, M.; Myers, J.L.; Richeldi, L.; Ryerson, C.J.; Lederer, D.J.; Behr, J.; Cottin, V.; Danoff, S.K.; Morell, F.; et al. American thoracic society documents diagnosis of idiopathic pulmonary fibrosis an official ATS/ERS/JRS/ALAT clinical practice guideline. *Am. J. Respir. Crit. Care Med.* **2018**, *198*, 44–68. [CrossRef]
3. Olson, A.L.; Swigris, J.J. Idiopathic pulmonary fibrosis: Diagnosis and epidemiology. *Clin. Chest Med.* **2012**, *33*, 41–50. [CrossRef]
4. Shumar, J.N.; Chandel, A.; King, C.S.; Bendstrup, M. Clinical medicine antifibrotic therapies and Progressive Fibrosing Interstitial Lung Disease (PF-ILD): Building on INBUILD. *J. Clin. Med.* **2021**, *10*, 2285. [CrossRef] [PubMed]
5. Parimon, T.; Hohmann, M.S.; Yao, C.; Marchioni, A.; Tonelli, R. Pathogenic mechanisms in lung fibrosis. *Int. J. Mol. Sci.* **2021**, *2021*, 6214. [CrossRef] [PubMed]
6. Noble, P.W.; Barkauskas, C.E.; Jiang, D. Review series pulmonary brosis: Patterns and perpetrators. *Am. J. Physiol. Lung Cell Mol. Physiol.* **2012**, *122*, 4–10. [CrossRef]

7. Sisson, T.H.; Mendez, M.; Choi, K.; Subbotina, N.; Courey, A.; Cunningham, A.; Dave, A.; Engelhardt, J.F.; Liu, X.; White, E.S.; et al. Targeted injury of type ii alveolar epithelial cells induces pulmonary fibrosis. *Am. J. Respir. Crit. Care Med.* 2010, *181*, 254–263. [CrossRef]
8. Yao, C.; Guan, X.; Carraro, G.; Parimon, T.; Liu, X.; Huang, G.; Mulay, A.; Soukiasian, H.J.; David, G.; Weigt, S.S.; et al. Senescence of alveolar type 2 cells drives progressive pulmonary fibrosis. *Am. J. Respir. Crit. Care Med.* 2021, *203*, 707–717. [CrossRef]
9. Camelo, A.; Dunmore, R.; Sleeman, M.A.; Clarke, D.L. The epithelium in idiopathic pulmonary fibrosis: Breaking the barrier. *Front. Pharmacol.* 2014, *4*, 1–11. [CrossRef]
10. Desai, T.J.; Brownfield, D.G.; Krasnow, M.A. Alveolar progenitor and stem cells in lung development, renewal and cancer. *Nature* 2014, *507*, 190–194. [CrossRef]
11. Zacharias, W.J.; Frank, D.B.; Zepp, J.A.; Morley, M.P.; Alkhaleel, F.A.; Kong, J.; Zhou, S.; Cantu, E.; Morrisey, E.E. Regeneration of the lung alveolus by an evolutionarily conserved epithelial progenitor. *Nature* 2018, *555*, 251–255. [CrossRef]
12. Haller, T.; Ortmayr, J.; Friedrich, F.; Voelkl, F.; Dietl, P. Dynamics of surfactant release in alveolar type II Cells. *Proc. Nat. Acad. Sci. USA* 1998, *95*, 1579–1584. [CrossRef]
13. Weaver, T.E. Synthesis, processing and secretion of surfactant proteins B and C. *Biochim. Biophys. Acta Mol. Basis Dis.* 1998, *1408*, 173–179. [CrossRef]
14. Korimilli, A.; Gonzales, L.W.; Guttentag, S.H. Intracellular localization of processing events in human surfactant protein B biosynthesis. *J. Biol. Chem.* 2000, *275*, 8672–8679. [CrossRef]
15. Sever, N.; Miličić, G.; Bodnar, N.O.; Wu, X.; Rapoport, T.A. Mechanism of lamellar body formation by lung surfactant protein, B. *Mol. Cell* 2021, *81*, 49–66. [CrossRef]
16. Strunz, M.; Simon, L.M.; Ansari, M.; Mattner, L.F.; Angelidis, I.; Mayr, C.H.; Kathiriya, J.; Yee, M.; Ogar, P.; Sengupta, A.; et al. Longitudinal single cell transcriptomics reveals Krt8+ alveolar epithelial progenitors in lung regeneration. *bioRxiv* 2019. [CrossRef]
17. Vaughan, A.E.; Brumwell, A.N.; Xi, Y.; Gotts, J.E.; Brownfield, D.G.; Treutlein, B.; Tan, K.; Tan, V.; Liu, F.C.; Looney, M.R.; et al. Lineage-negative progenitors mobilize to regenerate lung epithelium after major injury. *Nature* 2015, *517*, 621–625. [CrossRef] [PubMed]
18. Liang, J.; Zhang, Y.; Xie, T.; Liu, N.; Chen, H.; Geng, Y.; Kurkciyan, A.; Mena, J.M.; Stripp, B.R.; Jiang, D.; et al. Hyaluronan and TLR4 promote surfactant-protein-C-positive alveolar progenitor cell renewal and prevent severe pulmonary fibrosis in mice. *Nat. Med.* 2016, *22*, 1285–1293. [CrossRef] [PubMed]
19. Lopez-Rodriguez, E.; Boden, C.; Echaide, M.; Perez-Gil, J.; Kolb, M.; Gauldie, J.; Maus, U.A.; Ochs, M.; Knudsen, L. Surfactant dysfunction during overexpression of TGF-B1 precedes profibrotic lung remodeling in vivo. *Am. J. Physiol. Lung Cell. Mol. Physiol.* 2016, *310*, L1260–L1271. [CrossRef] [PubMed]
20. Beike, L.; Wrede, C.; Hegermann, J.; Lopez-Rodriguez, E.; Kloth, C.; Gauldie, J.; Kolb, M.; Maus, U.A.; Ochs, M.; Knudsen, L. Surfactant dysfunction and alveolar collapse are linked with fibrotic septal wall remodeling in the TGF-B1-induced mouse model of pulmonary fibrosis. *Lab. Investig.* 2019, *99*, 830–852. [CrossRef]
21. Mulugeta, S.; Nureki, S.I.; Beers, M.F. Lost after translation: Insights from pulmonary surfactant for understanding the role of alveolar epithelial dysfunction and cellular quality control in fibrotic lung disease. *Am. J. Physiol. Lung Cell. Mol. Physiol.* 2015, *309*, L507–L525. [CrossRef] [PubMed]
22. Wasnick, R.M.; Korfei, M.; Piskulak, K.; Henneke, I.; Wilhelm, J.; Mahavadi, P.; von der Beck, D.; Koch, M.; Shalashova, I.; Klymenko, O.; et al. Restored alveolar epithelial differentiation and reversed human lung fibrosis upon notch inhibition. *bioRxiv* 2019, 580498. [CrossRef]
23. Watanabe, S.; Markov, N.S.; Lu, Z.; Aillon, R.P.; Soberanes, S.; Runyan, C.E.; Ren, Z.; Grant, R.A.; Maciel, M.; Abdala-Valencia, H.; et al. Resetting Proteostasis with ISRIB promotes epithelial differentiation to attenuate pulmonary fibrosis. *Proc. Nat. Acad. Sci. USA* 2021, *118*, e2101100118. [CrossRef]
24. Chapman, H.A.; Li, X.; Alexander, J.P.; Brumwell, A.; Lorizio, W.; Tan, K.; Sonnenberg, A.; Wei, Y.; Vu, T.H. Integrin A6β4 identifies an adult distal lung epithelial population with regenerative potential in mice. *J. Clin. Investig.* 2011, *121*, 2855–2862. [CrossRef]
25. Watson, J.K.; Sanders, P.; Dunmore, R.; Rosignoli, G.; Julé, Y.; Rawlins, E.L.; Mustelin, T.; May, R.; Clarke, D.; Finch, D.K. Distal lung epithelial progenitor cell function declines with age. *Sci. Rep.* 2020, *10*, 1–12. [CrossRef]
26. Yee, M.; Domm, W.; Gelein, R.; de Mesy Bentley, K.L.; Kottmann, R.M.; Sime, P.J.; Lawrence, B.P.; O'Reilly, M.A. Alternative progenitor lineages regenerate the adult lung depleted of alveolar epithelial type 2 cells. *Am. J. Respir. Cell Mol. Biol.* 2017, *56*, 453–464. [CrossRef] [PubMed]
27. Smirnova, N.F.; Schamberger, A.C.; Nayakanti, S.; Hatz, R.; Behr, J.; Eickelberg, O. Detection and quantification of epithelial progenitor cell populations in human healthy and IPF lungs. *Respri. Res.* 2016, *17*, 1–11. [CrossRef]
28. Xu, Y.; Mizuno, T.; Sridharan, A.; Du, Y.; Guo, M.; Tang, J.; Wikenheiser-Brokamp, K.A.; Perl, A.-K.T.; Funari, V.A.; Gokey, J.J.; et al. Single-cell RNA sequencing identifies diverse roles of epithelial cells in idiopathic pulmonary fibrosis. *JCI Insight* 2016, *1*, 1–18. [CrossRef]
29. Travaglini, K.J.; Nabhan, A.N.; Penland, L.; Sinha, R.; Gillich, A.; Sit, R.V.; Chang, S.; Conley, S.D.; Mori, Y.; Seita, J.; et al. A molecular cell atlas of the human lung from single-cell RNA sequencing. *Nature* 2020, *587*, 619–625. [CrossRef]

30. Reyfman, P.A.; Walter, J.M.; Joshi, N.; Anekalla, K.R.; McQuattie-Pimentel, A.C.; Chiu, S.; Fernandez, R.; Akbarpour, M.; Chen, C.-I.; Ren, Z.; et al. Single-cell transcriptomic analysis of human lung provides insights into the pathobiology of pulmonary fibrosis. *Am. J. Respir. Crit. Care Med.* **2019**, *199*, 1517–1536. [CrossRef]
31. Adams, T.S.; Schupp, J.C.; Poli, S.; Ayaub, E.A.; Neumark, N.; Ahangari, F.; Chu, S.G.; Raby, B.A.; DeIuliis, G.; Januszyk, M.; et al. Single-Cell RNA-seq reveals ectopic and aberrant lung-resident cell populations in idiopathic pulmonary fibrosis. *Sci. Adv.* **2020**, *6*. [CrossRef]
32. Habermann, A.C.; Gutierrez, A.J.; Bui, L.T.; Yahn, S.L.; Winters, N.I.; Calvi, C.L.; Peter, L.; Chung, M.I.; Taylor, C.J.; Jetter, C.; et al. Single-Cell RNA sequencing reveals profibrotic roles of distinct epithelial and mesenchymal lineages in pulmonary fibrosis. *Sci. Adv.* **2020**, *6*, eaba1972. [CrossRef]
33. McDonough, J.E.; Ahangari, F.; Li, Q.; Jain, S.; Verleden, S.E.; Herazo-Maya, J.; Vukmirovic, M.; DeIuliis, G.; Tzouvelekis, A.; Tanabe, N.; et al. Transcriptional regulatory model of fibrosis progression in the human lung. *JCI Insight* **2019**, *4*, 131597. [CrossRef]
34. American Thoracic Society. Idiopathic Pulmonary Fibrosis: Diagnosis and Treatment International Consensus Statement. *Am. J. Respir. Crit. Care Med.* **2000**, *161*, 646–664. [CrossRef]
35. Teisanu, R.M.; Lagasse, E.; Whitesides, J.F.; Stripp, B.R. Prospective isolation of bronchiolar stem cells based upon immunophenotypic and autofluorescence characteristics. *Stem Cells* **2009**, *27*, 612–622. [CrossRef] [PubMed]
36. Teisanu, R.M.; Chen, H.; Matsumoto, K.; Mcqualter, J.L.; Potts, E.; Foster, W.M.; Bertoncello, I.; Stripp, B.R. Functional Analysis of Two Distinct Bronchiolar Progenitors during Lung Injury and Repair. *Am. J. Respir. Cell Mol. Biol.* **2011**, *44*, 794–803. [CrossRef] [PubMed]
37. Tighe, R.M.; Redente, E.F.; Yu, Y.-R.; Herold, S.; Sperling, A.I.; Curtis, J.L.; Duggan, R.; Swaminathan, S.; Nakano, H.; Zacharias, W.J.; et al. American thoracic society documents improving the quality and reproducibility of flow cytometry in the lung an official american thoracic society workshop report. *Am. J. Respir. Cell Mol. Biol.* **2019**, *61*, 150–161. [CrossRef]
38. Smyth, G.K. *Limma: Linear Models for Microarray Data*; Springer: New York, NY, USA, 2005; pp. 397–420. [CrossRef]
39. Gentleman, R.C.; Carey, V.J.; Bates, D.M.; Bolstad, B.; Dettling, M.; Dudoit, S.; Ellis, B.; Gautier, L.; Ge, Y.; Gentry, J.; et al. Bioconductor: Open software development for computational biology and bioinformatics. *Genome Biol.* **2004**, *5*, 1–16. [CrossRef]
40. Smyth, G.K.; Speed, T. Normalization of cDNA microarray data. *Methods* **2003**, *31*, 265–273. [CrossRef]
41. Smyth, G.K. Linear models and empirical bayes methods for assessing differential expression in microarray experiments. *Stat. Appl. Genet. Mol. Biol.* **2004**, *3*. [CrossRef]
42. van der Velden, J.L.; Bertoncello, I.; McQualter, J.L. LysoTracker is a marker of differentiated alveolar type II cells. *Respir. Res.* **2013**, *14*, 123. [CrossRef]
43. Strunz, M.; Simon, L.M.; Ansari, M.; Kathiriya, J.J.; Angelidis, I.; Mayr, C.H.; Tsidiridis, G.; Lange, M.; Mattner, L.F.; Yee, M.; et al. Alveolar regeneration through a Krt8+ transitional stem cell state that persists in human lung fibrosis. *Nat. Commun.* **2020**, *11*, 1–20. [CrossRef] [PubMed]
44. Williamson, J.D.; Sadofsky, L.R.; Hart, S.P. The pathogenesis of bleomycin-induced lung injury in animals and its applicability to human idiopathic pulmonary fibrosis. *Exp. Lung Res.* **2015**, *41*, 57–73. [CrossRef]
45. Gonzalez, R.F.; Allen, L.; Gonzales, L.; Ballard, P.L.; Dobbs, L.G. HTII-280, a biomarker specific to the apical plasma membrane of human lung alveolar type II cells. *J. Histochem. Cytochem.* **2010**, *58*, 891–901. [CrossRef] [PubMed]
46. Schiller, H.B.; Montoro, D.T.; Simon, L.M.; Rawlins, E.L.; Meyer, K.B.; Strunz, M.; Vieira Braga, F.A.; Timens, W.; Koppelman, G.H.; Scott Budinger, G.R.; et al. The human lung cell atlas: A high-resolution reference map of the human lung in health and disease. *Am. J. Respir. Cell Mol. Biol.* **2019**, *61*, 31–41. [CrossRef]
47. Konda, B.; Mulay, A.; Yao, C.; Beil, S.; Israely, E.; Stripp, B.R. Isolation and enrichment of human lung epithelial progenitor cells for organoid culture. *J. Vis. Exp.* **2020**, 1–17. [CrossRef] [PubMed]
48. Rock, J.R.; Onaitis, M.W.; Rawlins, E.L.; Lu, Y.; Clark, C.P.; Xue, Y.; Randell, S.H.; Hogan, B.L.M. Basal cells as stem cells of the mouse trachea and human airway epithelium. *Proc. Nat. Acad. Sci. USA* **2009**, *106*, 12771–12775. [CrossRef] [PubMed]
49. Ayre, D.C.; Christian, S.L. CD24: A rheostat that modulates cell surface receptor signaling of diverse receptors. *Front. Cell Develop. Biol.* **2016**, *4*, 146. [CrossRef]
50. Sinjab, A.; Han, G.; Treekitkarnmongkol, W.; Hara, K.; Brennan, P.M.; Dang, M.; Hao, D.; Wang, R.; Dai, E.; Dejima, H.; et al. Resolving the spatial and cellular architecture of lung adenocarcinoma by multiregion single-cell sequencing. *Cancer Discov.* **2021**, *11*, 2506–2523. [CrossRef] [PubMed]
51. Barkal, A.A.; Brewer, R.E.; Markovic, M.; Kowarsky, M.; Barkal, S.A.; Zaro, B.W.; Krishnan, V.; Hatakeyama, J.; Dorigo, O.; Barkal, L.J.; et al. CD24 signalling through macrophage siglec-10 is a target for cancer immunotherapy. *Nature* **2019**, *572*, 392–396. [CrossRef] [PubMed]
52. Treutlein, B.; Brownfield, D.G.; Wu, A.R.; Neff, N.F.; Mantalas, G.L.; Espinoza, F.H.; Desai, T.J.; Krasnow, M.A.; Quake, S.R. Reconstructing lineage hierarchies of the distal lung epithelium using single-cell RNA-Seq. *Nature* **2014**, *509*, 371–375. [CrossRef] [PubMed]
53. Perl, A.-K.T.; Kist, R.; Shan, Z.; Scherer, G.; Whitsett, J.A. Normal lung development and function after Sox9 inactivation in the respiratory epithelium. *Genesis* **2005**, *41*, 23–32. [CrossRef]
54. Rockich, B.E.; Hrycaj, S.M.; Shih, H.P.; Nagy, M.S.; Ferguson, M.A.H.; Kopp, J.L.; Sander, M.; Wellik, D.M.; Spence, J.R. Sox9 plays multiple roles in the lung epithelium during branching morphogenesis. *Proc. Nat. Acad. Sci. USA* **2013**, *110*, E4456–E4464. [CrossRef] [PubMed]

55. Danopoulos, S.; Alonso, I.; Thornton, M.E.; Grubbs, B.H.; Bellusci, S.; Warburton, D.; al Alam, D. Human lung branching morphogenesis is orchestrated by the spatiotemporal distribution of ACTA2, SOX2, and SOX9. *Am. J. Physiol. Lung Cell. Mol. Physiol.* **2018**, *314*, L144–L149. [CrossRef] [PubMed]
56. Ludbrook, L.; Alankarage, D.; Bagheri-Fam, S.; Harley, V. Dataset of differentially expressed genes from SOX9 over-expressing NT2/D1 cells. *Data Brief* **2016**, *9*, 194–198. [CrossRef]
57. Alankarage, D.; Lavery, R.; Svingen, T.; Kelly, S.; Ludbrook, L.; Bagheri-Fam, S.; Koopman, P.; Harley, V. SOX9 regulates expression of the male fertility gene Ets Variant Factor 5 (ETV5) during mammalian sex development. *Int. J. Biochem. Cell Biol.* **2016**, *79*, 41–51. [CrossRef]
58. Reginensi, A.; Clarkson, M.; Neirijnck, Y.; Lu, B.; Ohyama, T.; Groves, A.K.; Sock, E.; Wegner, M.; Costantini, F.; Chaboissier, M.-C.; et al. SOX9 controls epithelial branching by activating RET effector genes during kidney development. *Hum. Mol. Genet.* **2011**, *20*, 1143–1153. [CrossRef]
59. Jones, M.R.; Lingampally, A.; Dilai, S.; Shrestha, A.; Stripp, B.; Helmbacher, F.; Chen, C.; Chao, C.M.; Bellusci, S. Characterization of Tg(Etv4-GFP)and Etv5RFP reporter lines in the context of fibroblast growth factor 10 signaling during mouse embryonic lung development. *Front. Genet.* **2019**, *10*, 1–12. [CrossRef]
60. Liu, Y.; Jiang, H.; Crawford, H.C.; Hogan, B.L.M. Role for ETS domain transcription factors Pea3/Erm in mouse lung development. *Develop. Biol.* **2003**, *261*, 10–24. [CrossRef]
61. Zhang, Z.; Newton, K.; Kummerfeld, S.K.; Webster, J.; Kirkpatrick, D.S.; Phu, L.; Eastham-Anderson, J.; Liu, J.; Lee, W.P.; Wu, J.; et al. Transcription factor Etv5 is essential for the maintenance of alveolar type II cells. *Proc. Nat. Acad. Sci. USA* **2017**, *114*, 3903–3908. [CrossRef] [PubMed]
62. Ahmadvand, N.; Khosravi, F.; Lingampally, A.; Wasnick, R.; Vazquez-Armendariz, A.I.; Carraro, G.; Heiner, M.; Rivetti, S.; Lv, Y.; Wilhelm, J.; et al. Identification of a novel subset of alveolar type 2 cells enriched in PD-L1 and expanded following pneumonectomy. *Eur. Respir. J.* **2021**, *58*, 2004168. [CrossRef] [PubMed]
63. Leach, J.P.; Morrisey, E.E. Repairing the lungs one breath at a time: How dedicated or facultative are you? *Genes Dev.* **2018**, *32*, 1461–1471. [CrossRef] [PubMed]

Article

FGF10 Therapeutic Administration Promotes Mobilization of Injury-Activated Alveolar Progenitors in a Mouse Fibrosis Model

Yu-Qing Lv [1,2,†], Ge-Fu Cai [3,†], Ping-Ping Zeng [2], Qhaweni Dhlamini [2], Le-Fu Chen [1], Jun-Jie Chen [1], Han-Deng Lyu [2], Majid Mossahebi-Mohammadi [2], Negah Ahmadvand [4], Saverio Bellusci [4], Xiaokun Li [2,*], Chengshui Chen [1,5,*] and Jin-San Zhang [1,5,*]

[1] Department of Pulmonary and Critical Care Medicine, The First Affiliated Hospital of Wenzhou Medical University, Wenzhou 325000, China; lyuyuqing@wmu.edu.cn (Y.-Q.L.); chenlefu915@outlook.com (L.-F.C.); chenjunjie@wzhospital.cn (J.-J.C.)

[2] International Collaborative Center on Growth Factor Research, School of Pharmaceutical Sciences, Wenzhou Medical University, Wenzhou 325035, China; zengpingping@wmu.edu.cn (P.-P.Z.); dhlaminiqhaweni@wmu.edu.cn (Q.D.); lyu.handeng@mayo.edu (H.-D.L.); majid.mossahebi@modares.ac.ir (M.M.-M.)

[3] Biomedical Collaborative Innovation Center of Zhejiang Province, Institute of Life Sciences, Wenzhou University, Wenzhou 325035, China; 194511382323@stu.wzu.edu.cn

[4] Department of Pulmonary and Critical Care Medicine and Infectious Diseases, Universities of Giessen and Marburg Lung Center, Justus-Liebig University Giessen, 35392 Giessen, Germany; negah.ahmadvand@innere.med.uni-giessen.de (N.A.); saverio.bellusci@innere.med.uni-giessen.de (S.B.)

[5] Department of Pulmonary and Critical Care Medicine, The Quzhou Affiliated Hospital of Wenzhou Medical University, Quzhou People's Hospital, Quzhou 324000, China

* Correspondence: xiaokunli@wmu.edu.cn (X.L.); chenchengshui@wmu.edu.cn (C.C.); zhang_jinsan@wmu.edu.cn (J.-S.Z.)

† These authors contributed equally to this work.

Abstract: Idiopathic pulmonary fibrosis (IPF) is a devastating interstitial lung disease with dire consequences and in urgent need of improved therapies. Compelling evidence indicates that damage or dysfunction of AT2s is of central importance in the development of IPF. We recently identified a novel AT2 subpopulation characterized by low SFTPC expression but that is enriched for PD-L1 in mice. These cells represent quiescent, immature AT2 cells during normal homeostasis and expand upon pneumonectomy (PNX) and were consequently named injury-activated alveolar progenitors (IAAPs). FGF10 is shown to play critical roles in lung development, homeostasis, and injury repair demonstrated in genetically engineered mice. In an effort to bridge the gap between the promising properties of endogenous Fgf10 manipulation and therapeutic reality, we here investigated whether the administration of exogenous recombinant FGF10 protein (rFGF10) can provide preventive and/or therapeutic benefit in a mouse model of bleomycin-induced pulmonary fibrosis with a focus on its impact on IAAP dynamics. C57BL/6 mice and $Sftpc^{CreERT2/+}$; $tdTomato^{flox/+}$ mice aged 8–10 weeks old were used in this study. To induce the bleomycin (BLM) model, mice were intratracheally (i.t.) instilled with BLM (2 μg/g body weight). BLM injury was induced after a 7-day washout period following tamoxifen induction. A single i.t. injection of rFGF10 (0.05 μg/g body weight) was given on days 0, 7, 14, and 21 after BLM injury. Then, the effects of rFGF10 on BLM-induced fibrosis in lung tissues were assessed by H&E, IHC, Masson's trichrome staining, hydroxyproline and Western blot assays. Immunofluorescence staining and flow cytometry was used to assess the dynamic behavior of AT2 lineage-labeled $Sftpc^{Pos}$ (IAAPs and mature AT2) during the course of pulmonary fibrosis. We observed that, depending on the timing of administration, rFGF10 exhibited robust preventive or therapeutic efficacy toward BLM-induced fibrosis based on the evaluation of various pathological parameters. Flow cytometric analysis revealed a dynamic expansion of IAAPs for up to 4 weeks following BLM injury while the number of mature AT2s was drastically reduced. Significantly, rFGF10 administration increased both the peak ratio and the duration of IAAPs expansion relative to $EpCAM^{Pos}$ cells. Altogether, our results suggest that the administration of rFGF10 exhibits therapeutic potential for IPF most likely by promoting IAAP proliferation and alveolar repair.

Keywords: pulmonary fibrosis; bleomycin; recombinant FGF10; alveolar epithelial progenitors; AT2 cells

1. Introduction

Idiopathic pulmonary fibrosis (IPF) is the most common form of interstitial lung disease, which almost inevitably leads to respiratory failure and patient death within five years after diagnosis [1,2]. IPF-associated respiratory failure results from the aberrant deposition of extracellular matrix (ECM) and progressive loss of lung architecture and function [3]. Activated myofibroblasts (MYF) and MYF-derived ECM have traditionally been considered central in IPF pathobiology, and hence the focus of numerous studies aimed at developing targeted anti-fibrotic therapies [4]. Pirfenidone and Nintedanib, two FDA-approved anti-fibrotic IPF therapeutics, have been shown to slow the progression of the disease [5–13]. However, accumulating evidence suggest a pivotal role for dysfunctional alveolar epithelial cells, particularly alveolar type 2 cells (AT2s), in the pathogenesis of several parenchymal diseases, including IPF [14,15]. In this context, AT2 loss or dysfunction due to chronic or repetitive injury may lead to the development of a profibrotic phenotype [16,17]. Therefore, mitigating AT2 loss and dysfunction may prove to be beneficial in combating IPF.

AT2 cells act as prime stem cells in adult lungs for alveolar maintenance, repair, and regeneration [18–20]. Accumulating studies have indicated that AT2 cells are heterogenous [21] and comprise various subpopulations defined based on multiple markers, including our recently identified AT2-Sftpc^{Low} (tdTom^{Low}, aka injury-activated alveolar progenitors, IAAPs) [22]. In contrast to mature AT2-Sftpc^{High} (tdTom^{High} cells, which account for the mature AT2s expressing higher levels of *Sftpc*, *Etv5*, and *Fgfr2b*), IAAPs express lower levels of AT2 differentiation markers such as *Sftpc* as well as lower levels of the FGFR2b signaling genes *Fgfr2b*, and *Etv5*, but are enriched for the immune checkpoint programmed death ligand 1 (PD-L1). IAAPs are quiescent during normal homeostasis but proliferate and are proposed to differentiate into bona fide AT2 following lung pneumonectomy (PNX). FACS-based quantification revealed that the ratio of IAAPs to total EpCAM^{Pos} cells was significantly increased upon PNX compared to sham, whereas the AT2-tdTom^{High} to total EpCAM^{Pos} ratio remained unchanged, suggesting that IAAPs are, in fact, the significant contributor to lung regeneration, rather than the previously thought mature AT2s [22].

Fibroblast growth factor 10 (FGF10) is a multifunctional growth factor that belongs to the FGF7 subfamily of the FGF family and mainly elicits biological responses through binding to and activating FGFR2b with heparan sulfate as cofactor [23,24]. In the lung, FGF10 and FGFR2b are expressed in both the mesenchymal and epithelial cell compartments, respectively, exerting a critical role for FGF10/FGFR2b in mesenchymal–epithelial crosstalk. In addition, mesenchymal FGF10 is crucial for the lineage commitment and proliferation of epithelial cells during embryonic and postnatal development and for driving epithelial cell regeneration after injury [25]. Gupte et al. reported that *Fgf10* overexpression during different stages of the bleomycin (BLM) model resulted in a significantly reduced extent of lung fibrosis, suggesting that FGF10 may be a potential candidate for treating pulmonary fibrosis [26].

Recently, we have identified the equivalent of the mouse IAAPs in the human lungs [27]. These cells were amplified in the context of end-stage IPF, concomitant with a significant decrease in the number of mature AT2s. In addition, an in vitro culture of precision cut lung slides from donor lungs demonstrated the emergence of HTII-280^{Neg} PD-L1^{Pos} cells (likely the IAAPs) and HTII-280^{Pos} PD-L1^{Pos} cells (IAAPs differentiating into AT2s) [27]. We also reported recently that in mice, IAAPs are activated upon injury, upregulate Fgfr2b expression and proliferate. This was observed following PNX to induce compensatory growth [22], as well as following *Fgfr2b* deletion in AT2 cells to robustly ablate the AT2 lineage [28]. In both cases, we observed either no change (for the PNX) or a decrease (for *Fgfr2b* deletion in AT2s) in the number of mature AT2s.

In an effort to bridge the gap between promising properties of endogenous *Fgf10* manipulation and therapeutic reality, we here investigated whether the administration of exogenous recombinant FGF10 protein (rFGF10) can provide preventive and/or therapeutic benefit in a mouse model of bleomycin-induced pulmonary fibrosis. In addition to the histopathological aspects, we mainly focused on establishing the dynamic profile of IAAPs following BLM injury. A combination of flow cytometry and genetic lineage tracing was used to reveal the relationship between IAAPs and mature AT2s during the fibrosis development and resolution processes and the impact of rFGF10.

2. Materials and Methods

2.1. Animals and Drug Administration

Male C57BL/6 mice and $Sftpc^{CreERT2/+}$; $tdTomato^{flox/+}$ mice at the age of 8 to 10 weeks old were used in this study [22]. According to the "Guide for the Care and Use of Laboratory Animals" prepared by the National Academy of Sciences and published by the National Institutes of Health (NIH publication 86-23 revised 1985). Mice were housed in a temperature-controlled facility with a 12 h light/dark cycle and allowed feeding ad libitum. All animal procedures were approved by the Institutional Animal Care and Use Committee of Wenzhou Medical University.

For bleomycin (BLM) injury, adult 8- to 12-week-old mice were intratracheally (i.t.) instilled with BLM (2 μg/g body weight) or saline for the control group. BLM injury was induced after a 7-day washout period following tamoxifen induction. For tamoxifen induction, mice were administered tamoxifen in corn oil (200 μg/g) every other day for a total of 3 intraperitoneal (i.p.) injections. For recombinant FGF10 protein (rFGF10) treatment, mice were i.t. instilled with rFGF10 (0.05 μg/g body weight) on day 0, 7, 14, 21 after BLM injury as specified, and control group mice were i.t. instilled with the same volume of saline solution.

2.2. Histology and Immunohistochemistry and Hydroxyproline Measurement

The lungs were embedded in paraffin wax, fixed in 10% formalin, and processed into sections. The sections were stained either with hematoxylin–eosin (H&E) or subjected to Masson's trichrome staining. For immunohistochemistry (IHC) staining, lung sections were subjected to deparaffinization and antigen retrieval at first, then blocked by using 10% bovine serum albumin (BSA; Solarbio, Beijing, China) at room temperature (RT) for 1 h. After incubating with primary antibodies of collagen (Abcam, Cambridge, UK; 1:100) and α-smooth muscle actin (αSMA) (Beyotime, Shanghai, China; 1:100) at 4 °C overnight, appropriate secondary antibodies conjugated with HRP were added and incubated at RT. Finally, sections were visualized using a metal-enhanced DAB substrate kit (Solarbio), followed by hematoxylin counterstaining. Pulmonary fibrosis was evaluated by measuring Masson staining and the percentage-positive area was quantified using the ImageJ software. The hydroxyproline content in the mouse lungs was determined using the Hydroxyproline assay kit (Nanjing Jiancheng Bioengineering Institute, Nanjing, China; A030-2-1) following the manufacturer's instructions.

2.3. Immunofluorescence

PBS perfused lung tissue was fixed in 4% PFA and incubated at 4 °C for 24 h before embedding in OCT cryostat medium (Sakura Finetek, Torrance, CA, USA) and storing at −80 °C until sectioning into 10 μm slices. The following primary antibodies were used for staining the frozen sections: Pro-SFTPC (rabbit, Abcam, 1:100), PDPN (mouse, Santa Cruz Biotechnology, Santa Cruz, CA, USA; 1:100), PD-L1(rabbit, Abcam, 1:100), Ki67 (mouse, Invitrogen, Waltham, MA, USA; 1:100), rabbit anti-FGF10 (AP14882PU-N; Acris, Rockville,

MD, USA; 1:200). The sections were first washed with PBS and incubated with antigen repair solution (Beyotime) for 5 min at RT and blocked with 5% Bovine Serum Albumin (BSA) for 30 min at RT. Then the sections were incubated with the above primary antibodies diluted in 1% BSA at 4 °C overnight. The slides were washed in PBS next day and incubated with the secondary antibodies diluted in 1% BSA for 2 h at RT. Finally, the cell nuclei were counter stained with DAPI. Images were visualized and captured by using an Olympus FV3000 confocal microscope. The ImageJ program was used to determine the positive cells.

2.4. Western Blot

Dissected lung tissues were placed in cell lysis buffer freshly supplemented with protease inhibitor cocktail (Sigma, Alexandria, VA, USA) and phosphatase inhibitors (Roche, Nutley, NJ, USA) and homogenized for protein extraction. The protein samples were quantitated with BCA (bicinchoninic acid) protein assay (Beyotime). Protein samples (20–50 μg) were resolved on a 10% SDS–polyacrylamide gel and transferred onto PVDF membranes (Roche, 3010040001). The membranes were blocked with 5% skimmed milk in Tris-buffered saline (TBS) at RT on a shaker for 1h and then incubated with the specific primary antibodies: Collagen I (Meridian, Beijing, China; no. 1:1000), α-SMA (Abcam, no. ab9588, 1:1000), and α-tubulin (Beyotime, AF0001 1:10,000) overnight at 4 °C. After washing with TBS-T buffer, the membrane was incubated with proper HRP-conjugated goat anti-mouse or goat anti-rabbit secondary antibody (1:10,000) at RT for 1h before detection by ECL reagent (Enhanced Chemiluminescence, Amersham, UK) and image acquisition.

2.5. Lung Dissociation and Preparation of Single Cells

The mice were euthanized with 4% chloral hydrate, and upon proper exposure following standard surgical procedures, the lungs were perfused with 5 mL of PBS. A 20G Angio catheter was used for i.t. instillation, via a tracheal cannula, of 1 mL dispase solution in DMEM (1 mg/mL). Then, 0.6 mL of 1% agarose was gently administered into the lungs via the catheter, and the lungs were allowed to cool down on ice for 2 min. Individual lung lobes were dissected and put in a 50 mL conical tube containing the dispase solution, incubated at RT for 45 min on a rocker at 150 rpm. Digested lungs were decanted into a 10 cm Petri dish and supplemented with complete DMEM medium containing DNase. The lung parenchyma was gently teased away from the large airways using sharp tweezers. The Petri dish was rocked at 60 rpm for another 10 min at RT. The airways were discarded by straining the lung crude single-cell prep sequentially through 70, 40, and 20 μm strainers. Cells were finally spun down at 300× g at 4 °C, and the corresponding pellet was resuspended in 500 μL complete DMEM.

2.6. Magnetic Cell Sorting (MACS) and Flow Cytometry Analysis

The MACS® Separator Kit was used to deplete CD45- and CD31-positive cells from lung single cell suspensions prepared above following recommended procedures by the manufacturers. Briefly, cell suspensions were centrifuged, with the supernatant completely aspirated before adding 100 μL of CD45 and/or CD31 MicroBeads (Miltenyi Biotec, Bergisch Gladbach, Germany) per 10 million cells in MACS buffer. The cells were gently mixed and incubated for 15 min at 4 °C, then washed in 1 mL of buffer, and resuspended in 500 μL of MACS buffer before applying on the column. Next, flow-through unlabeled cells were collected and centrifuged to pellet the cells and resuspended in 500 μL of MACS buffer containing anti-EpCAM (APC-conjugated, 1:50; Biolegend, San Diego, CA, USA) for 45 min on ice in the dark. APC-conjugated rat IgG2a (Biolegend, 1:50) was used as the isotype control. Flow cytometry analysis and data acquisition were carried out using the ACEA NovoCyte flow cytometer. Data were analyzed using FlowJo software version X (FlowJo, LLC, Ashland, OR, USA).

2.7. Quantification and Statistical Analysis

For quantification of immunofluorescence, cells were counted in 10 independent 20× fields per sample. For H&E staining, fibrosis was evaluated by the Ashcroft score. For Masson and IHC staining, positive areas were isolated and calculated by ImageJ. Statistical analysis and graph assembly were carried out using GraphPad Prism 8 (GraphPad Prism Software, San Diego, CA, USA). Unpaired two-tailed Student's t-tests determined significance. Data are presented as mean ± standard error of mean (SEM). Values of $p < 0.05$ were considered significant. The number of biological samples (n) for each group is stated in the corresponding figure legends. *: $p < 0.05$; **: $p < 0.01$; ***: $p < 0.001$; ****: $p < 0.0001$.

3. Results

3.1. Preventative rFGF10 Delivery Decreases Fibrosis Formation

First, we examined FGF10 expression in tissue sections at three and six weeks after bleomycin injury. The immunofluorescence results showed that FGF10 expression was significantly increased in the bleomycin-injured group when compared to the control group (Figure S1). To determine the effect of exogenous FGF10 on fibrosis formation, we validated in our experimental conditions in the widely used bleomycin (BLM) model of lung fibrosis [29]. Our experimental scheme is depicted in Figure 1A. BLM-induced lung fibrosis is characterized by an acute injury, followed by localized inflammation (0–7 days), and subsequent fibrosis within four weeks [30]. We could recapitulate critical features of human IPF by i.t. instillation of BLM in mice and observed that the administration of rFGF10 at 7 days post-injury (dpi) significantly reduced collagen accumulation and fibrotic scarring induced by BLM in mice (Figure 1B). Histologic analysis of mouse lungs by H&E staining showed the gross destruction of normal lung tissue morphology due to chronic injury and pathologic scarring at 28 dpi in the BLM group. However, when compared with the BLM alone group, lung tissues from BLM + rFGF10 mice had much less architectural destruction and fibrosis (Figure 1B). We further analyzed the H&E sections to compare the extent of fibrosis in BLM + rFGF10 versus BLM lungs according to Ashcroft's method [31]. As anticipated, rFGF10 treatment reduced the Ashcroft's fibrosis score in response to BLM treatment (Figure 1C,D). Treatment with rFGF10 alone had no apparent effects on normal mouse lung tissue, as visualized by H&E and Masson staining (Figure S3). To further evaluate the extent of fibrosis, Masson's trichrome and IHC staining were performed to determine collagen deposition and α-smooth muscle actin (α-SMA) expression in mouse lungs. In addition, hydroxyproline, the major constituent of collagen, was also measured. As shown in Figure 1B,E,F, i.t. instillation of BLM led to a significant increase in collagen deposition and α-SMA expression, whereas rFGF10 administration significantly attenuated the BLM-induced damage. Consistent with these findings, the hydroxyproline content was also found to be markedly increased in BLM-alone mice, but was significantly lowered in BLM + rFGF10 mice, suggesting that treatment with rFGF10 inhibited the BLM-induced hydroxyproline accumulation (Figure S2). Furthermore, coadministration of rFGF10 at day zero also significantly reduced collagen accumulation and fibrotic scarring induced by BLM in mice (Figure S4), suggesting that i.t administration of rFGF10 at an early phase of BLM injury attenuates fibrosis formation.

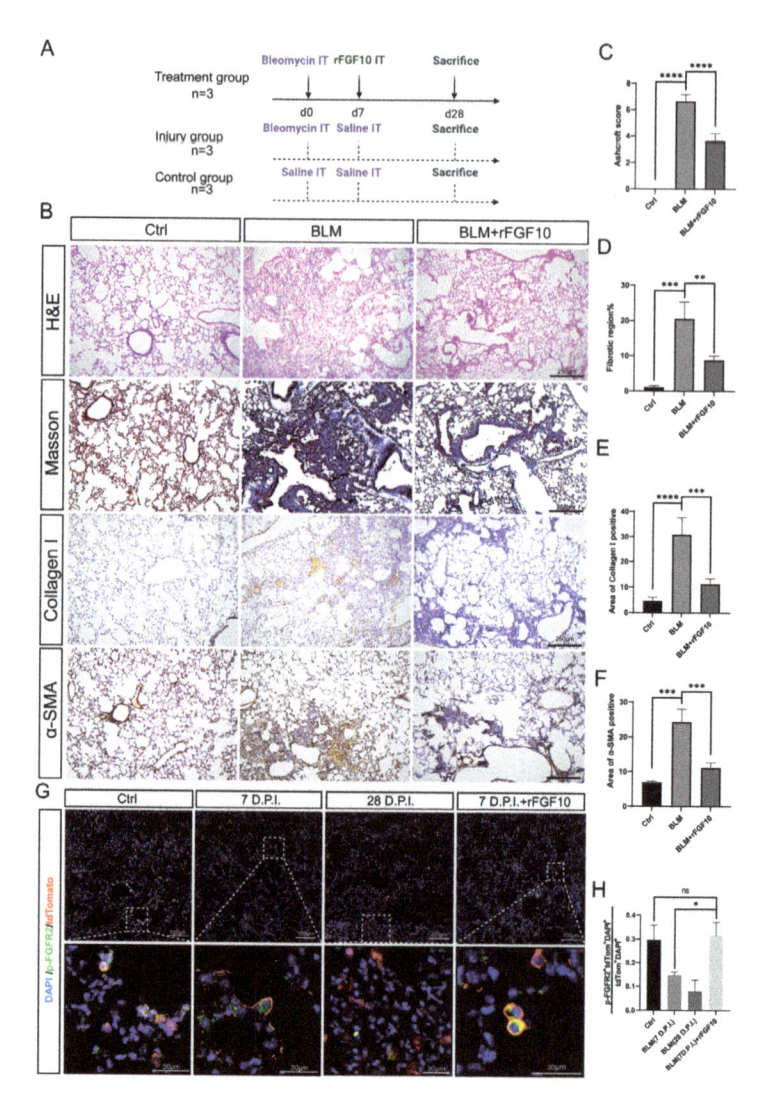

Figure 1. rFGF10 exhibits preventive efficacy toward BLM-induced injury. (**A**) Timelines of BLM and rFGF10 administration with saline as control; all the mice were euthanized 28 days after BLM administration (designated as Day 0). Histological analysis and quantitative fibrosis scoring of lung sections. (**B**) H&E, Masson's trichrome and IHC staining (α-SMA, collagen) of lung tissue from control, BLM, and BLM + rFGF10 group mice. (**C**) Semi-quantitative analyses of lung tissue using the Ashcroft score ($n = 3$). Note the significantly decreased score in the BLM + rFGF10 group compared to BLM alone. (**D**) ImageJ quantification of fibrotic regions based on Masson's trichrome staining ($n = 3$). (**E,F**), Quantification of collagen and α-SMA IHC staining in the lung sections of each mouse group ($n = 3$). (**G**) Immunostaining for p-FGFR2 on $Sftpc^{CreERT2/+}$; $tdTomato^{flox/+}$ mouse lungs that received BLM at 2 months of age and were harvested at 7, 28 and 7 dpi with rFGF10 administered for 12 h, as indicated. (**H**) Quantification of immunofluorescence, showing the expression of p-FGFR2 in lineage labeled cells of the indicated groups. Data are presented as mean ± SEM. *: $p < 0.05$; **: $p < 0.01$; ***: $p < 0.001$; ****: $p < 0.0001$.

To verify whether the effects of rFGF10 were mediated via FGFR2b activation, we used the [$Sftpc^{CreERT2}$/+; $tdTomato^{flox/+}$] mice to examine AT2-lineage labeled cells across different groups. In our experimental approach, mice received three i.p. injections of 200 μg tamoxifen/g (body weight) every other day to induce CreERT2 translocation to the nucleus and subsequent Cre-mediated recombination of the *Lox-STOP-Lox-tdTomato* allele located in the *Rosa26* locus, thereby leading to constitutive tdTomato expression in all Sftpc^{Pos} cells. After one week of washout following tamoxifen induction, BLM injury was performed. Mice were sacrificed at 7 dpi (Sham and BLM group), 7 dpi + 12 h (BLM + rFGF10 group), and 28 dpi (BLM group). A quantitative analysis of pFGFR2b^{Pos} tdTom^{Pos} DAPI^{Pos}/tdTom^{Pos}DAPI^{Pos} by immunofluorescence staining was carried out (Figure 1G,H). Note that it is not technically possible to distinguish between IAAPs and AT2s based on tdTomato expression by immunofluorescence [22]. Our results indicated that in the non-injured lung, around 30% of the lineage-traced cells are positive for pFGFR2b, indicating that FGFR2b signaling is active during homeostasis. Following BLM administration, this percentage fell to 15% and 10% at 7 and 28 dpi, respectively, suggesting the loss of FGFR2b signaling. Interestingly, rFGF10 administration at 7 dpi maintained FGFR2b signaling at close to normal levels in lineage-labeled cells 12 h later. Taken together, these results suggest that the administration of rFGF10 during the early phase of BLM-induced injury (0–7 days) prevents the decrease in lineage-labeled cells undergoing FGFR2b signaling and is associated with decreased fibrosis formation.

3.2. Therapeutic rFGF10 Delivery at 21 dpi Accelerates Fibrosis Resolution

Fibrosis formation is usually observed by day 14 following BLM exposure in the mice, with the maximal pathological responses around 14–21 dpi. Therefore, to explore the therapeutic potential of exogenous rFGF10 on BLM-induced pulmonary injury following fibrosis formation, mice were administered rFGF10 at 21 dpi and sacrificed at 28 dpi, as depicted in Figure S5A. H&E staining of lung sections revealed that exogenous rFGF10 treatment significantly attenuated the BLM-induced pathological changes, such as the distortion of lung morphology and fibrotic scarring. This result was further supported by an improved Ashcroft score, indicating the alleviated severity of fibrosis (Figure S5B,C) and the reduced area of fibrotic lesions in the BLM + rFGF10 group versus the BLM-only group (Figure S5B,D). To further evaluate the effects of rFGF10 in pulmonary fibrosis, we next determined the expression of collagen and α-SMA in different groups by Masson's trichrome, IHC, and WB. As expected, collagen and α-SMA expression levels were increased in the BLM injury group. In contrast, treatment with rFGF10 markedly reduced the BLM-induced increases in fibrotic markers α-SMA and collagen in vivo (Figure S5B,E–G). These data suggest a therapeutic potential of exogenous rFGF10 in the treatment of IPF.

3.3. rFGF10 Promotes Alveolar Epithelial Progenitor Cell Proliferation and Alveolar Repair

Using the $Sftpc^{CreERT2}$; *tdTomato* lineage-traced mice, we recently reported a novel AT2-IAAP subpopulation characterized by low *Sftpc* expression but that is enriched for PD-L1 expression [22]. IAAP cells, which represent quiescent and immature epithelial progenitors, undergo activation and expansion following PNX injury [22]. We recently reported the deletion of *Fgfr2b* in Sftpc^{Pos} cells and demonstrated that FGFR2b signaling is necessary for the survival of mature AT2s (tdTom^{High}). Interestingly, IAAPs were concomitantly activated and proliferated [28]. Furthermore, IAAPs displayed upregulated *Fgfr2b* and *Etv5* expression, suggesting that these cells not only escaped *Fgfr2b* deletion by a mechanism that remains to be identified but responded to FGFR2b signaling. To explore whether IAAPs can also be activated by rFGF10 to play a progenitor role after BLM injury, $Sftpc^{CreERT2/+}$; $tdTomato^{flox/+}$ mice were used to label the AT2 lineage, rFGF10 was administered at 14 dpi, and all mice were sacrificed at 28 dpi (Figure 2A). Co-staining for the canonical AT1 marker PDPN and PD-L1 showed that labeled AT2s distributed sporadically throughout the alveolar region in the control group, as shown in Figure 2B. BLM administration caused gross damage to both AT1 (PDPN) and AT2 (SFTPC) cells relative to the control group.

However, rFGF10 administration showed a reparative re-organization effect on both cell types and alveolar structures. Furthermore, we identified tdTomato^{Pos} cells that co-stained for PDL1 and PDPN in BLM + rFGF10 mice, suggestive of a PD-L1-positive precursor to these cells, presumably IAAPs (Figure 2B). Figure 2C shows the ratio of PDPN$^+$IAAPs in total IAAPs in the BLM group, which remained statistically higher, although in the BLM + rFGF10 group compared to the BLM group, no statistical significance was observed. In addition, co-staining of lung sections for tdTomato, PD-L1, and the proliferation marker Ki67 revealed an increased number of ki67-enriched clusters of PD-L1^{Pos} tdTomato^{Pos} cells in BLM + rFGF10 mice when compared to BLM-alone and control mice, suggesting that the clustering may have been a result of a proliferative response. In contrast, under the action of rFGF10, cells co-expressing SFTPC, PD-L1 and Ki67 were statistically enriched in areas of alveolar damage (Figure 2D–F). Altogether, these results suggest that in the context of BLM injury, rFGF10 may promote the proliferation of IAAPs, which will later differentiate into AT1s.

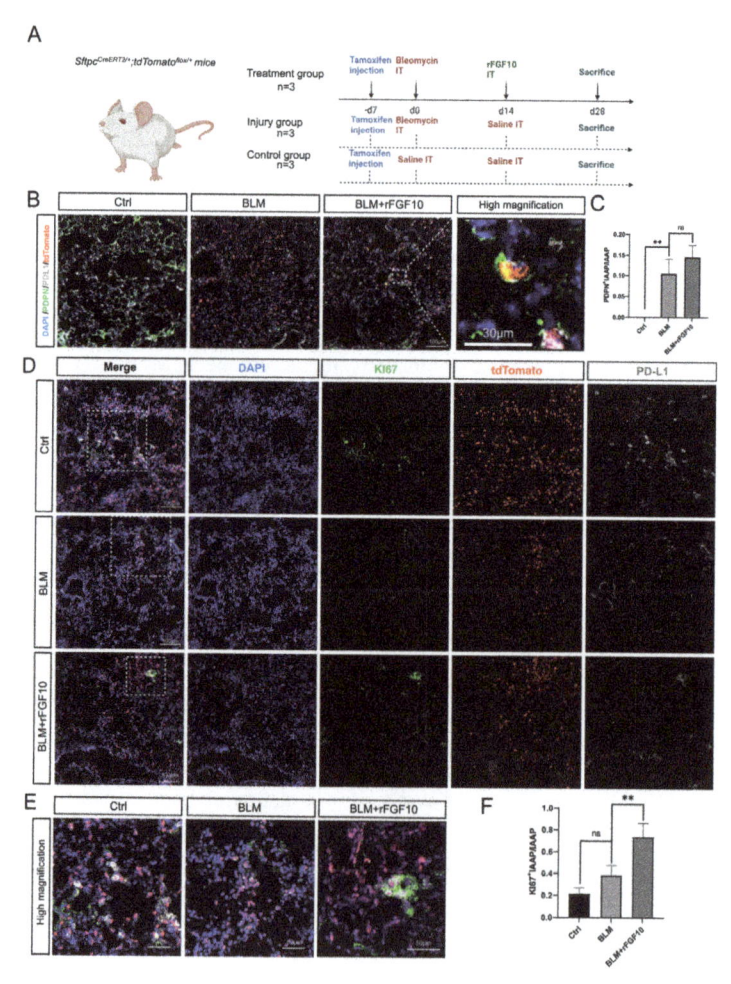

Figure 2. rFGF10 promotes alveolar epithelial progenitor cell proliferation and alveolar repair. (**A**) Timeline of tamoxifen, BLM and rFGF10 treatment of Sftpc^{Pos} lineage-labeled mice. BLM was

administered in 2-month-old $Sftpc^{CreERT2/+}$; $tdTomato^{flox/+}$ mice (n = 3). rFGF10 was administered 14 days after BLM administration in the treatment group (n = 3). Control mice were administered saline (n = 3). These mice were sacrificed at 28 dpi of BLM or saline administration (designated as Day 0). (**B**) Immunostaining of control, BLM, and BLM + rFGF10 groups of mouse lungs for PDPN (green) and PD-L1 (grey) at 28 dpi of BLM injury. (**C**) Quantification and ratio of PDPN$^+$IAAPs in total IAAP cells. (**D**) Immunostaining of lung sections from mice for KI67 (green) and PD-L1 (grey) at 28 dpi. (**E**) Magnification of figure D. (**F**) Quantification and ratio of KI67$^+$IAAPs in total IAAP cells. **: $p < 0.01$; ns: no significance.

3.4. Dynamic Alteration of IAAP Population during BLM-Induced Lung Fibrosis and Resolution

Next, we sought to determine whether the mature AT2s and IAAPs are differentially involved in BLM-induced injury using the $Sftpc^{CreERT2/+}$; $tdTomato^{flox/+}$ mice to label the AT2 lineage (Figure 3A). The lungs of euthanized mice were processed for single-cell suspensions at 14, 21, and 28 dpi. After removing CD31^{Pos} and CD45^{Pos} cells by MACS to enrich for the epithelial population, the cells were stained with APC-EpCAM antibodies and subjected to FACS analysis. We showed that the proportion of EpCAM^{Pos} cells as a percentage of total cells was 32.2%, of which the percentage of tdTom^{Pos} cells was 80.2% in the control mice. IAAPs and mature AT2s represented 24.0% and 75.3%, respectively, of the overall tdTom^{Pos} cells in the control mice (Figure 3B). Interestingly, the relative ratio of IAAPs to tdTom^{Pos} AT2s was increased to 47.0% in the 14 dpi group, and this ratio decreased to 38.5% at 21 dpi, then 31.7% at 28 dpi, which is still higher than that of the control group. In contrast, the tdTom^{High} AT2 population decreased to 51.0% at 14 dpi, rebounded to 59.6% at 21 dpi, and continued to rise at 28 dpi (66.5%) (Figure 3C). Our data suggest that, when compared to the tdTom^{High} AT2s, IAAPs are more resistant to BLM injury and are rapidly activated to proliferate. To determine whether this ratio peaked at 14 dpi and whether it was likely to return to normal ratios over time, we further sacrificed the post-BLM mice at 10, 16, and 60 dpi (Figure 3C). FACS results showed the ratio of IAAPs was also increased at 10 dpi (47.0%), peaked at 16 dpi (62.3%) and returned to normal levels at 60 dpi (18.7%) as shown in Figure 3C,D. Consistent with our flow cytometry data, immunofluorescence staining for PD-L1 revealed more IAAPs at 16 dpi in the lungs of BLM-treated mice when compared to the control and 28 dpi groups (Figure 3E,F). Altogether, our data reveal that tdTom^{High} AT2 cells represent the majority of total AT2s during homeostasis. However, the situation changes in response to BLM, whereby IAAPs become activated and the IAAP/tdTom^{High} ratio dynamically changes.

3.5. rFGF10 Administration Triggers Further IAAPs Expansion

Given the potent effect of rFGF10 in promoting alveolar epithelial progenitor cell proliferation and alveolar repair, whether IAAPs are further activated in the presence of rFGF10 is a critical question. Post-BLM mice were administered rFGF10 at 14 dpi and sacrificed 2 weeks later at 28 dpi. The entire lungs were then sectioned for immunostaining or processed for cell isolation and FACS analysis. Our treatment scheme is depicted in Figure 4A. Consistent with the beneficial effect of rFGF10 shown in Figures 1B and 2B, rFGF10 given at 14 dpi similarly attenuated pulmonary fibrosis as indicated by the significantly lower Ashcroft score (Figure 4B,C). Also, our immunofluorescence staining data revealed marginally increased IAAPs in BLM-treated mice when compared to the saline control, as well as the BLM + rFGF10 group compared to the BLM group, albeit no statistical significance was observed (Figure 4D,F). The ratio of tdTomato$^+$ cells in total cells shows that BLM administration caused gross damage to AT2 (SFTPC) cells relative to the control group and rFGF10 administration showed a reparative re-organization effect in the AT2 cells (Figure 4E). Flow results showed that IAAPs and tdTom^{High}-AT2s represented 17.7% and 81.4%, respectively, of the overall AT2 cells in the control group, whereas in the BLM group, IAAPs and tdTom^{High}-AT2s represented 25.7% and 73.2%, respectively, of the overall tdTom^{Pos}-AT2s, reflecting a significant increase in the IAAP subpopulation with a concomitant decrease of tdTom^{High}-AT2s. Additionally, in the BLM + rFGF10 group, out of total AT2s, 40.4% were IAAPs and 57.9% were tdTom^{High}-AT2s (Figure 4G) which represents a further and persistent increase in the ratio of IAAPs over tdTom^{High}-AT2s in the post-BLM mice by rFGF10 treatment (Figure 4H). When combined with the histological and immunofluorescence results, we hypothesized that IAAPs, rather than tdTom^{High}-AT2s, are the significant contributors during lung repair, and rFGF10 has a significant and sustained impact on the relative and dynamic change between the two subpopulations.

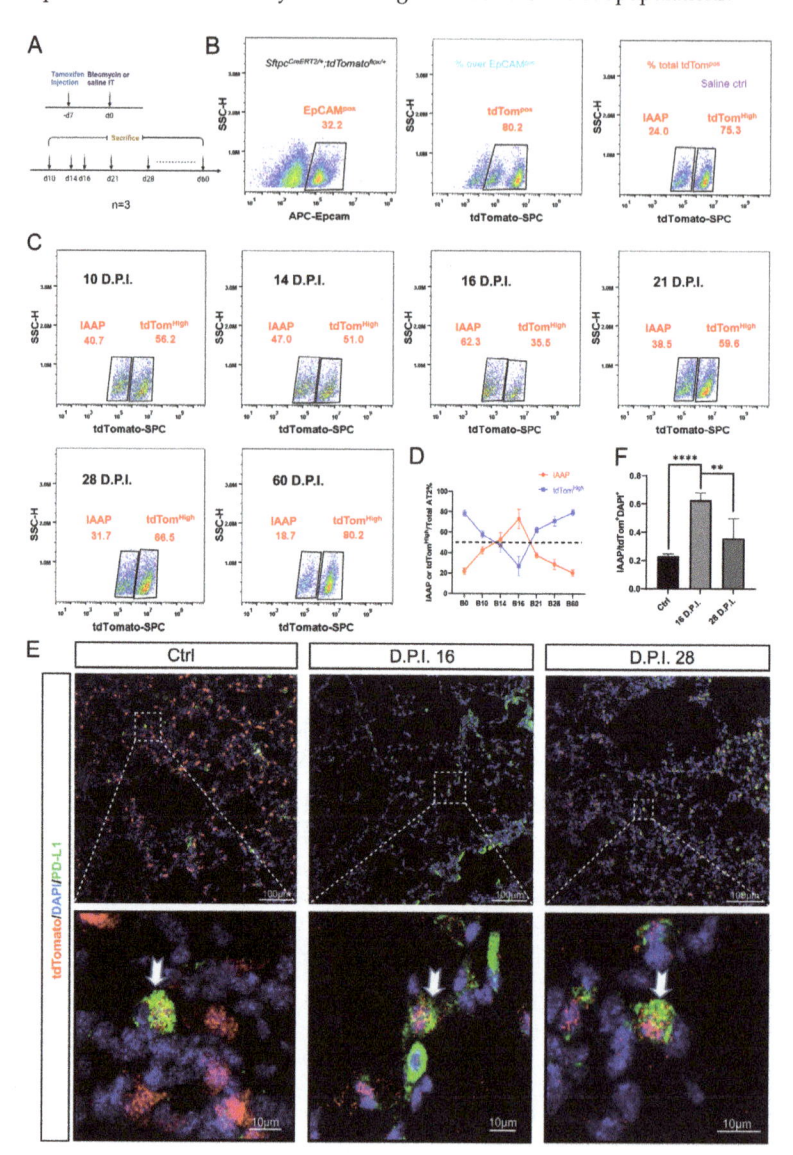

Figure 3. IAAPs are activated in response to BLM. (**A**) Timeline of tamoxifen treatment of *Sftpc$^{CreERT2/+}$, tdTomato$^{flox/+}$* mice (*n* = 4). BLM was i.t. administered in 2-month-old *Sftpc$^{CreERT2/+}$, tdTomato$^{flox/+}$* mice. Control mice were administered saline. For analysis, these mice were sacrificed

28 days after BLM (BLM) or saline administration (designated as Day 0). (**B**) Representative flow cytometry of EpCAM-positive population selection and the identification of IAAPs and mature AT2s in the control group. Flow chart shows the percentage of IAAPs and AT2s in total tdTomato^{Pos} cells. (**C**) Representative flow cytometry analysis of IAAPs and AT2s populations at 10, 14, 16, 21, 28 60 days after BLM administration. (**D**) Dynamic ratio change based on the quantification of IAAPs and AT2s percentages in total tdTomato^{Pos} cells at different times after BLM-induced injury ($n = 3$). (**E**) Immunostaining for PD-L1 on $Sftpc^{CreERT2/+}$; $tdTomato^{flox/+}$ mouse lungs that received i.t. BLM at 2 months of age and were harvested at 16 and 28 dpi. (**F**) Quantification of the immunofluorescence showing a ratio of IAAPs in AT2 cells at 16 and 28 dpi compared to the control group. Data are presented as mean ± SEM. **: $p < 0.01$; ****: $p < 0.0001$.

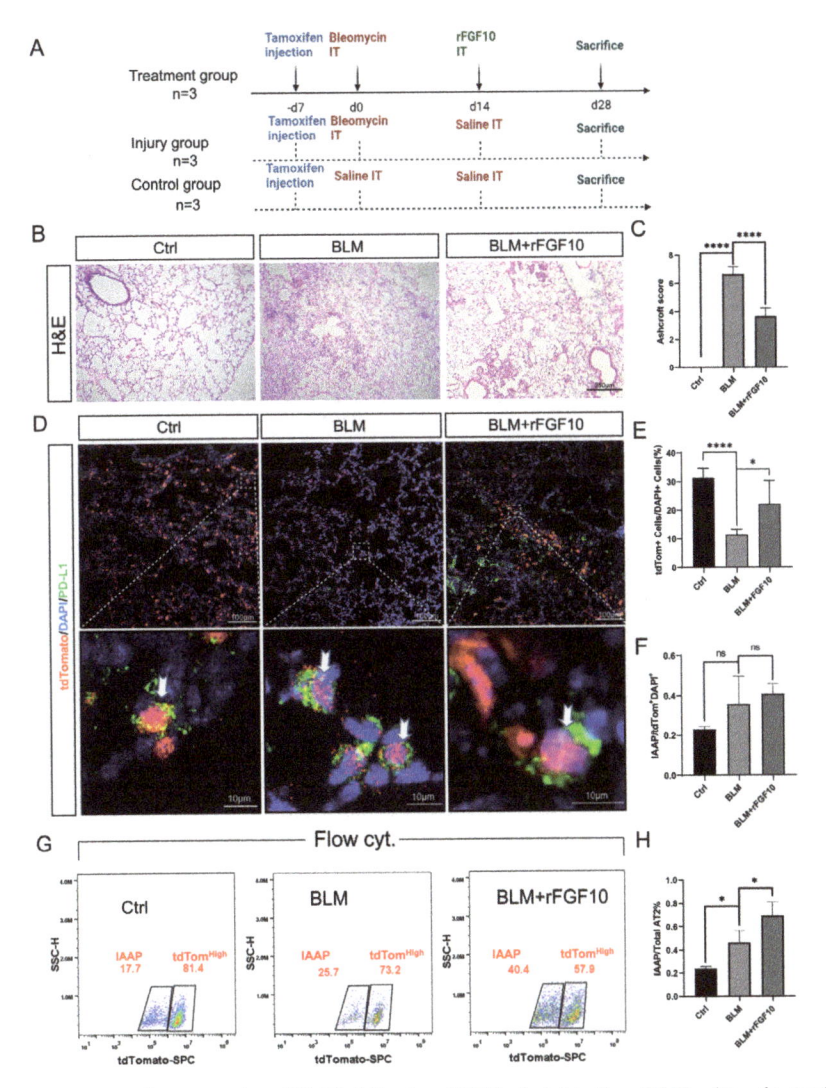

Figure 4. Further expansion of IAAPs following rFGF10 administration. (**A**) Timeline of tamoxifen treatment of *Sftpc* lineage traced mice ($n = 3$). BLM was administered in 2-month-old Sftpc$^{CreERT2/+}$, tdTomato$^{flox/+}$ mice (BLM). rFGF10 was administered at 14 dpi in post-BLM mice (BLM + rFGF10).

Control mice were administered saline (Ctrl). For analysis, these mice were sacrificed at 28 dpi. (**B**) H&E staining of lung sections (original magnification, ×20) of ctrl, BLM, BLM + rFGF10 group. (**C**) Semi-quantitative analyses of lung tissue using Ashcroft score ($n = 3$). Note the score was markedly decreased in the BLM + rFGF10 group ($p < 0.0001$). (**D**) Immunostaining for PD-L1 on control, BLM, and BLM + rFGF10 of $Sftpc^{CreERT2/+}$; $tdTomato^{flox/+}$ lungs. (**E**) Quantification and ratio of tdTomato$^+$ cells in total cells. (**F**) Quantification of the immunofluorescence showing the expression of PD-L1 in lineage-labeled cells for the indicated mouse groups. (**G**) Representative FACS analysis of IAAP and tdTom^{High}-AT2 populations of ctrl, BLM and BLM + rFGF10 at 28 dpi. (**H**) The quantification of IAAPs/tdTom^{High}-AT2s ratio of all tdTom^{Pos} cells. Data are presented as mean ± SEM. *: $p < 0.05$; ****: $p < 0.0001$.

3.6. rFGF10 Increases the Duration of IAAP/AT2 Population Ratio

The results shown in Figure 4 indicated that rFGF10 administration enhanced the magnitude of the IAAPs to tdTom^{High}-AT2 cell ratio when compared to the BLM-alone group, which was not restored to the control level at 28 dpi. We, therefore, further extended our observation of the potential impact of rFGF10 administration on IAAP and mature AT2(tdTom^{High}) dynamic change to 60 dpi. Our experimental scheme is depicted in Figure 5A. Histological analysis revealed apparent remaining lung scarring at 60 dpi in the BLM-alone group. Although these scars were incompletely resolved in the BLM + rFGF10 lungs, the remaining fibrosis was less severe, as evidenced by the significantly lower Ashcroft score than the BLM-alone group (Figure 5B,C). Furthermore, immunofluorescence analysis showed that rFGF10 administration at 14 dpi greatly enhanced the duration and the magnitude of the IAAPs to overall tdTom^{Pos}-AT2s ratio when compared to the BLM-alone control at 60 dpi in the region of injury (Figure 5D–F). Notably, although the relative proportion of IAAPs over tdTom^{Pos}-AT2 returned to normal levels in the BLM-alone group (19.5%), such ratios in the BLM + rFGF10 group were 35.7% (Figure 5G), which remained statistically higher than the BLM-alone group suggesting a persistent IAAPs activation (Figure 5H). Altogether, these results indicate that rFGF10 may exert beneficial effects in the context of BLM injury via enhancing IAAPs' proliferation and mediated regeneration.

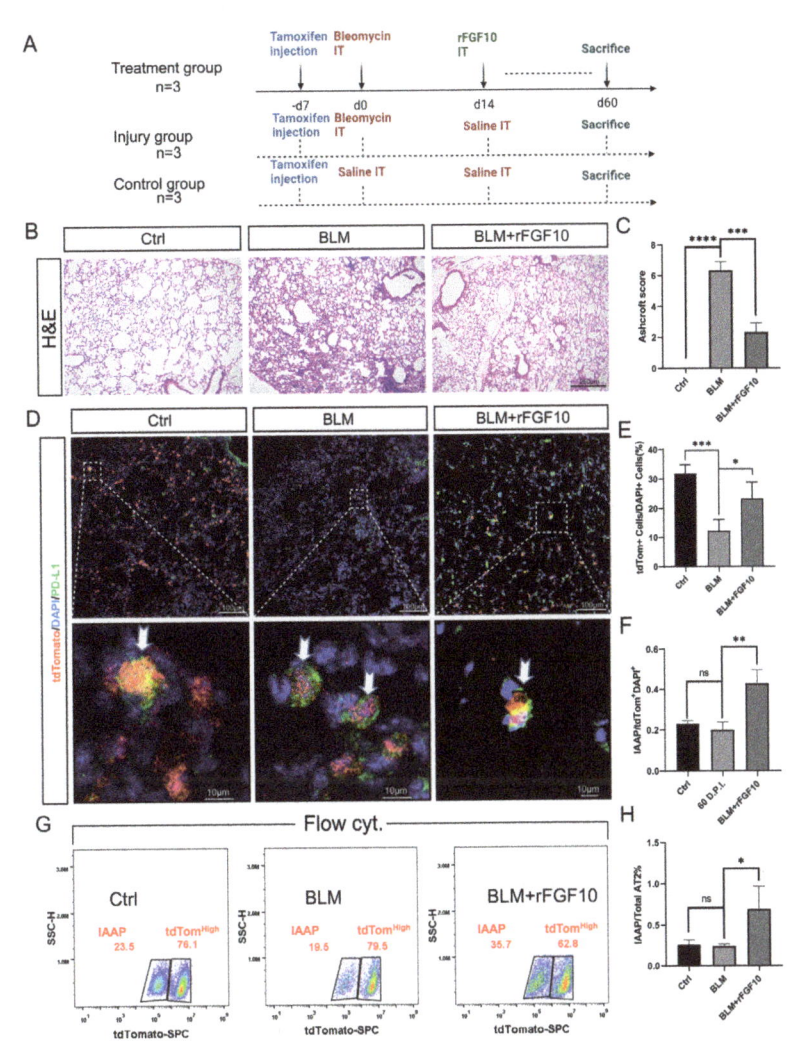

Figure 5. rFGF10 leads to a persistent increase in the IAAPs/AT2s ratio. (**A**) Timeline and treatment scheme of $Sftpc^{Pos}$ lineage-labeled mice (n = 3). BLM was administered in 2-month-old $Sftpc^{CreERT2/+}$, $tdTomato^{flox/flox}$ mice. For the BLM + rFGF10 group, rFGF10 was administered in post-BLM mice at 14 dpi. For analysis, these mice were sacrificed at 60 dpi after BLM or saline administration (designated as Day 0). (**B**) H&E staining of 5-μm-thick lung sections (original magnification, ×20) of ctrl, BLM, BLM + rFGF10 group. (**C**) Semi-quantitative analyses of lung tissue using Ashcroft score (n = 3). Note the markedly decreased score in the BLM + rFGF10 group (p < 0.001). (**D**) Immunostaining for PD-L1 on control, BLM, and BLM + rFGF10 of $Sftpc^{CreERT2/+}$; $tdTomato^{flox/+}$ lungs. (**E**) Quantification and ratio of tdTomato+ cells in total cells. (**F**) Quantification of the immunofluorescence showing the expression of PD-L1 in $Sftpc^{Pos}$ lineage-labeled cells for the indicated mouse groups. (**G**) Representative FACS analysis results of IAAPs and tdTom^{High}-AT2s subpopulations at 60 dpi of control and post-BLM administration. (**H**) Quantification and ratio of IAAPs/ tdTomato^{High}-AT2s ratio in total tdTom^{Pos} cells. Data are presented as mean ± SEM. *: p < 0.05; **: p < 0.01; ***: p < 0.001; ****: p < 0.0001.

4. Discussion

Herein, we demonstrated that, depending on the timing of administration, exogenous rFGF10 exhibited robust preventative or significant therapeutical efficacy toward BLM-induced fibrosis. Therefore, our findings provide fundamental preclinical data for the potential clinical uses of rFGF10 in IPF. While this work is ongoing, another line of our research revealed an essential role of FGFR2b signaling in maintaining the AT2 lineage during adult lung homeostasis. In this model of AT2 injury, we observed a drastic drop in mature AT2s, which underwent apoptosis upon the targeted deletion of $Fgfr2b$ in the $Sftpc^{Pos}$ lineage [28]. On the contrary, IAAPs not only managed to survive and expand (despite being also targeted for $Fgfr2b$ deletion) but also displayed enhanced alveolosphere formation in vitro [28]. How IAAPs responded to FGFR2b signaling and escaped $Fgfr2b$ deletion remains to be further investigated. Our most recent study further identified the human equivalent of the IAAPs, which were amplified in IPF patients [27]. These findings are consistent with our initial description of this newly identified AT2 subpopulation as becoming activated and proliferative in the context of PNX-induced injury [22]. Overall, our results using rFGF10 as a therapeutic approach are highly consistent with the previously reported beneficial properties of endogenous FGF10/FGFR2b signaling in promoting epithelial repair and regeneration from various injuries such as naphthalene, hyperoxia in neonates (to mimic a bronchoalveolar dysplasia-like phenotype) and BLM-induced fibrosis [25]. The beneficial effects of rFGF10 likely reflect the net outcome of its impact on different epithelial cell types and their interplay with the surrounding mesenchymal cells, as exemplified by AT2/lipofibroblast interactions that we recently reviewed [32].

As a newly identified AT2 subpopulation, the regulation of IAAPs remains to be further characterized molecularly and functionally. Given the critical importance of AT2s in injury repair and fibrosis and the progenitor-like properties of IAAPs, we tested the hypothesis that IAAPs would be responsive and dynamically regulated in the course of BLM injury. We first attempted to determine whether IAAPs can be mobilized after BLM-induced injury and, for the first time, established the dynamic profile of IAAPs versus the canonical mature AT2s in the course of BLM-induced fibrosis development and resolution. Indeed, contrary to the drastic loss of mature AT2s following BLM injury, the relative proportions of the IAAPs were markedly amplified, with the ratio of IAAPs/EpCAM peaking at 16 dpi, reflecting a six-fold increase in the ratio of IAAPs/tdTom^{High}-AT2s when compared to the non-injured controls. BLM injury elicited an initial rise in the IAAPs/EpCAM ratio, which was apparent at 10 dpi, peaking at 16 dpi before slowly returning to baseline by 2 months. In contrast, tdTom^{High}-AT2 exhibited the opposite trend concurrently, reflecting the loss of mature AT2s. Significantly, although tdTom^{High}-AT2 cells express higher levels of $Fgfr2b$, rFGF10 administration preferentially enhanced the duration and extent of the IAAPs/EpCAM ratio. Together with previous studies, the current data suggest that IAAPs may be the primary source of regenerative activity in the alveolar region, rather than the previously thought mature bona fide Sftpc^{High}-AT2s. Further studies will be required to validate the relative importance of these two distinct AT2 subpopulations. Although our findings reveal a potential therapeutic role for exogenous rFGF10 in IPF, as well as new insight about IAAP/mature AT2 ratio dynamic alterations in response to BLM injury, whether the beneficial effects of rFGF10 on BLM-induced fibrosis are indeed mediated through the enhancement of IAAP proliferation is not entirely conclusive. It is vital to generate novel lineage-tracing strategies that allow for the specific labeling of $Sftpc/Pd-l1$ double-positive cells to address these questions. In this regard, a dual recombinase-mediated genetic lineage tracing system to specifically track $Pd-l1^{Pos}$ $Sftpc^{Pos}$ AT2 subpopulations will be needed to gain deeper insights into the various biological aspects of IAAPs in the normal and diseased lung.

A puzzling question related to the behavior of IAAPs in end-stage IPF is their lack of contribution to the mature AT2 lineage. These cells are indeed amplified in IPF but seem to be stalled in their differentiation status [27]. One possibility explaining this failure to differentiate could be linked to the high inflammatory status of these lungs. Inflammation has been shown to prevent the differentiation of KRT8[Pos] intermediate AT2s into AT1 in mice [33]. Similar intermediate populations of human AT2 have recently been reported upon co-culture with human mesenchymal cells [34]. These cells are defined by the differential expression of a set of epithelial markers including SFTPC, KRT5, KRT8, KRT17, as well as TP63, in response to fibrotic signaling. Such a mechanism is proposed to underlie the functional AT2 loss and expansion of alveolar metaplastic KRT5[Pos] basal cells, which are highly pertinent to human IPF pathogenesis. The potential relationship of these human AT2 intermediate populations with IAAPs in response to lung injuries and whether the same process is at work in IAAPs remains to be illustrated in the future. Exogenous rFGF10 treatment, which delivered a significant therapeutic efficacy toward BLM-induced fibrosis, likely accelerated the restoration of AT2 homeostasis, whereas the mobilization of IAAPs, as indicated by both increased peak ratio and the duration of IAAP expansion relative to EpCAM[Pos] cells, may contribute to such a process. Additionally, upon in vitro co-culture with Sca1[Pos] residential mesenchyme, these IAAP cells displayed enhanced alveolosphere formation and increased their AT2 signature drastically, suggesting their differentiation towards mature AT2s [28].

Another puzzling question is whether the IAAPs have a direct impact on fibroblast behaviors and expansion. The precise nature of the interaction between alveolar epithelial stem cells (AT2s or IAAPs) and relevant mesenchymal cells during homeostasis is still largely unknown. In addition, how alveolar epithelial cells impact mesenchymal niches that have undergone a transition towards the activated myofibroblast phenotype present in fibrotic foci, to trigger their differentiation towards a benign phenotype, is largely unknown. In this context, co-culturing IAAPs with lung fibroblasts could be considered. However, a first difficulty to carry out this experiment deals with the IAAPs themselves. We have previously isolated IAAPs from non-injured lungs [22] and from lungs displaying deletion of $Fgfr2b$ in AT2s [27]. The deletion of Fgfr2b in AT2s leads to a situation similar to what we showed in the context of bleomycin treatment: we observed a significant drop in Tom[High] (mature) AT2s and an increase in IAAPs. An in vitro culture of the IAAPs from the non-injured lung with Sca1[Pos]-resident mesenchymal cells (rMC, CD31/CD45/EpCAM triple negative) from wild-type lungs shows that IAAPs display very low level of proliferative capability, therefore confirming the results obtained in vivo that these cells are quiescent. On the other hand, an in vitro culture of the IAAPs from lungs displaying deletion of $Fgfr2b$ in AT2s with resident Sca1[Pos] mesenchymal cells from wild-type lungs shows that injured IAAPs display an enhanced proliferative capability, albeit at a much lower level of what was expected to compensate for the loss of AT2s. This leads to the question as to whether the 3D model used (IAAPs with Sca1[Pos] rMC) is sufficient to capture the full behavior of the IAAPs. Among the missing components potentially allowing a full response are immune cells, as well as the damage associated molecular patterns (DAMPs) released by dying AT2 cells. Without these components, any attempt to carry out in vitro co-culture experiments between IAAPs and lung fibroblasts is bound to be disappointing.

Another challenge linked to the in vitro co-culture experiment deals with the nature of the fibroblasts to be used. The fibroblasts still constitute a big black box and are made of many subtypes. The alveolar fibroblasts, and in particular the Fgf10[Pos] Sca1[Pos] rMC, which likely represent the so-called lipofibroblasts, are likely the ones undergoing a transition towards the activated myofibroblast phenotype present in fibrotic conditions [35,36]. Ideally, this is the mesenchymal cell subtype that needs to be isolated from bleomycin lungs to co-culture them with the IAAPs. A major problem is that activated myofibroblasts do not support the proliferation of non-injured AT2s (or IAAPs for that matter), limiting the use of this in vitro model. Therefore new in vitro models need to be established. Such models include, for example, human embryonic lung cell lines as well as primary cultures of human lung fibroblasts from either donor or IPF lungs to study the impact of signals inducing their differentiation towards the alveolar fibroblasts/lipofibroblast phenotype, such as with metformin [37] or towards the activated myofibroblasts phenotype (for example, upon treatment with TGF-β1). Once the cellular, transcriptional and metabolic readouts have been clearly delineated, co-culture experiments with either AT2s or IAAPs can be carried out.

Interestingly, the fact that the IAAPs responded to rFGF10, indicated by the increase in their *Fgfr2b* expression following injury, can be translated into increased FGFR2b signaling. Therefore, FGFR2b signaling likely contributes to compensate for the lost mature AT2s caused by BLM injury. However, further studies using, for instance, IAAP-specific lineage-tracing and targeted cell ablation, are needed to determine the causal role of IAAPs in lung injury/repair, and whether FGF10 is a causal factor in IAAP expansion after injury. Elucidating the molecular mechanisms underlying IAAPs' activation, proliferation, and differentiation into mature AT2s, and their sequential capacity for further differentiation into AT1 cells, will be critical to promote optimal injury repair. Overall, the present study suggests that the exogenous administration of rFGF10 as well as harnessing the reparative capacity of IAAPs holds potential as a future therapeutic strategy in the treatment of IPF.

Supplementary Materials: The following supporting information can be downloaded at: https://www.mdpi.com/article/10.3390/cells11152396/s1, Figure S1: FGF10 is overexpressed in bleomycin injury group; Figure S2: rFGF10 reduces hydroxyproline content; Figure S3: rFGF10 have no effect on normal lung tissue; Figure S4: rFGF10 exhibits preventive efficacy toward BLM-induced injury; Figure S5: rFGF10 exhibits therapeutic efficacy toward BLM-induced fibrosis.

Author Contributions: Conceptualization, S.B., C.C. and J.-S.Z.; Data acquisition and analysis, Y.-Q.L., G.-F.C., P.-P.Z., Q.D., L.-F.C., J.-J.C., H.-D.L., M.M.-M., N.A., S.B., X.L., C.C. and J.-S.Z.; Methodology and investigation, Y.-Q.L., G.-F.C., P.-P.Z., Q.D., L.-F.C., J.-J.C., H.-D.L., M.M.-M. and N.A.; Funding and resource, X.L., C.C., S.B. and J.-S.Z.; Supervision, S.B., C.C. and J.-S.Z.; Writing—original draft, Y.-Q.L. and Q.D.; Writing—review and editing, S.B. and J.-S.Z. All authors have read and agreed to the published version of the manuscript.

Funding: This study was supported, in part, by a start-up package from The First Affiliated Hospital of Wenzhou Medical University to J.-S.Z., the Interventional Pulmonary Key Laboratory of Zhejiang Province, the National Natural Science Foundation of China (8217011045 to C.C.), the Chinese Academy of Medical Sciences (CAMS) Innovation Fund for Medical Sciences (2019-I2M-5-028) to X.L., and the Deutsche Forschungsgemeinschaft (DFG; BE4443/1-1, BE4443/4-1, BE4443/6-1, DFG4443/22-1, KFO309 P7 and SFB1213-projects A02 and A04 to S.B.).

Institutional Review Board Statement: The study was conducted according to the guidelines of the Declaration of Helsinki and was approved by the Animal Care and Use Committee of the Wenzhou Medical University (Ethics number: wydw2019-0510).

Informed Consent Statement: Not applicable.

Data Availability Statement: The data presented in this study are available on request from the corresponding author.

Conflicts of Interest: The authors declare no conflict of interest.

References

1. King, T.E., Jr.; Pardo, A.; Selman, M. Idiopathic pulmonary fibrosis. *Lancet* **2011**, *378*, 1949–1961. [CrossRef]
2. Steele, M.P.; Schwartz, D.A. Molecular Mechanisms in Progressive Idiopathic Pulmonary Fibrosis. *Annu. Rev. Med.* **2013**, *64*, 265–276. [CrossRef] [PubMed]
3. Barkauskas, C.E.; Noble, P.W. Cellular Mechanisms of Tissue Fibrosis. 7. New insights into the cellular mechanisms of pulmonary fibrosis. *Am. J. Physiol. Physiol.* **2014**, *306*, C987–C996. [CrossRef] [PubMed]
4. Glass, D.S.; Grossfeld, D.; Renna, H.A.; Agarwala, P.; Spiegler, P.; DeLeon, J.; Reiss, A.B. Idiopathic pulmonary fibrosis: Current and future treatment. *Clin. Respir. J.* **2022**, *16*, 84–96. [CrossRef]
5. Karimi-Shah, B.A.; Chowdhury, B.A. Forced Vital Capacity in Idiopathic Pulmonary Fibrosis — FDA Review of Pirfenidone and Nintedanib. *New Engl. J. Med.* **2015**, *372*, 1189–1191. [CrossRef] [PubMed]
6. Noble, P.W.; Albera, C.; Bradford, W.Z.; Costabel, U.; Glassberg, M.K.; Kardatzke, D.; King, T.E., Jr.; Lancaster, L.; Sahn, S.A.; Szwarcberg, J.; et al. Pirfenidone in patients with idiopathic pulmonary fibrosis (CAPACITY): Two randomised trials. *Lancet* **2011**, *377*, 1760–1769. [CrossRef]

7. King, T.E., Jr.; Bradford, W.Z.; Castro-Bernardini, S.; Fagan, E.A.; Glaspole, I.; Glassberg, M.K.; Gorina, E.; Hopkins, P.M.; Kardatzke, D.; Lancaster, L.; et al. A Phase 3 Trial of Pirfenidone in Patients with Idiopathic Pulmonary Fibrosis. *N. Engl. J. Med.* **2014**, *370*, 2083–2092. [CrossRef]
8. Noble, P.W.; Albera, C.; Bradford, W.Z.; Costabel, U.; Du Bois, R.M.; Fagan, E.A.; Fishman, R.S.; Glaspole, I.; Glassberg, M.K.; Lancaster, L.; et al. Pirfenidone for idiopathic pulmonary fibrosis: Analysis of pooled data from three multinational phase 3 trials. *Eur. Respir. J.* **2015**, *47*, 243–253. [CrossRef]
9. Richeldi, L.; Costabel, U.; Selman, M.; Kim, D.S.; Hansell, D.M.; Nicholson, A.G.; Brown, K.K.; Flaherty, K.R.; Noble, P.W.; Raghu, G.; et al. Efficacy of a Tyrosine Kinase Inhibitor in Idiopathic Pulmonary Fibrosis. *N. Engl. J. Med.* **2011**, *365*, 1079–1087. [CrossRef] [PubMed]
10. Richeldi, L.; Du Bois, R.M.; Raghu, G.; Azuma, A.; Brown, K.K.; Costabel, U.; Cottin, V.; Flaherty, K.R.; Hansell, D.M.; Inoue, Y.; et al. Efficacy and Safety of Nintedanib in Idiopathic Pulmonary Fibrosis. *N. Engl. J. Med.* **2014**, *370*, 2071–2082. [CrossRef]
11. Azuma, A.; Nukiwa, T.; Tsuboi, E.; Suga, M.; Abe, S.; Nakata, K.; Taguchi, Y.; Nagai, S.; Itoh, H.; Ohi, M.; et al. Double-blind, Placebo-controlled Trial of Pirfenidone in Patients with Idiopathic Pulmonary Fibrosis. *Am. J. Respir. Crit. Care Med.* **2005**, *171*, 1040–1047. [CrossRef] [PubMed]
12. Corte, T.J.; Bonella, F.; Crestani, B.; Demedts, M.G.; Richeldi, L.; Coeck, C.; Pelling, K.; Quaresma, M.; Lasky, J.A. Safety, tolerability and appropriate use of nintedanib in idiopathic pulmonary fibrosis. *Respir. Res.* **2015**, *16*, 1–10. [CrossRef] [PubMed]
13. Costabel, U.; Inoue, Y.; Richeldi, L.; Collard, H.R.; Tschoepe, I.; Stowasser, S.; Azuma, A. Efficacy of Nintedanib in Idiopathic Pulmonary Fibrosis across Prespecified Subgroups in INPULSIS. *Am. J. Respir. Crit. Care Med.* **2016**, *193*, 178–185. [CrossRef] [PubMed]
14. Ruaro, B.; Salton, F.; Braga, L.; Wade, B.; Confalonieri, P.; Volpe, M.C.; Baratella, E.; Maiocchi, S.; Confalonieri, M. The History and Mystery of Alveolar Epithelial Type II Cells: Focus on Their Physiologic and Pathologic Role in Lung. *Int. J. Mol. Sci.* **2021**, *22*, 2566. [CrossRef] [PubMed]
15. Calkovska, A.; Kolomaznik, M.; Calkovsky, V. Alveolar Type II Cells and Pulmonary Surfactant in COVID-19 Era. *Physiol. Res.* **2021**, S195–S208. [CrossRef]
16. Parimon, T.; Yao, C.; Stripp, B.R.; Noble, P.W.; Chen, P. Alveolar Epithelial Type II Cells as Drivers of Lung Fibrosis in Idiopathic Pulmonary Fibrosis. *Int. J. Mol. Sci.* **2020**, *21*, 2269. [CrossRef]
17. Katzen, J.; Beers, M.F. Contributions of alveolar epithelial cell quality control to pulmonary fibrosis. *J. Clin. Investig.* **2020**, *130*, 5088–5099. [CrossRef] [PubMed]
18. Barkauskas, C.E.; Cronce, M.J.; Rackley, C.R.; Bowie, E.J.; Keene, D.R.; Stripp, B.R.; Randell, S.H.; Noble, P.W.; Hogan, B.L.M. Type 2 alveolar cells are stem cells in adult lung. *J. Clin. Investig.* **2013**, *123*, 3025–3036. [CrossRef]
19. Desai, T.J.; Brownfield, D.; Krasnow, M.A. Alveolar progenitor and stem cells in lung development, renewal and cancer. *Nature* **2014**, *507*, 190–194. [CrossRef]
20. Evans, M.J.; Cabral, L.J.; Stephens, R.J.; Freeman, G. Transformation of alveolar Type 2 cells to Type 1 cells following exposure to NO2. *Exp. Mol. Pathol.* **1975**, *22*, 142–150. [CrossRef]
21. Chen, Q.; Liu, Y. Heterogeneous groups of alveolar type II cells in lung homeostasis and repair. *Am. J. Physiol. Physiol.* **2020**, *319*, C991–C996. [CrossRef] [PubMed]
22. Ahmadvand, N.; Khosravi, F.; Lingampally, A.; Wasnick, R.; Vazquez-Armendariz, A.I.; Carraro, G.; Heiner, M.; Rivetti, S.; Lv, Y.; Wilhelm, J.; et al. Identification of a novel subset of alveolar type 2 cells enriched in PD-L1 and expanded following pneumonectomy. *Eur. Respir. J.* **2021**, *58*, 2004168. [CrossRef] [PubMed]
23. Itoh, N.; Ohta, H. Fgf10: A paracrine-signaling molecule in development, disease, and regenerative medicine. *Curr. Mol. Med.* **2014**, *14*, 504–509. [CrossRef] [PubMed]
24. Itoh, N. FGF10: A multifunctional mesenchymal-epithelial signaling growth factor in development, health, and disease. *Cytokine Growth Factor Rev.* **2016**, *28*, 63–69. [CrossRef] [PubMed]
25. Yuan, T.; Volckaert, T.; Chanda, D.; Thannickal, V.J.; De Langhe, S.P. Fgf10 Signaling in Lung Development, Homeostasis, Disease, and Repair After Injury. *Front. Genet.* **2018**, *9*. [CrossRef]
26. Gupte, V.V.; Ramasamy, S.K.; Reddy, R.; Lee, J.; Weinreb, P.H.; Violette, S.M.; Guenther, A.; Warburton, D.; Driscoll, B.; Minoo, P.; et al. Overexpression of Fibroblast Growth Factor-10 during Both Inflammatory and Fibrotic Phases Attenuates Bleomycin-induced Pulmonary Fibrosis in Mice. *Am. J. Respir. Crit. Care Med.* **2009**, *180*, 424–436. [CrossRef] [PubMed]
27. Ahmadvand, N.; Carraro, G.; Jones, M.R.; Shalashova, I.; Wilhelm, J.; Baal, N.; Kosravi, F.; Chen, C.; Zhang, J.; Ruppert, C.; et al. Cell-surface PD-L1 expression identifies a sub-population of distal epithelial cells enriched in idiopathic pulmonary fibrosis. *Biorxiv* **2022**. [CrossRef]
28. Ahmadvand, N.; Lingampally, A.; Khosravi, F.; Vazquez-Armendariz, I.; Rivetti, S.; Wilhelm, J.; Herold, S.; Barreto, G.; Koepke, J.; Samakovlis, C.; et al. Fgfr2b signaling is essential for the maintenance of the alveolar epithelial type 2 lineage during lung homeostasis in mice. *Cell. Mol. Life Sci.* **2022**, *79*, 302. [CrossRef] [PubMed]
29. Carrington, R.; Jordan, S.; Pitchford, S.C.; Page, C.P. Use of animal models in IPF research. *Pulm. Pharmacol. Ther.* **2018**, *51*, 73–78. [CrossRef] [PubMed]
30. Liu, T.; De Los Santos, F.G.; Phan, S.H. The Bleomycin Model of Pulmonary Fibrosis. *Methods Mol. Biol.* **2017**, *1627*, 27–42. [CrossRef]

31. Ashcroft, T.; Simpson, J.M.; Timbrell, V. Simple method of estimating severity of pulmonary fibrosis on a numerical scale. *J. Clin. Pathol.* **1988**, *41*, 467–470. [CrossRef] [PubMed]
32. Lv, Y.-Q.; Dhlamini, Q.; Chen, C.; Li, X.; Bellusci, S.; Zhang, J.-S. FGF10 and Lipofibroblasts in Lung Homeostasis and Disease: Insights Gained From the Adipocytes. *Front. Cell Dev. Biol.* **2021**, *9*. [CrossRef] [PubMed]
33. Choi, J.; Park, J.-E.; Tsagkogeorga, G.; Yanagita, M.; Koo, B.-K.; Han, N.; Lee, J.-H. Inflammatory Signals Induce AT2 Cell-Derived Damage-Associated Transient Progenitors that Mediate Alveolar Regeneration. *Cell Stem Cell* **2020**, *27*, 366–382. [CrossRef] [PubMed]
34. Kathiriya, J.J.; Wang, C.; Zhou, M.; Brumwell, A.; Cassandras, M.; Le Saux, C.J.; Cohen, M.; Alysandratos, K.-D.; Wang, B.; Wolters, P.; et al. Human alveolar type 2 epithelium transdifferentiates into metaplastic KRT5+ basal cells. *Nature* **2021**, *24*, 10–23. [CrossRef] [PubMed]
35. El Agha, E.; Moiseenko, A.; Kheirollahi, V.; De Langhe, S.; Crnkovic, S.; Kwapiszewska, G.; Szibor, M.; Kosanovic, D.; Schwind, F.; Schermuly, R.T.; et al. Two-Way Conversion between Lipogenic and Myogenic Fibroblastic Phenotypes Marks the Progression and Resolution of Lung Fibrosis. *Cell Stem Cell* **2017**, *20*, 571. [CrossRef]
36. Nouri-Keshtkar, M.; Taghizadeh, S.; Farhadi, A.; Ezaddoustdar, A.; Vesali, S.; Hosseini, R.; Totonchi, M.; Kouhkan, A.; Chen, C.; Zhang, J.-S.; et al. Potential Impact of Diabetes and Obesity on Alveolar Type 2 (AT2)-Lipofibroblast (LIF) Interactions After COVID-19 Infection. *Front. Cell Dev. Biol.* **2021**, *9*, 676150. [CrossRef] [PubMed]
37. Kheirollahi, V.; Wasnick, R.M.; Biasin, V.; Vazquez-Armendariz, A.I.; Chu, X.; Moiseenko, A.; Weiss, A.; Wilhelm, J.; Zhang, J.-S.; Kwapiszewska, G.; et al. Metformin induces lipogenic differentiation in myofibroblasts to reverse lung fibrosis. *Nat. Commun.* **2019**, *10*, 2987. [CrossRef] [PubMed]

Review

3D In Vitro Models: Novel Insights into Idiopathic Pulmonary Fibrosis Pathophysiology and Drug Screening

Ana Ivonne Vazquez-Armendariz *, Margarida Maria Barroso, Elie El Agha and Susanne Herold

Department of Medicine V, Internal Medicine, Infectious Diseases and Infection Control, Universities of Giessen and Marburg Lung Center (UGMLC), Cardio-Pulmonary Institute (CPI), Institute for Lung Health (ILH), Member of the German Center for Lung Research (DZL), Justus-Liebig University Giessen, 35392 Giessen, Hessen, Germany; margarida.barroso@innere.med.uni-giessen.de (M.M.B.); elie.el-agha@innere.med.uni-giessen.de (E.E.A.); susanne.herold@innere.med.uni-giessen.de (S.H.)
* Correspondence: ana.i.vazquez-armendariz@innere.med.uni-giessen.de

Abstract: Idiopathic pulmonary fibrosis (IPF) is a progressive and often lethal interstitial lung disease of unknown aetiology. IPF is characterised by myofibroblast activation, tissue stiffening, and alveolar epithelium injury. As current IPF treatments fail to halt disease progression or induce regeneration, there is a pressing need for the development of novel therapeutic targets. In this regard, tri-dimensional (3D) models have rapidly emerged as powerful platforms for disease modelling, drug screening and discovery. In this review, we will touch on how 3D in vitro models such as hydrogels, precision-cut lung slices, and, more recently, lung organoids and lung-on-chip devices have been generated and/or modified to reveal distinct cellular and molecular signalling pathways activated during fibrotic processes. Markedly, we will address how these platforms could provide a better understanding of fibrosis pathophysiology and uncover effective treatment strategies for IPF patients.

Keywords: 3D cultures; IPF modelling; drug screening

1. Introduction

Idiopathic pulmonary fibrosis (IPF) is a chronic progressive interstitial lung disease associated with ageing and DNA damage that particularly affects adult males between 60 and 70 years old with a history of smoking [1]. While IPF aetiology remains unknown, environmental exposure to contaminants (e.g., dust or mould) and viral infections have been shown to increase the risk of contracting the disease [2]. Depending on the method used, IPF's reported incidence and prevalence in Europe and North America varies between three and nine cases per 100,000 people per year [3]. Clinically, IPF is a devastating disease that displays a progressive lung function decline with a median survival of only 3 to 4 years [1]. Patients present persistent dyspnoea and dry cough while, at a cellular level, IPF is characterised by epithelial cell hyperplasia, alveolar consolidation, and myofibroblast activation [4,5].

Current diagnosis relies on typical radiology imaging with high-resolution computed tomography [6]. Until now, only nintedanib and pirfenidone, both anti-fibrotic medications, have shown promise in the amelioration of IPF progression [7]. Nintedanib is an intracellular suppressor of tyrosine kinases that acts as an inhibitor of fibroblast recruitment, proliferation, and differentiation, therefore negatively affecting extracellular matrix (ECM) deposition [8]. Alternatively, pirfenidone slows fibrosis generation by modulation of procollagen transcription and reduction of transforming growth factor (TGF)-β-induced fibroblast activation and differentiation [9].

Despite significant research being conducted, the majority of drug targets shown to attenuate induced fibrosis in pre-clinical models have failed in human clinical trial phases II or III [10]. A probable reason for these setbacks may be that animal models of IPF are generated artificially (e.g., application of bleomycin, silica and asbestos, age-related models, and cytokine overexpression) while the direct cause of the disease is still unknown [11]. Consequently, the identification of specific cellular and molecular mechanisms activated during IPF is essential for the understanding of crucial events that trigger unusual fibroblast outgrowth, progressive tissue scaring, and/or abnormal epithelial repair. Three-dimensional (3D) cultures have quickly become prominent tools for disease modelling, regenerative medicine, and drug development. Regarding the lung, hydrogels, precision cut lung slices (PCLS), lung organoids, and lung-on-chip have shown to be valuable techniques for the discovery and test of drugs in a variety of pulmonary diseases, including cystic fibrosis (CF), lung cancer, and chronic obstructive pulmonary disease [12–14].

In this review, we outline current 3D models used to elucidate cellular and molecular cues involved in IPF. We also discuss how each of these systems recapitulate specific elements of lung fibrosis and, to which extent, these systems and other cutting-edge in vitro technologies can be exploited to aid in the discovery of novel molecular targets for the treatment of IPF patients (Figure 1).

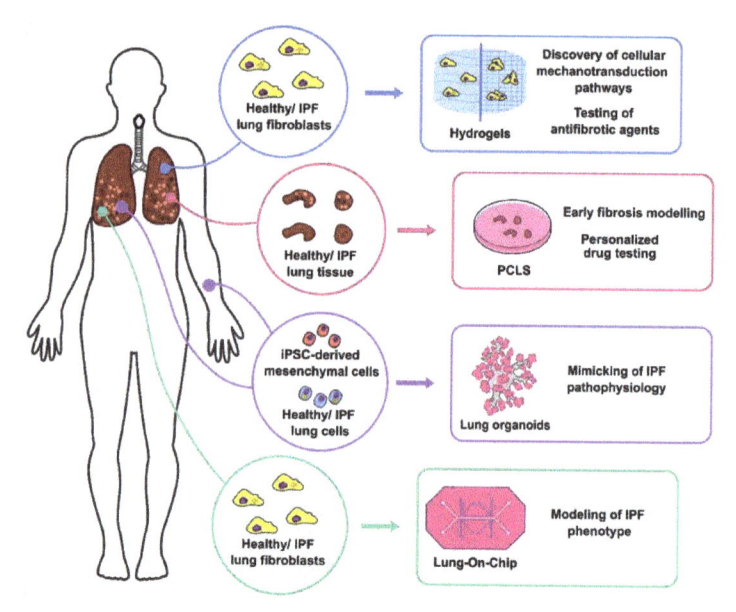

Figure 1. Current human 3D in vitro systems used in IPF research. Lung fibroblasts obtained from healthy donors and IPF patients can be cultured in hydrogels with different stiffness to study cellular mechanotransduction and drug testing. PCLS obtained from patients are being used for modelling early fibrosis and drug screening. In addition, lung organoids derived from lung epithelial stem cells and iPSCs-derived mesenchymal cells have been proven to model IPF pathophysiology, therefore, potentially aiding personalised medicine. Lastly, lung-on-chip devices recapitulate IPF phenotype by culture of fibroblasts isolated from donors and IPF lung tissues together with vascular and lung epithelial cells.

2. 3D Lung Culture Systems

3D culture systems display the cell-to-matrix and cell-to-cell communication lacking in common two-dimensional (2D) monolayer cultures. Mimicking the lung microenvironment in vitro enables 3D systems to assess cell structure and function during homeostatic and pathological conditions. In line with this, hydrogels are defined as water-swollen networks of polymers that allow cells to grow in a more physiological 3D shape. Hydrogels can be customised to better simulate the homeostatic or disease microenvironments by modifying the culture´s stiffness [15]. Another relevant in vitro model is the culture of PCLS obtained from ex vivo lung explants. PCLS contain nearly all cell types present in the lung, including epithelial cells, endothelial cells, smooth muscle cells, and fibroblasts. In culture, PCLS have a 3D configuration, remain metabolically active, and respond to cell-specific stimuli [16]. Alternatively, organoids derived from embryonic progenitors (ESC), induced pluripotent stem cells (iPSC), or adult tissue-resident stem cells have the capacity to proliferate and differentiate into 3D structures that resemble the organ of origin [17]. Notably, lung organoid systems have recently become valuable methods for investigating developmental organogenesis, disease, and regeneration [18,19]. Lastly, lung-on-chip systems introduce another level of complexity by implementing microfluidics. This technique recapitulates some of the organ functions by recreating lung, biochemical, and biomechanical microenvironments through continuous media perfusion and controlled mechanical stress [20]. In the next sections, we describe in more detail the applicability of each of these 3D lung in vitro systems for pulmonary fibrosis modelling and regenerative medicine (Table 1).

2.1. Hydrogels: Modelling of Human Lung Fibroblast Migration and Differentiation

Fibroblast foci and tissue stiffening are considered key pathological markers of IPF [4]. To implement more targeted studies, hydrogels with tunable matrix rigidities that allow fibroblast migration, myofibroblast differentiation, and ECM deposition have been employed to model how fibroblast phenotypes deviate in IPF patients. For example, cultures of human lung fibroblasts in stiff cultures promote upregulation of the transcription factor *megakaryoblastic leukaemia-1* (*MKL1*) and α-smooth muscle actin (αSMA) expression, resulting in myofibroblast differentiation and actin polymerisation. In this study, the mechanotransduction mechanisms that regulate myofibroblast differentiation were investigated by culturing fibroblasts in polyacrylamide (PA) hydrogels with different stiffnesses to mimic normal and fibrotic lung rigidities [21]. Notably, overexpression of nuclear *MKL1* was shown to promote fibroblast differentiation on soft matrixes, suggesting that actin polymerisation-dependent MKL1 nuclear accumulation is sufficient to override matrix stiffness-mediated cell differentiation. Furthermore, Asano et al. also showed higher expression of αSMA in primary human lung fibroblasts when PA hydrogels with higher stiffnesses were employed. In addition, fibroblasts stimulated with the chemotactic factor platelet-derived growth factor (PDGF) rapidly migrated and grew with dendritic extensions when cultured on stiffer gels. Interestingly, blockage of αSMA by short interfering RNA inhibited PDGF-mediated cell migration, indicating that αSMA is not only involved in human lung fibroblast differentiation but also regulates cell migration processes [22].

TGF-β is a potent pro-fibrotic cytokine secreted by myofibroblasts involved in the induction of lung fibrosis, particularly IPF [23]. In this regard, the relation between TGF-β and matrix stiffness was investigated by the culture of primary pulmonary fibroblasts isolated from healthy and IPF patients, in collagen-rich hydrogels with diverse rigidities and in the absence or presence of TGF-β. After culture of control and IPF fibroblasts in pro-fibrotic rigidities, TGF-β stimulation led to FAK/Akt signalling pathway activation, initiating collagen deposition by gene upregulation of *collagen type I alpha 1 chain* (*COL1A1*) along with inhibition of matrix metalloproteinase (*MMP*)-1 expression [24]. The authors' results corroborate the role of the FAK/Akt pathway in collagen deposition in both normal and fibrotic environments. Accordingly, prostaglandin E2 (PGE2), a bioactive prostanoid, has been shown to prevent myofibroblast proliferation and differentiation by reducing the expression of *COL1A1* and αSMA in myofibroblasts [25]. PGE2 is synthesised from endogenous arachidonic acid through the cyclo-oxygenase (COX) pathway, particularly via COX2 after inflammatory stimuli such as TGF-β [26]. Remarkably, levels of both PGE2 and COX2 are considerably reduced in the lungs of patients with IPF compared to control individuals [27]. In concordance, PGE2 and COX2 expression in fibroblasts was also reduced when cultured in stiff matrixes, implying a direct correlation between matrix rigidity and PGE2-COX2 axis modulation [28]. In a recent study, terminal PGE2 synthetic enzyme prostaglandin E synthase (PTGES) was also reduced in the lungs of patients with IPF. Notably, human lung fibroblasts cultured in soft collagen hydrogels and spheroids showed a significant induction of the eicosanoid biosynthetic enzymes COX2, PTGES, and cytosolic phospholipase A2 compared to fibroblasts cultured in stiff plastic plates. These data indicate that lung stiffness in fibrotic regions may negatively affect the expression of multiple eicosanoid biosynthetic enzymes, halting PGE2 synthesis and, consequently, supporting fibrosis progression [29].

In another study, IPF-derived lung fibroblasts were shown to overexpress α6-integrin when cultured on stiff PA matrices. Data showed that upregulation of α6-integrin gene expression on stiff matrices was dependent on ROCK activation of the c-Fos and c-Jun transcription complex. Moreover, blockage of c-Fos/c-Jun-dependent α6-integrin-promoter activation by CRISPR interference technology or pharmacological inhibitors prevented stiff matrix-induced α6-integrin expression. Interestingly, along with other in vitro and in vivo models, the authors showed that α6-integrin mediates myofibroblasts invasion and lung fibrosis after injury, indicating that targeting this pathway might represent an attractive anti-fibrotic therapeutic strategy [30].

While hydrogels are not suitable in vitro models for the study of cellular interactions (e.g., epithelial-mesenchymal cell crosstalk), these studies demonstrate that the platforms are rather useful to recapitulate fibroblast cellular and molecular mechanisms occurring in vivo during fibrosis and are ideal for driving cell-specific therapeutic strategies.

2.2. PCLS: Uncovering Antifibrotic/Regenerative Pathways to Treat IPF

Besides myofibroblast activation and ECM deposition, it has been proposed that repetitive lung epithelial cell damage and reprogramming are closely involved in IPF pathogenesis [31]. In line with this, PCLS models are well-established methods that can be used to investigate the effect of potential drugs for the treatment of IPF patients [32]. For instance, Marudamuthu et al. used PCLS to demonstrate that a 7-mer deletion fragment of calveolin-1 scaffolding domain (CSP7) attenuates fibroblast activation. In vivo, CSP7 delivered systemically or locally improved the overall survival of bleomycin-injured mice by inhibiting not only the expression of ECM proteins but also by reducing the apoptosis of alveolar epithelial cells (AEC). Further, human end-stage IPF lung tissues treated with CSP7 showed a clear inhibition of the expression of pro-fibrotic proteins COL1A1 and α-SMA, supporting the potential use of CSP7 as a therapeutic target for IPF [33].

Given that IPF lung explants are rare and belong mostly to the end-stage of the disease, there was a need for human PCLS models that represent initial fibrosis to investigate early-stage pathomechanisms. In this regard, Alsafadi et al. used a cytokine cocktail containing TGF-β, PDGF-AB, tumour necrosis factor-α, and lysophosphatidic acid to create a model of early fibrosis using human PCLS derived from donors without IPF [34]. PCLS treatment with the fibrotic media upregulated the expression of pro-fibrotic (i.e., Actin alpha 2 (ACTA2), MMP7, and Serpin family E member 1 (SERPINE1)) and pro-inflammatory markers (Interleukin (IL-)1β and Wnt Family Member 5A) without affecting cell viability. In addition, pro-fibrotic treatment-induced ECM deposition while reducing *surfactant protein C (SFTPC)* and *homeodomain-only protein homeobox* expression in AECII and AECI, respectively. In a follow-up study, 14 days after bleomycin or saline administration, PCLS obtained from injured mice was characterised by upregulation of mesenchymal fibrotic markers, fibronectin 1 (*Fn1*), and *Col1a1*, as well as increased secretion of total collagen and Wnt1-inducible signalling protein 1 (Wisp1). Moreover, treatment of control and bleomycin-treated PCLS with nintedanib showed increased *Sftpc* expression in fibrotic PCLS and attenuated *Wisp1* expression in both fibrotic and normal PCLS. Notably, pirfenidone treatment did not trigger *Sftpc* expression nor reduced Wisp1 secretion. For the human model, PCLS obtained from tumour-free lung tissue were treated with the mentioned pro-fibrotic cocktail to induce early fibrosis. Nintedanib treatment restored both *Sftpc* expression and SPC secretion, implying that recovery of AECII function might be a relevant feature of the anti-fibrotic mechanisms of nintedanib [35].

In the pursuit of novel molecular targets for IPF treatment, the role of senescence in lung epithelial cells after fibrosis was investigated by the measurement of SA-β-galactosidase activity, a surrogate marker for the detection of senescence cells, on PCLS obtained from

PBS or bleomycin-challenged mice [36]. The authors showed a higher number of senescent AECs in fibrotic lungs, while treatment with senolytic drugs, dasatinib, and quercetin, resulted in reduced SA-β-galactosidase activity. In addition, treated AECs displayed a lower expression of the fibrotic markers, *Col1a1* and *Wisp1*, leading to the decline of the fibrotic burden and increased AECII marker expression [36]. These findings suggest a potential role of AEC senescence in the development of lung fibrosis and, if further confirmed in humans, identify senolytic drugs as possible candidates for IPF pre-clinical trials. Similarly, it was shown that metformin, an antidiabetic drug and an AMP-activated protein kinase (AMPK) activator, has a dual anti-fibrotic and lipogenic effect in murine and human models of IPF [37,38]. For instance, metformin was able to macroscopically attenuate fibrosis in human PCLS by relaxing the lung structure while increasing the number of lipid-containing cells and decreasing collagen deposition. These observations imply a transition from myofibroblast to lipofibroblast phenotype in metformin-treated PCLS. In combination with in vivo murine models, the authors showed that metformin activates AMPK signalling, which downregulates TGFβ-induced *COL1A1* expression. Along with AMPK upregulation, activation of a separate signalling pathway prompts lipogenic trans-differentiation of myofibroblasts by boosting bone morphogenetic protein 2 expression and peroxisome proliferator-activated receptor-gamma phosphorylation. These data highlight metformin as a promising and safe option for therapies that aim to accelerate fibrosis resolution.

In another recent study, the receptor-like protein tyrosine phosphatase eta (CD148/PTPRJ) mediated by its ligand syndecan-2 (SDC2) has been shown to also have anti-fibrotic effects in murine and human models of IPF. For instance, CD148-deficient mouse fibroblasts highly upregulated PI3K/Akt/mTOR signalling, suppressed autophagy, and promoted p62 expression, leading to nuclear factor kappa B activation and pro-fibrotic markers, *Fn1* and *Col1a1*, upregulation. Additionally, PCLS obtained from IPF and control individuals and treated with a pro-fibrotic mix presented an attenuated pro-fibrotic response when SDC2-based mimetic peptide was added to the media [39]. Furthermore, PCLS obtained from IPF patients, and bleomycin-injured mouse lungs treated with an inhibitor for the TGF-β regulators, αvβ6 and αvβ1 integrins, lead to lower *COL1A1* and *SERPINE1* expression [40]. Future studies will clarify if therapies focused on targeting CD148 ligands and/or αvβ integrins could become alternative clinical approaches to halt fibrosis progression in IPF patients.

Even though obtaining lung tissue is challenging, especially from patients, PCLS offers substantial advantages over traditional 2D cultures by preserving the lung architecture, harbouring multiple cell types, and being metabolically active in culture. Markedly, PCLSs support the identification of unknown molecular mechanisms underlying lung fibrosis and regeneration and aid the screening and discovery of anti-fibrotic/regenerative medications.

2.3. Lung Organoids: Mimicking of Pulmonary Fibrosis Pathophysiology for Personalised Medicine

Over the last decade, major progress has been made in organoid technology to develop structures that closely mimic the cellular and structural complexity of the in vivo scenario [41]. For instance, Sachs et al. generated human airway organoids (AO) from non-small cell lung cancer epithelial cells to create a model that could be applied to a variety of pulmonary diseases such as CF, lung cancer, and respiratory syncytial virus infection. AO contained polarised pseudostratified airway epithelium comprising basal, club, multi-ciliated, and secretory cells. Notably, passaged organoids retain similar cell frequencies independently of the number of passages, thus allowing long-term expansion. Regarding CF, AO lines obtained from the broncho-alveolar lavage of CF patients were characterised and proved to have a thicker layer of apical mucus, which was comparable to the in vivo phenotype [42]. As for translational approaches, Sette et al. described novel in vitro models, including organoids derived from primary airway epithelial cells obtained by nasal brushing of CF patients. Following treatment with CF transmembrane conductance regulator (CFTR) modulators, the drugs' efficacy was confirmed by downregulation of CFTR protein expression, while treatment effectiveness was evaluated by Forskolin-induced swelling functional assays. Given the limited accessibility to patient primary airway epithelial cells, these data strongly support the use of this model for CF pre-clinical studies [43]. In the future, these systems could be adapted to model other types of fibrotic diseases and provide more opportunities for personalised medicine. In another study, a lung organoid model was used to investigate the expression of innate immune receptor, Toll-like receptor 4 (TLR4), and ECM component glycosaminoglycan hyaluronan (HA), are relevant for AECII renewal and repair by limiting fibrosis progression. In vivo, bleomycin treatment of TLR4-/- animals or mice with a HA synthase 2 targeted deletion in AECII were more susceptible to injury when compared with WT mice. For the organoid model, isolated AECII were co-cultured with mouse lung fibroblasts in Matrigel to generate alveolospheres that contain SFTPC positive AECII at the periphery and podoplanin-positive AECI in the interior. Compared to WT alveolospheres, TLR4- and HA-deficient AECII formed fewer and smaller organoids, suggesting that their AECII renewal capacity was compromised. Interestingly, treatment of alveolospheres with exogenous HA increased colony formation efficiency (CFE) in AECII obtained from bleomycin-challenged WT mice. Moreover, 3D cultures of human HTII-280 positive AECII obtained from IPF patients showed lower cell surface HA and reduced CFE compared to AECII isolated from healthy individuals. As with the murine alveolospheres, CFE could be increased by the addition of HA into the media. Ultimately, these results emphasise HAs role in AECII renewal capacity, inferring that future studies will focus on dissecting the molecular mechanisms involved in the loss of HA during pro-fibrotic processes and, if successful, develop strategies for HA restoration on the AECII of IPF patients [44].

Lung organoids are particularly useful to model epithelial-mesenchymal interactions occurring during disease [45–49]. Accordingly, Wilkinson et al. developed a method for the generation of human lung organoids reproducing the distal lung alveolar sac compartment by scaffolding mesenchymal cells into the interstitial space. In this model, alginate beads were coated with polydopamine/collagen 1 and inserted in a bioreactor together with mesenchymal cells allowing an even covering of the epithelial cell types and prompting organoid formation. Notably, mesenchymal cells were indispensable for organoid formation due to their ability to form bead-to-bead bridges. To recreate an IPF environment, TGF-β was added into fetal and iPSC-derived mesenchymal organoid culture. Following TGF-β treatment, highly condensed and smaller organoids grew and exhibited enhanced proliferation markers and *COL1A1* expression with broader α-SMA patches. All these findings were representative of activated myofibroblasts, and subsequent fibroblastic foci formation present in IPF. Importantly, in this study, iPSC-derived mesenchymal cells were successfully transduced with a lentivirus to express mCherry under the control of an ACTA2 promoter that would allow better visualisation, modelling, and analysis of the fibrotic cues occurring during severe fibrosis [50]. In another study, 3D pulmospheres characterised by the presence of multicellular structures embedded in ECM proteins were employed for IPF modelling. Pulmospheres were generated from controls or IPF-derived primary lung cells and contained multiple cell types, including AECII, endothelial cells, macrophages, vascular smooth muscle cells, and myofibroblasts. The presence of an IPF phenotype was confirmed by the increase of α-SMA positive cells radiating outward from the pulmospheres. Interestingly, the extension of invading fibroblasts outside of the organoids' core provided the authors with a measurement of injury defined as the "zone of invasion" (ZOI) percentage. Following treatment with TGF-β, control lung pulmospheres showed increased ZOI% while treatment of IPF pulmospheres with nintedanib or pirfenidone lowered the invasion area, suggesting that the degree of fibrosis can be modulated using known treatments. Notably, patients with progressive end-stage disease had higher ZOI%, while patients with non-progressive disease but treated with nintedanib or pirfenidone exhibited lower ZOI%, indicating that pulmospheres could reflect, at least to some extent, the in vivo situation [51]. Furthermore, Strikoudis et al. generated a human lung organoid model of fibrosis, employing CRISPR/Cas9 gene-editing technology. In this model, human ESC with engineered mutations in several HPS (Hermansky–Pudlak syndrome) genes caused deformed lysosome-related organelles leading to the development of fibrosis. ESC mutations in HPS1, HPS2, and HPS4 genes generate structurally abnormal organoids characterised by mesenchymal cell aggregation and collagen deposition. Of note, IL-11 was overexpressed in epithelial and mesenchymal cells obtained from HPS1-/- and HPS2-/- organoids. Treatment with IL-11 led to a significant increase of the fibrotic markers, PDGFRα and αSMA, in WT organoids, while deletion of IL-11 in HPS4-/- organoids displayed a morphology similar to WT organoids, implying that prolonged IL-11 exposure may have a significant role in fibrosis induction [52].

Overall, lung organoid systems provide a deeper understanding of physiologically relevant molecular mechanisms of fibrosis that are especially difficult to study in vivo. Importantly, lung organoids derived from patients could be used for high throughput drug screening and prompt the generation of effective and affordable personalised medicine for IPF patients.

2.4. Lung in a Chip: Development of Complex Ex Vivo Systems for Pulmonary Fibrosis Modelling

In the last few years, several advances in micro-bioengineering have been achieved to create sophisticated organ-on-a-chip devices containing hollow microchannels lined by living cells. These devices recapitulate certain structural and functional features of tissues and organs, including cell–cell and cell–matrix crosstalk, physical microenvironment, and vascular perfusion [53]. Considering that the human lung is one of the most difficult organs to model in vitro due to its structural and cellular complexity, lung-on-a-chip models are rapidly becoming powerful tools to mimic human lung physiology and pathology [54–58]. For instance, Barkal et al. developed a microscale organotypic model of a human bronchiole to assess fungal and bacterial infection. In this model, pulmonary fibroblasts, primary bronchial epithelial cells, and lung microvascular cells were embedded within a 3D collagen matrix and cultured in a lung-on-chip device with two adjacent lumens to recapitulate the microvascular and airway compartment of the in vivo bronchiole. Notably, this model allows the addition of an interchangeable microbial culture and leucocytes in separate channels that incites an immune response towards the microbial agents via volatile compounds and enables tracking of recruited immune cells [59].

Regarding fibrotic disease modelling, a lung-on-chip model called a "CF-airway-chip" containing primary human CF bronchial epithelial cells, including differentiated ciliated, basal, club, and goblet cells, and pulmonary microvascular endothelial cells, was developed to study CF pathology. Compared to devices containing healthy epithelial cells, the CF-airway-chip recapitulated important features of CF pathology such as increased mucus built-up, cilia density, and beating frequency. After the addition of polymorphonuclear leukocytes (PMNs), circulating PMNs adhered to the endothelium and transmigrated into the airway compartment. In this model, *Pseudomonas aeruginosa* infection led to IL-6, tumour necrosis factor-α, and granulocyte macrophage-colony stimulating factor release in both healthy and CF-airway-chips, while IL-8, a potent PMN chemo-attractant, was significantly higher in CF-airway-chips. Although this model lacks the fibroblast compartment, this model could be a valuable system for the study of pulmonary fibrosis pathophysiology [58]. Another fibrotic model aimed to mimic the human lung upper respiratory airways and model IPF by culturing small airway epithelial cells (SAECs) in one channel and an endothelial-fibroblast-fibrin gel mixture in the outer/central channels. This 3D lung-on-chip design permits the culture of SAECs above a vascular compartment composed of endothelium and fibroblasts. TGF-β treatment of chips containing the healthy or IPF fibroblasts led to upregulation of αSMA expression and downregulation of club and ciliated cell markers, recreating an important component of IPF phenotype. Nevertheless, treatment with the anti-fibrotic agent pirfenidone failed to reduce the fibrotic phenotype in this model, suggesting that further model adaptations are still needed to more closely resemble IPF physiology [60,61].

In a more complex approach, Varone et al. developed a flexible "Open-Top Alveolus-Chip" to mimic the human alveoli by generating a chambered-organotypic epithelium surrounded by two vacuum channels that allow stretch. The top of the chamber contained a removable microchannel capable of being perfused with air or liquid, while the bottom contained a porous flexible membrane permitting transport diffusion. To build vasculature, endothelial cells were cultured in the top chamber and formed a tight monolayer expressing von Willebrand factor, vascular endothelial-cadherin, and platelet and endothelial cell adhesion molecule-1. Epithelial cells (stratified keratinocytes and AEC) could also be cultured in the top chamber. Upon seeding, AECI and II and microvilli were detected, and when cultured with fibroblasts under mechanical stretch, AECII produced surfactant protein C, confirming that exposure to both factors stimulates surfactant production. To study stromal-epithelial crosstalk, the device was challenged with lipopolysaccharide, resulting in upregulation of intracellular adhesion molecule-1 on endothelial cells and production of IL-6, IL-8, and mitochondrial pyruvate carrier-1 on the vascular channel. Notably, this immune response was only detectable when the stromal, vascular, and epithelial cell layers were present. While this device has not been proven to reproduce fibrotic processes, given its complexity and the presence of an alveolar and stromal compartment, it could certainly represent an attractive approach to studying fibrotic diseases [61].

Since lung-on-chip technology is relatively new, further studies are still needed to fully evaluate if such models could be employed to model pulmonary fibrosis. Nonetheless, these devices hold great promise, and it is likely a matter of time until more complex systems can mimic other main features of IPF pathophysiology.

Table 1. 3D in vivo models employed to study pulmonary fibrosis.

3D Culture System	Species	Source	Cellular Composition	Applicability/Main Finding	Reference
PA hydrogels	Human	Healthy donors		Cellular mechanotransduction	Tse et al. [21] Asano et al. [22] Chen et al. [30]
	Mouse	IPF patients Saline/Bleomycin-treated mice		PGE2-COX2 axis modulation in stiff matrixes	Liu et al. [28]
Collagen-rich hydrogels	Human	Healthy donors/ IPF patients		FAK/Akt signalling pathway activation promoting collagen deposition	Giménez et al. [24]
			Lung fibroblasts	Eicosanoid biosynthetic enzymes upregulation in fibrotic conditions	Berhan et al. [29]
PCLS	Mouse	Saline/ Bleomycin-treated lung tissue	Distal lung epithelial cells, vascular and mesenchymal compartment	Drug testing: CSP7	Marudamuthu et al. [33]
				Drug testing: senolytic drugs	Lehmann et al. [36]
				Drug testing: αvβ integrins	Tsoyi et al. [39]
	Human			Disease modelling: early fibrosis	Alsafadi et al. [34]
		Healthy donors/ IPF lung tissue		Drug testing: metformin	Kheirollahi et al. [37]
				Drug testing: SDC2 ligands	Decaris et al. [40]
	Human /Mouse	Healthy lung tissue/Bleomycin-treated lung tissue		Disease modelling: early fibrosis	Lehmann et al. [35]
Lung organoids	Human	CF patients broncho-alveolar lavage	Airway organoids: basal, ciliated, secretory, and club cells	Disease modelling: CF pathophysiology	Sachs et al. [42]
		CF patient nasal brushing	Airway organoids: basal, ciliated, and secretory cells	Personalised medicine: discovery of therapeutic targets and more effective CFTR modulators	Sette et al. [43].
		Healthy donors	Distal alveolar organoids: AECII, AECI, iPSC derived-mesenchymal cells	Disease modelling: epithelial-mesenchymal interactions during fibrosis	Wilkinson et al. [50]
		Healthy/ IPF lung tissue	Pulmospheres: AECII, endothelial cells, macrophages, mesenchymal cells	Disease modelling: myofibroblast activation	Surolia et al. [51]
		Healthy donors	ESC-derived lung organoids–epithelial cells and mesenchymal cells	Disease modelling: mutation in HPS1, HPS2 and HPS4 genes to induce fibrosis	Strikoudis et al. [52]
	Mouse/ Human	HA- and TLR4-deficient mice/ IPF patients	Alveolospheres: AECI, AECII, fibroblasts	Disease modelling: AECII regeneration after fibrosis	Liang et al. [44]

Table 1. Cont.

3D Culture System	Species	Source	Cellular Composition	Applicability/ Main Finding	Reference
Lung-on-chip	Human	CF patients	CF bronchial epithelial cells and pulmonary microvascular endothelial cells	Disease modelling: CF pathology	Plebani et al. [58]
		Healthy Donors/ IPF patients	SAEC, endothelial cells, fibroblast	Disease modelling: IPF phenotype	Mejías et al. [60]

3. Conclusions

As shown above, 3D in vitro lung models have advantages as well as disadvantages that largely depend on the scientific question that needs to be addressed (Figure 1 and Table 2). Regarding IPF, the most used models rely on mouse experimentation, namely, bleomycin-induced pulmonary injury. Although this model mimics certain aspects of IPF pathophysiology, it has been heavily criticized partly due to the presence of inflammation/acute lung injury preceding the fibrotic phase, self-resolution after a few weeks, number of mice needed, strong age- and gender-dependency, among others [62]. Several of these drawbacks can be circumvented or even diminished by the inclusion of 3D in vitro/ex vivo systems. For example, primary human-derived samples such as fibroblasts, iPSC-derived mesenchymal cells, and PCLS can be used after patient consent, therefore, alleviating the ethical concerns of animal experimentation. In addition, these models provide the opportunity to more accurately dissect the cellular and molecular players involved in lung fibrosis, as well as the possibility of high-throughput analyses. One interesting novel and non-invasive approach would be to employ liquid biopsies from IPF patients to facilitate drug testing [63]. The aim of this method would be to evaluate if circulating cells or/and soluble mediators added onto lung-on-chip devices could drive a fibrotic phenotype and then be used to identify specific therapeutic targets.

Table 2. Main strengths and weaknesses of hydrogels, PCLS, lung organoids, and lung-on-chip systems.

3D Culture System	Strengths	Weaknesses
Hydrogels	✓ Tunable matrix stiffness allows mimicking homeostatic and fibrotic microenvironments ✓ Fibroblasts can be obtained from donors and patients	• In most instances, not suitable to study intercellular interactions
PCLS	✓ Presence of several lung cell types ✓ Preservation of native lung architecture, microenvironment, and metabolic activity ✓ Patient-derived-PCLS can be used for drug-testing	• Cultures are difficult to maintain • Analyses involving cell migration are limited
Lung organoids	✓ Progenitor cells from donors and patients can be employed ✓ Suitable to study mesenchymal-epithelial crosstalk ✓ High throughput analyses are possible	• Lack vasculature • Lack immune cells
Lung-on-chip	✓ Relatively cheap ✓ Mimic lung biochemical microenvironment ✓ Vascular and immune cells can be integrated	• Culture and analysis require special equipment • Low experimental throughput

Ultimately, as these models advance in cellular and structural complexity, their central challenge would be to reveal hidden molecular and cellular signals governing pulmonary fibrosis, which could lead to the discovery and implementation of effective therapies for the treatment and resolution of fibrotic lung diseases.

Author Contributions: A.I.V.-A. and M.M.B. designed and wrote the manuscript. A.I.V.-A., M.M.B., E.E.A. and S.H. contributed to the interpretation and discussion of the manuscript. All authors have read and agreed to the published version of the manuscript.

Funding: This work was supported by the German Research Foundation (DFG; SFB 1021 C05 and Z02, SFB-TR84 B9, and A6, SFB CRC1213 project-A04, KFO 309 P2/P7/P8/Z01; and EL 931/4-1, excellence cluster Cardio-Pulmonary Institute [CPI]), University Hospital Giessen and Marburg (FOKOOPV), Institute for Lung Health (ILH), and the German Center for Lung Research (DZL).

Conflicts of Interest: The authors declare no conflict of interest.

References

1. Hyldgaard, C.; Hilberg, O.; Bendstrup, E. How Does Comorbidity Influence Survival in Idiopathic Pulmonary Fibrosis? *Respir. Med.* **2014**, *108*, 647–653. [CrossRef] [PubMed]
2. Olson, A.L.; Swigris, J.J. Idiopathic Pulmonary Fibrosis: Diagnosis and Epidemiology. *Clin. Chest Med.* **2012**, *33*, 41–50. [CrossRef] [PubMed]
3. Wuyts, W.A.; Wijsenbeek, M.; Bondue, B.; Bouros, D.; Bresser, P.; Robalo Cordeiro, C.; Hilberg, O.; Magnusson, J.; Manali, E.D.; Morais, A.; et al. Idiopathic Pulmonary Fibrosis: Best Practice in Monitoring and Managing a Relentless Fibrotic Disease. *Respiration* **2020**, *99*, 73–82. [CrossRef]
4. Wolters, P.J.; Collard, H.R.; Jones, K.D. Pathogenesis of Idiopathic Pulmonary Fibrosis. *Annu. Rev. Pathol.* **2014**, *9*, 157. [CrossRef] [PubMed]
5. Moore, B.B.; Lawson, W.E.; Oury, T.D.; Sisson, T.H.; Raghavendran, K.; Hogaboam, C.M. Animal Models of Fibrotic Lung Disease. *Am. J. Respir. Cell Mol. Biol.* **2013**, *49*, 167–179. [CrossRef]
6. Raghu, G.; Remy-Jardin, M.; Myers, J.L.; Richeldi, L.; Ryerson, C.J.; Lederer, D.J.; Behr, J.; Cottin, V.; Danoff, S.K.; Morell, F.; et al. Diagnosis of Idiopathic Pulmonary Fibrosis An Official ATS/ERS/JRS/ALAT Clinical Practice Guideline. *Am. J. Respir. Crit. Care Med.* **2018**, *198*, e44–e68. [CrossRef]
7. Maher, T.M.; Strek, M.E. Antifibrotic Therapy for Idiopathic Pulmonary Fibrosis: Time to Treat. *Respir. Res.* **2019**, *20*, 205. [CrossRef]
8. Wollin, L.; Wex, E.; Pautsch, A.; Schnapp, G.; Hostettler, K.E.; Stowasser, S.; Kolb, M. Mode of Action of Nintedanib in the Treatment of Idiopathic Pulmonary Fibrosis. *Eur. Respir. J.* **2015**, *45*, 1434–1445. [CrossRef]
9. Meyer, K.C.; Decker, C.A. Role of Pirfenidone in the Management of Pulmonary Fibrosis. *Ther. Clin. Risk Manag.* **2017**, *13*, 427–437. [CrossRef]
10. Sgalla, G.; Cocconcelli, E.; Tonelli, R.; Richeldi, L. Novel Drug Targets for Idiopathic Pulmonary Fibrosis. *Expert Rev. Respir. Med.* **2016**, *10*, 393–405. [CrossRef]
11. Tashiro, J.; Rubio, G.A.; Limper, A.H.; Williams, K.; Elliot, S.J.; Ninou, I.; Aidinis, V.; Tzouvelekis, A.; Glassberg, M.K. Exploring Animal Models That Resemble Idiopathic Pulmonary Fibrosis. *Front. Med.* **2017**, *4*, 1. [CrossRef] [PubMed]
12. de Hilster, R.H.J.; Sharma, P.K.; Jonker, M.R.; White, E.S.; Gercama, E.A.; Roobeek, M.; Timens, W.; Harmsen, M.C.; Hylkema, M.N.; Burgess, J.K. Human Lung Extracellular Matrix Hydrogels Resemble the Stiffness and Viscoelasticity of Native Lung Tissue. *Am. J. Physiol.-Lung Cell. Mol. Physiol.* **2020**, *318*, L698–L704. [CrossRef] [PubMed]
13. Alsafadi, H.N.; Uhl, F.E.; Pineda, R.H.; Bailey, K.E.; Rojas, M.; Wagner, D.E.; Königshoff, M. Applications and Approaches for Three-Dimensional Precision-Cut Lung Slices. Disease Modeling and Drug Discovery. *Am. J. Respir. Cell Mol. Biol.* **2020**, *62*, 692–698. [CrossRef] [PubMed]
14. Kim, J.-H.; An, G.H.; Kim, J.-Y.; Rasaei, R.; Kim, W.J.; Jin, X.; Woo, D.-H.; Han, C.; Yang, S.-R.; Kim, J.-H.; et al. Human Pluripotent Stem Cell-Derived Alveolar Organoids for Modeling Pulmonary Fibrosis and Drug Testing. *Cell Death Discov.* **2021**, *7*, 48. [CrossRef]
15. Ahmed, E.M. Hydrogel: Preparation, Characterization, and Applications: A Review. *J. Adv. Res.* **2015**, *6*, 105–121. [CrossRef]
16. Liu, G.; Betts, C.; Cunoosamy, D.M.; Åberg, P.M.; Hornberg, J.J.; Sivars, K.B.; Cohen, T.S. Use of Precision Cut Lung Slices as a Translational Model for the Study of Lung Biology. *Respir. Res.* **2019**, *20*, 162. [CrossRef]
17. Lancaster, M.A.; Knoblich, J.A. Organogenesis in a Dish: Modeling Development and Disease Using Organoid Technologies. *Science* **2014**, *345*, 1247125. [CrossRef]
18. Miller, A.J.; Spence, J.R. In Vitro Models to Study Human Lung Development, Disease and Homeostasis. *Physiology* **2017**, *32*, 246–260. [CrossRef]
19. Gkatzis, K.; Taghizadeh, S.; Huh, D.; Stainier, D.Y.R.; Bellusci, S. Use of Three-Dimensional Organoids and Lung-on-a-Chip Methods to Study Lung Development, Regeneration and Disease. *Eur. Respir. J.* **2018**, *52*, 1800876. [CrossRef]
20. Artzy-Schnirman, A.; Hobi, N.; Schneider-Daum, N.; Guenat, O.T.; Lehr, C.M.; Sznitman, J. Advanced in Vitro Lung-on-Chip Platforms for Inhalation Assays: From Prospect to Pipeline. *Eur. J. Pharm. Biopharm.* **2019**, *144*, 11–17. [CrossRef]
21. Tse, J.R.; Engler, A.J. Preparation of Hydrogel Substrates with Tunable Mechanical Properties. *Curr. Protoc. Cell Biol.* **2010**, *10*, 10–16. [CrossRef] [PubMed]
22. Asano, S.; Ito, S.; Takahashi, K.; Furuya, K.; Kondo, M.; Sokabe, M.; Hasegawa, Y. Matrix Stiffness Regulates Migration of Human Lung Fibroblasts. *Physiol. Rep.* **2017**, *5*, e13281. [CrossRef] [PubMed]

23. Wei, P.; Xie, Y.; Abel, P.W.; Huang, Y.; Ma, Q.; Li, L.; Hao, J.; Wolff, D.W.; Wei, T.; Tu, Y. Transforming Growth Factor (TGF)-B1-Induced MiR-133a Inhibits Myofibroblast Differentiation and Pulmonary Fibrosis. *Cell Death Dis.* **2019**, *10*, 670. [CrossRef] [PubMed]
24. Giménez, A.; Duch, P.; Puig, M.; Gabasa, M.; Xaubet, A.; Alcaraz, J. Dysregulated Collagen Homeostasis by Matrix Stiffening and TGF-B1 in Fibroblasts from Idiopathic Pulmonary Fibrosis Patients: Role of FAK/Akt. *Int. J. Mol. Sci.* **2017**, *18*, 2431. [CrossRef]
25. Wettlaufer, S.H.; Scott, J.P.; McEachin, R.C.; Peters-Golden, M.; Huang, S.K. Reversal of the Transcriptome by Prostaglandin E2 during Myofibroblast Dedifferentiation. *Am. J. Respir. Cell Mol. Biol.* **2016**, *54*, 114–127. [CrossRef] [PubMed]
26. Keerthisingam, C.B.; Jenkins, R.G.; Harrison, N.K.; Hernandez-Rodriguez, N.A.; Booth, H.; Laurent, G.J.; Hart, S.L.; Foster, M.L.; McAnulty, R.J. Cyclooxygenase-2 Deficiency Results in a Loss of the Anti-Proliferative Response to Transforming Growth Factor-β in Human Fibrotic Lung Fibroblasts and Promotes Bleomycin-Induced Pulmonary Fibrosis in Mice. *Am. J. Pathol.* **2001**, *158*, 1411–1422. [CrossRef]
27. Coward, W.R.; Watts, K.; Feghali-Bostwick, C.A.; Knox, A.; Pang, L. Defective Histone Acetylation Is Responsible for the Diminished Expression of Cyclooxygenase 2 in Idiopathic Pulmonary Fibrosis. *Mol. Cell. Biol.* **2009**, *29*, 4325–4339. [CrossRef]
28. Liu, F.; Mih, J.D.; Shea, B.S.; Kho, A.T.; Sharif, A.S.; Tager, A.M.; Tschumperlin, D.J. Feedback Amplification of Fibrosis through Matrix Stiffening and COX-2 Suppression. *J. Cell Biol.* **2010**, *190*, 693–706. [CrossRef]
29. Berhan, A.; Harris, T.; Jaffar, J.; Jativa, F.; Langenbach, S.; Lönnstedt, I.; Alhamdoosh, M.; Ng, M.; Lee, P.; Westall, G.; et al. Cellular Microenvironment Stiffness Regulates Eicosanoid Production and Signaling Pathways. *Am. J. Respir. Cell Mol. Biol.* **2020**, *63*, 819–830. [CrossRef]
30. Chen, H.; Qu, J.; Huang, X.; Kurundkar, A.; Zhu, L.; Yang, N.; Venado, A.; Ding, Q.; Liu, G.; Antony, V.B.; et al. Mechanosensing by the A6-Integrin Confers an Invasive Fibroblast Phenotype and Mediates Lung Fibrosis. *Nat. Commun.* **2016**, *7*, 12564. [CrossRef]
31. Selman, M.; Pardo, A. The Leading Role of Epithelial Cells in the Pathogenesis of Idiopathic Pulmonary Fibrosis. *Cell. Signal.* **2020**, *66*, 109482. [CrossRef] [PubMed]
32. Cedilak, M.; Banjanac, M.; Belamarić, D.; Paravić Radičević, A.; Faraho, I.; Ilić, K.; Čužić, S.; Glojnarić, I.; Eraković Haber, V.; Bosnar, M. Precision-Cut Lung Slices from Bleomycin Treated Animals as a Model for Testing Potential Therapies for Idiopathic Pulmonary Fibrosis. *Pulm. Pharmacol. Ther.* **2019**, *55*, 75–83. [CrossRef] [PubMed]
33. Marudamuthu, A.S.; Bhandary, Y.P.; Fan, L.; Radhakrishnan, V.; MacKenzie, B.A.; Maier, E.; Shetty, S.K.; Nagaraja, M.R.; Gopu, V.; Tiwari, N.; et al. Caveolin-1-Derived Peptide Limits Development of Pulmonary Fibrosis. *Sci. Transl. Med.* **2019**, *11*, eaat2848. [CrossRef] [PubMed]
34. Alsafadi, H.N.; Staab-Weijnitz, C.A.; Lehmann, M.; Lindner, M.; Peschel, B.; Königshoff, M.; Wagner, D.E. An Ex Vivo Model to Induce Early Fibrosis-like Changes in Human Precision-Cut Lung Slices. *Am. J. Physiol.-Lung Cell. Mol. Physiol.* **2017**, *312*, L896–L902. [CrossRef]
35. Lehmann, M.; Buhl, L.; Alsafadi, H.N.; Klee, S.; Hermann, S.; Mutze, K.; Ota, C.; Lindner, M.; Behr, J.; Hilgendorff, A.; et al. Differential Effects of Nintedanib and Pirfenidone on Lung Alveolar Epithelial Cell Function in Ex Vivo Murine and Human Lung Tissue Cultures of Pulmonary Fibrosis 11 Medical and Health Sciences 1102 Cardiorespiratory Medicine and Haematology 06 Biologica. *Respir. Res.* **2018**, *19*. [CrossRef]
36. Lehmann, M.; Korfei, M.; Mutze, K.; Klee, S.; Skronska-Wasek, W.; Alsafadi, H.N.; Ota, C.; Costa, R.; Schiller, H.B.; Lindner, M.; et al. Senolytic Drugs Target Alveolar Epithelial Cell Function and Attenuate Experimental Lung Fibrosis Ex Vivo. *Eur. Respir. J.* **2017**, *50*. [CrossRef]
37. Kheirollahi, V.; Wasnick, R.M.; Biasin, V.; Vazquez-Armendariz, A.I.; Chu, X.; Moiseenko, A.; Weiss, A.; Wilhelm, J.; Zhang, J.S.; Kwapiszewska, G.; et al. Metformin Induces Lipogenic Differentiation in Myofibroblasts to Reverse Lung Fibrosis. *Nat. Commun.* **2019**, *10*, 2987. [CrossRef]
38. Rangarajan, S.; Bone, N.B.; Zmijewska, A.A.; Jiang, S.; Park, D.W.; Bernard, K.; Locy, M.L.; Ravi, S.; Deshane, J.; Mannon, R.B.; et al. Metformin Reverses Established Lung Fibrosis in a Bleomycin Model. *Nat. Med.* **2018**, *24*, 1121–1127. [CrossRef]
39. Tsoyi, K.; Liang, X.; De Rossi, G.; Ryter, S.W.; Xiong, K.; Chu, S.G.; Liu, X.; Ith, B.; Celada, L.J.; Romero, F.; et al. Cd148 Deficiency in Fibroblasts Promotes the Development of Pulmonary Fibrosis. *Am. J. Respir. Crit. Care Med.* **2021**, *204*, 312–325. [CrossRef]
40. Decaris, M.L.; Schaub, J.R.; Chen, C.; Cha, J.; Lee, G.G.; Rexhepaj, M.; Ho, S.S.; Rao, V.; Marlow, M.M.; Kotak, P.; et al. Dual Inhibition of Avβ6 and Avβ1 Reduces Fibrogenesis in Lung Tissue Explants from Patients with IPF. *Respir. Res.* **2021**, *22*, 265. [CrossRef]
41. Kim, J.; Koo, B.K.; Knoblich, J.A. Human Organoids: Model Systems for Human Biology and Medicine. *Nat. Rev. Mol. Cell Biol.* **2020**, *21*, 571–584. [CrossRef] [PubMed]
42. Sachs, N.; Papaspyropoulos, A.; Ommen, D.D.Z.; Heo, I.; Böttinger, L.; Klay, D.; Weeber, F.; Huelsz-Prince, G.; Iakobachvili, N.; Amatngalim, G.D.; et al. Long-Term Expanding Human Airway Organoids for Disease Modeling. *EMBO J.* **2019**, *38*, e100300. [CrossRef] [PubMed]
43. Sette, G.; Cicero, S.L.; Blaconà, G.; Pierandrei, S.; Bruno, S.M.; Salvati, V.; Castelli, G.; Falchi, M.; Fabrizzi, B.; Cimino, G.; et al. Theratyping Cystic Fibrosis in Vitro in ALI Culture and Organoid Models Generated from Patient-Derived Nasal Epithelial Conditionally Reprogrammed Stem Cells. *Eur. Respir. J.* **2021**, *58*. [CrossRef] [PubMed]
44. Liang, J.; Zhang, Y.; Xie, T.; Liu, N.; Chen, H.; Geng, Y.; Kurkciyan, A.; Mena, J.M.; Stripp, B.R.; Jiang, D.; et al. Hyaluronan and TLR4 Promote Surfactant-Protein-C-Positive Alveolar Progenitor Cell Renewal and Prevent Severe Pulmonary Fibrosis in Mice. *Nat. Med.* **2016**, *22*, 1285–1293. [CrossRef]

45. Moiseenko, A.; Vazquez-Armendariz, A.I.; Kheirollahi, V.; Chu, X.; Tata, A.; Rivetti, S.; Günther, S.; Lebrigand, K.; Herold, S.; Braun, T.; et al. Identification of a Repair-Supportive Mesenchymal Cell Population during Airway Epithelial Regeneration. *Cell Rep.* **2020**, *33*. [CrossRef]
46. Vazquez-Armendariz, A.I.; Heiner, M.; El Agha, E.; Salwig, I.; Hoek, A.; Hessler, M.C.; Shalashova, I.; Shrestha, A.; Carraro, G.; Mengel, J.P.; et al. Multilineage Murine Stem Cells Generate Complex Organoids to Model Distal Lung Development and Disease. *EMBO J.* **2020**, *39*. [CrossRef]
47. Moore, B.B.; Moore, T.A. Viruses in Idiopathic Pulmonary Fibrosis Etiology and Exacerbation. *Ann. Am. Thorac. Soc.* **2015**, *12*, S186–S192. [CrossRef]
48. Barkauskas, C.E.; Cronce, M.J.; Rackley, C.R.; Bowie, E.J.; Keene, D.R.; Stripp, B.R.; Randell, S.H.; Noble, P.W.; Hogan, B.L.M. Type 2 Alveolar Cells Are Stem Cells in Adult Lung. *J. Clin. Investig.* **2013**, *123*, 3025–3036. [CrossRef]
49. Vazquez-Armendariz, A.I.; Seeger, W.; Herold, S.; El Agha, E. Protocol for the Generation of Murine Bronchiolospheres. *STAR Protoc.* **2021**, *2*, 100594. [CrossRef]
50. Wilkinson, D.C.; Alva-Ornelas, J.A.; Sucre, J.M.S.; Vijayaraj, P.; Durra, A.; Richardson, W.; Jonas, S.J.; Paul, M.K.; Karumbayaram, S.; Dunn, B.; et al. Development of a Three-Dimensional Bioengineering Technology to Generate Lung Tissue for Personalized Disease Modeling. *Stem Cells Transl. Med.* **2017**, *6*, 622–633. [CrossRef]
51. Surolia, R.; Li, F.J.; Wang, Z.; Li, H.; Liu, G.; Zhou, Y.; Luckhardt, T.; Bae, S.; Liu, R.M.; Rangarajan, S.; et al. 3D Pulmospheres Serve as a Personalized and Predictive Multicellular Model for Assessment of Antifibrotic Drugs. *JCI Insight* **2017**, *2*. [CrossRef] [PubMed]
52. Strikoudis, A.; Cieślak, A.; Loffredo, L.; Chen, Y.W.; Patel, N.; Saqi, A.; Lederer, D.J.; Snoeck, H.W. Modeling of Fibrotic Lung Disease Using 3D Organoids Derived from Human Pluripotent Stem Cells. *Cell Rep.* **2019**, *27*, 3709–3723.e5. [CrossRef] [PubMed]
53. Wu, Q.; Liu, J.; Wang, X.; Feng, L.; Wu, J.; Zhu, X.; Wen, W.; Gong, X. Organ-on-a-Chip: Recent Breakthroughs and Future Prospects. *Biomed. Eng. OnLine* **2020**, *19*, 9. [CrossRef]
54. Azadi, S.; Aboulkheyr Es, H.; Razavi Bazaz, S.; Thiery, J.P.; Asadnia, M.; Ebrahimi Warkiani, M. Upregulation of PD-L1 Expression in Breast Cancer Cells through the Formation of 3D Multicellular Cancer Aggregates under Different Chemical and Mechanical Conditions. *Biochim. Biophys. Acta-Mol. Cell Res.* **2019**, *1866*, 118526. [CrossRef] [PubMed]
55. Neužil, P.; Giselbrecht, S.; Länge, K.; Huang, T.J.; Manz, A. Revisiting Lab-on-a-Chip Technology for Drug Discovery. *Nat. Rev. Drug Discov.* **2012**, *11*, 620–632. [CrossRef]
56. Si, L.; Bai, H.; Oh, C.Y.; Jin, L.; Prantil-Baun, R.; Ingber, D.E. Clinically Relevant Influenza Virus Evolution Reconstituted in a Human Lung Airway-on-a-Chip. *Microbiol. Spectr.* **2021**, *9*, e00257-21. [CrossRef] [PubMed]
57. Huang, D.; Liu, T.; Liao, J.; Maharjan, S.; Xie, X.; Pérez, M.; Anaya, I.; Wang, S.; Mayer, A.T.; Kang, Z.; et al. Reversed-Engineered Human Alveolar Lung-on-a-Chip Model. *Proc. Natl. Acad. Sci. USA* **2021**, *118*. [CrossRef]
58. Plebani, R.; Potla, R.; Soong, M.; Bai, H.; Izadifar, Z.; Jiang, A.; Travis, R.N.; Belgur, C.; Dinis, A.; Cartwright, M.J.; et al. Modeling Pulmonary Cystic Fibrosis in a Human Lung Airway-on-a-Chip: Cystic Fibrosis Airway Chip. *J. Cyst. Fibros.* **2021**. [CrossRef]
59. Barkal, L.J.; Procknow, C.L.; Álvarez-García, Y.R.; Niu, M.; Jiménez-Torres, J.A.; Brockman-Schneider, R.A.; Gern, J.E.; Denlinger, L.C.; Theberge, A.B.; Keller, N.P.; et al. Microbial Volatile Communication in Human Organotypic Lung Models. *Nat. Commun.* **2017**, *8*. [CrossRef]
60. Mejías, J.C.; Nelson, M.R.; Liseth, O.; Roy, K. A 96-Well Format Microvascularized Human Lung-on-a-Chip Platform for Microphysiological Modeling of Fibrotic Diseases. *Lab Chip* **2020**, *20*, 3601–3611. [CrossRef]
61. Varone, A.; Nguyen, J.K.; Leng, L.; Barrile, R.; Sliz, J.; Lucchesi, C.; Wen, N.; Gravanis, A.; Hamilton, G.A.; Karalis, K.; et al. A Novel Organ-Chip System Emulates Three-Dimensional Architecture of the Human Epithelia and the Mechanical Forces Acting on It. *Biomaterials* **2021**, *275*, 120957. [CrossRef] [PubMed]
62. Moeller, A.; Ask, K.; Warburton, D.; Gauldie, J.; Kolb, M. The Bleomycin Animal Model: A Useful Tool to Investigate Treatment Options for Idiopathic Pulmonary Fibrosis? *Int. J. Biochem. Cell Biol.* **2008**, *40*, 362–382. [CrossRef] [PubMed]
63. Stella, G.M.; D'Agnano, V.; Piloni, D.; Saracino, L.; Lettieri, S.; Mariani, F.; Lancia, A.; Bortolotto, C.; Rinaldi, P.; Falanga, F.; et al. The Oncogenic Landscape of the Idiopathic Pulmonary Fibrosis: A Narrative Review. *Transl. Lung Cancer Res.* **2022**, *11*, 472–496. [CrossRef] [PubMed]

Review
Emerging Roles of Airway Epithelial Cells in Idiopathic Pulmonary Fibrosis

Ashesh Chakraborty, Michal Mastalerz, Meshal Ansari, Herbert B. Schiller and Claudia A. Staab-Weijnitz *

Member of the German Center for Lung Research (DZL), Institute of Lung Health and Immunity and Comprehensive Pneumology Center with the CPC-M BioArchive, Helmholtz Zentrum München GmbH, 81377 Munich, Germany; ashesh.chakraborty@helmholtz-muenchen.de (A.C.); michal.mastalerz@helmholtz-muenchen.de (M.M.); meshal.ansari@helmholtz-muenchen.de (M.A.); herbert.schiller@helmholtz-muenchen.de (H.B.S.)
* Correspondence: staab-weijnitz@helmholtz-muenchen.de; Tel.: +49-(0)89-3187-4681

Abstract: Idiopathic pulmonary fibrosis (IPF) is a fatal disease with incompletely understood aetiology and limited treatment options. Traditionally, IPF was believed to be mainly caused by repetitive injuries to the alveolar epithelium. Several recent lines of evidence, however, suggest that IPF equally involves an aberrant airway epithelial response, which contributes significantly to disease development and progression. In this review, based on recent clinical, high-resolution imaging, genetic, and single-cell RNA sequencing data, we summarize alterations in airway structure, function, and cell type composition in IPF. We furthermore give a comprehensive overview on the genetic and mechanistic evidence pointing towards an essential role of airway epithelial cells in IPF pathogenesis and describe potentially implicated aberrant epithelial signalling pathways and regulation mechanisms in this context. The collected evidence argues for the investigation of possible therapeutic avenues targeting these processes, which thus represent important future directions of research.

Keywords: basal cells; bronchial epithelium; airway epithelium; lung fibrosis; MUC5B; single cell RNA sequencing; epithelial populations; IPF

1. Introduction: An Emerging Role of the Airway Epithelium in IPF Aetiology

Idiopathic pulmonary fibrosis (IPF) is characterized by excessive deposition of extracellular matrix (ECM) within the alveolar compartment of the lung, leading to impairment of gas exchange, increased stiffness and, ultimately, loss of lung function. Despite approval of the two first effective antifibrotic drugs more than six years ago [1,2] and intensive sustained efforts in clinical drug development, IPF remains associated with high mortality rates. Current therapeutic options do not halt disease progression and prevalence of IPF appears to be rising worldwide [3].

The aetiology of IPF is incompletely understood. Traditionally, IPF was believed to be mainly caused by repetitive injuries to the alveolar epithelium. A growing body of evidence, however, based on genome-wide association studies (GWAS), molecular profiling of patient samples, high-resolution micro-CT imaging, and single cell RNA-Sequencing (scRNA-Seq), suggests that IPF equally involves an aberrant response of the bronchial and bronchiolar epithelium, which contributes significantly to disease development and progression. In this review, we summarize known alterations in airway structure, function, and cell type composition in IPF. We furthermore give a comprehensive overview on the genetic and mechanistic evidence pointing towards an essential role of the airway epithelium in IPF pathogenesis. Potential mechanisms of aberrant airway epithelial regeneration and, finally, possible therapeutic avenues targeting these processes are discussed.

2. General Airway Structure

The lung is structurally and functionally categorized into two regions, the conducting zone and the respiratory zone. The conducting airways consist of the trachea, the bronchi, and the conducting bronchioles, whereas the respiratory zone contains the areas of gas exchange, the terminal (respiratory) bronchioles and the alveoli (Figure 1A). The conducting airways are lined with a pseudostratified epithelium composed primarily of basal, club, goblet and ciliated cells, which play an essential role in the first-line defence against inhaled toxins, particles, and pathogens. Structure and cell type composition of the conducting airway epithelium gradually changes with increasing airway generations from a pseudostratified appearance with mainly ciliated cells next to secretory and basal cells over a simple columnar to a simple cuboidal epithelium, which harbours fewer ciliated cells and more secretory cells, particularly club cells. In contrast, the alveolar epithelium in the respiratory airways is lined with alveolar type 1 (AT1) and type 2 (AT2) cells, which, together with endothelial cells below and the interjacent basement membrane, make up the blood-air barrier for O_2/CO_2 exchange [4,5] (Figure 1A). Basal cells are established as the main human progenitor cells for all cell types in the pseudostratified epithelium lining the conducting airways [6] while AT2 cells give rise to AT1 cells in the alveoli [7]. More recently, in the murine lung, the bronchoalveolar duct junction at the transition between bronchioles and alveoli has been described to harbour additional multipotent stem cells, the so-called bronchoalveolar stem cells (BASCs). These can give rise to club and ciliated cells on the one hand and AT1 and AT2 cells on the other hand, in particular in response to injury [8]. Whether such a population exists in the human lung, however, is unclear to date.

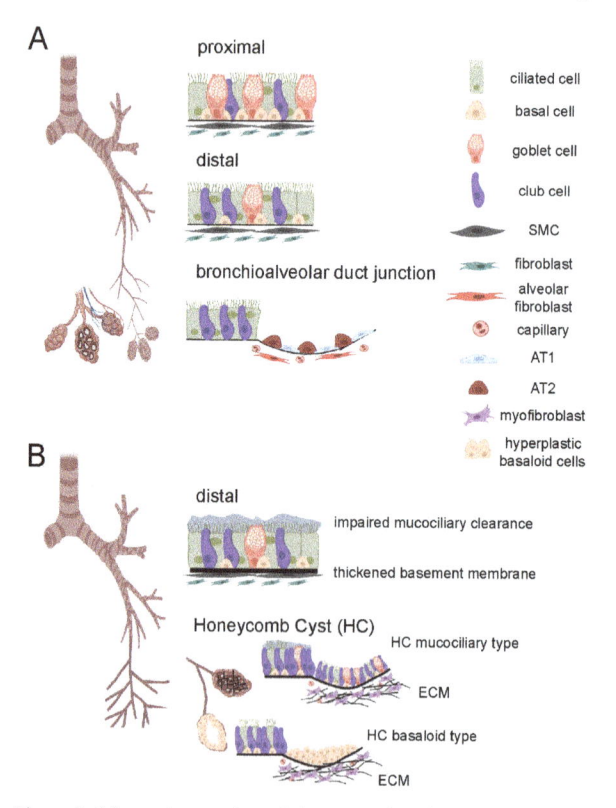

Figure 1. Schematic overview of airways in healthy lung and idiopathic pulmonary fibrosis (IPF). (**A**) Airways in the healthy lung, depicting normal cell type distribution in the proximal and distal

airways as well as in the bronchioalveolar duct junction. (**B**) Airways in the IPF lung, depicting dilated bronchioles, impaired mucociliary clearance and the thickened basement membrane in the distal airways, two types of honeycomb cysts (HC, mucociliary, basaloid), and accumulation of extracellular matrix (ECM) in the alveolar region. AT1, alveolar cell type 1; AT2, alveolar cell type II; ECM, extracellular matrix; SMC, smooth muscle cell. Figure was created with biorender.com.

3. Changes in Airway Morphology in IPF

3.1. Airway Dilation

In recent years, multiple evidence has emerged that strongly argues for considerable changes in airway morphology and physiology in IPF, which contribute to disease progression. For instance, clinical CT findings in IPF patients as well as experimental micro-CT imaging of explanted IPF lungs demonstrate that proximal and distal airways are dilated [9–12], which may explain why FEV_1/FVC ratios for IPF patients are higher than expected [13,14]. This is in agreement with aerosol-derived airway morphometry and capnographic measurements, which equally show increased airway volumes in IPF patients [15,16]. While changes in conducting airway volumes seem independent of disease severity [16], they appear to facilitate the distinction between stable and progressive disease, hence bear prognostic value [9]. The underlying mechanisms for airway dilation in IPF are not fully understood. Traditionally, traction bronchiectasis and bronchiolectasis, caused by increased collagen deposition and contraction of the peripheral fibrotic areas, have been thought to "pull open" the bronchi and bronchioles, respectively [17,18]. This concept is supported by the observation that the quantity of fibroblast foci correlates with traction bronchiectasis in high-resolution CT (HRCT) scans [19]. However, considering the comparatively distant location of fibrotic areas relative to the affected airways in IPF, and recent findings on emerging proliferative epithelial cell type populations in IPF (discussed below in Section 4), it has been suggested that the HRCT pattern of traction bronchiectasis in IPF is rather caused by bronchiolar proliferation than by mechanical traction alone [20].

3.2. Increased Airway Wall Thickness (AWT)

Recent studies report increases in airway wall thickness (AWT). Verleden et al. performed clinical CT and micro-CT of IPF explant and donor lungs, in combination with matched histological examinations. The authors observed that, due to increased AWT, more small airways are visible in CT scans of IPF specimens [21], a finding which was very recently confirmed by Ikezoe et al. [12] (Figure 2A). Additionally, a retrospective analysis of clinical chest CT images by Miller et al. suggested that lungs of IPF patients display significant increases in AWT, notably already in early disease stages [22]. Here, the authors performed so-called Pi10 measurements, which rely on a series of experimental determinations of total airway and luminal airway areas at different luminal perimeters. For each patient, the airway wall areas are calculated by subtraction of the luminal airway from the total airway area and the square root of these values is plotted against the perimeter. Regression analysis allows for the determination of the airway wall thickness of a hypothetical airway with an internal perimeter of 10 mm, the Pi10, a measure, which can then be directly compared between patients and disease cohorts. Interestingly, and explicitly mentioned by the authors as a limitation of their study, the way Pi10 is determined implies that changes in the internal luminal area, e.g., altered mucus layers, may have impacted the findings. As altered mucociliary clearance and increased MUC5B expression indeed are important features of IPF airways (discussed in Section 5), this raises the question whether Pi10 measurements are affected by increased levels of airway MUC5B, for example.

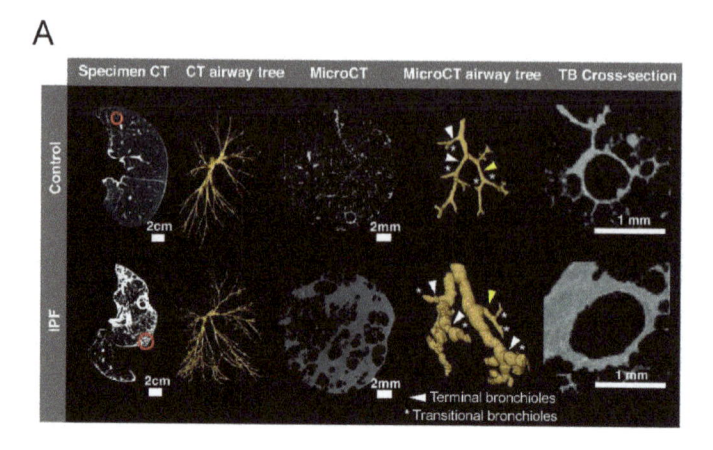

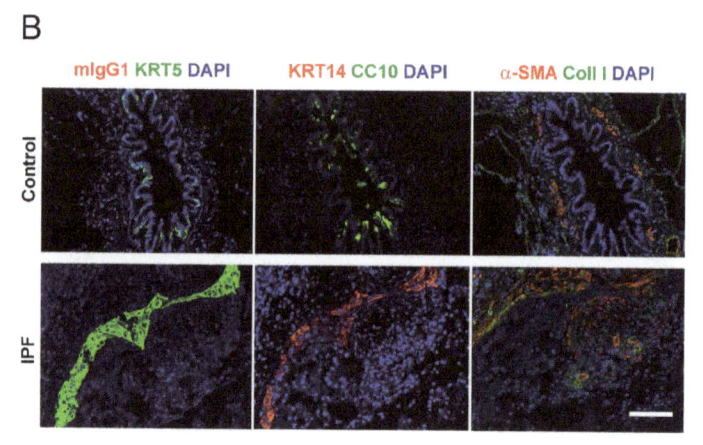

Figure 2. Airway epithelial abnormalities in IPF. (**A**) Comparison of airway features in control and IPF lungs as monitored by computed tomography (CT, adapted from Ikezoe et al. [12] with permission of the American Thoracic Society). Computed tomography (CT) scans from lungs of a control subject (upper row) and a case of IPF (lower row). The panels show from left to right: (1) Axial midslice multidetector computed tomography (MDCT) scans indicating where a random tissue sample was obtained for microCT (red circles); (2) reconstructed airway tree for the same scan from the lateral perspective; (3) midslice microCT scans of the tissue sample circled in red; (4) small airway tree segmentations obtained from the microCT scans visualized in three dimensions, identifying terminal bronchioles (TB, white arrowheads) and transitional bronchioles (asterisks); (5) representative cross-sectional image of the terminal bronchiole (TB) highlighted by the yellow arrowhead. This figure panel is adapted from Ikezoe et al. [12] with permission of the American Thoracic Society. Copyright © 2022 American Thoracic Society. All rights reserved. The American Journal of Respiratory and Critical Care Medicine is an official journal of the American Thoracic Society. Readers are encouraged to read the entire article for the correct context at https://www.atsjournals.org/doi/10.1164/rccm.202103-0585OC (last accessed 8 March 2022). The authors, editors, and The American Thoracic Society are not responsible for errors or omissions in adaptations. (**B**) Immunofluorescent stainings of serial lung sections of a representative control subject (upper row) and a case of IPF (lower row) with mouse isotype control antibody (mIgG1) and antibodies directed towards keratin 5 (KRT5), keratin 14 (KRT14), club cell-specific protein 10 (CC10), α-smooth muscle actin (α-SMA) as a marker for smooth muscle cells and myofibroblasts, and type I collagen (Coll I). Scale bar 100 µm.

3.3. Bronchiolar Abnormalities

Bronchiolar lesions involving abnormal bronchiolar proliferation and migration are typical features of IPF and represent regions of injury and active regeneration [23–25]. While the observed increase in bronchiolar proliferation has been interpreted to result in an increased number of bronchioles in IPF [14,23], recent evidence based on micro-CT imaging and histology suggests it more likely leads to dilation and distortion of the small airways [10–12,21] (Figure 2A). In contrast, the number of terminal bronchioles is even reduced in IPF [10,12,21]. Importantly, the latter observation was made in areas of mild fibrosis and the number of terminal bronchioles did not further decline in areas with more severe fibrosis, indicating that loss of terminal bronchioles is an early event in IPF [21]. In addition, it was demonstrated in two very recent independent studies that loss of terminal bronchioles correlates with honeycomb formation and that conducting airways directly lead into honeycomb cysts [10,12]. In agreement, early studies have demonstrated that peripheral cystic air spaces are ventilated, but represent physiological dead-space because they are not perfused [26]. This supports the concept that small airways are the origin of honeycomb cysts, abnormal peripheral airway spaces that will be discussed in more detail in the following.

3.4. Honeycomb Formation and Bronchiolization

In thoracic radiology, the term "honeycombing" refers to clustered cystic airspaces which typically are located in the subpleural region of the lung [27]. While clinical HRCT only detects honeycomb cysts with a diameter of about 1 mm and bigger, smaller honeycomb cysts are usually observed in histology [28]. Typical microscopic honeycomb cysts in IPF are small, subpleural, and localized in vicinity to fibrotic areas. Figure 2B (lower row, IPF) shows a collapsed honeycomb cyst characterized by $KRT5^+$ $KRT14^+$ $CC10^-$ cells in close proximity to fibroblast foci. On a cellular level, these honeycomb cysts are characterized by $p63^+$ $KRT5^+$ airway epithelial-like cell types replacing the normal alveolar epithelium, a process termed bronchiolization [29]. Some honeycomb cysts appear to be composed of stratified layers of hyperplastic $p63^+$ $KRT5^+$ $KRT14^+$ cells [25] (e.g., Figure 2B), while others display a pseudostratified mucociliary epithelium, containing ciliated, $p63^+$ $KRT5^+$ basal, and goblet cells expressing *MUC5B* as the main mucin component [25,30,31]. Whether honeycomb cysts derive from the small airways or from the alveolar epithelium as a result of ectopic bronchiolar differentiation is still controversially discussed. Considering the current knowledge about epithelial progenitor cells in the distal lung, bronchiolization could be a result of AT2 cells committing to an aberrant differentiation program [7], or derive from migrating basal cells [6] or BASCs [8,32] originating from the small airway or of bronchoalveolar duct junction, respectively. BASCs, at least in the mouse, can give rise to AT2 and club cells upon injury [32], but there is, to the best of our knowledge, no evidence that they can give rise to $p63^+$ $KRT5^+$ basal cell-like populations, which most frequently line bronchiolized areas in the IPF lung [23,25,30,33]. This, in contrast, has been unambiguously demonstrated for airway stem cells in distal lung regeneration after injury: After influenza infection of mice, for example, $p63^+$ cells emerge in the bronchioles and form extra-bronchiolar parenchymal clusters of $p63^+$ $Krt5^+$ basal cells, despite of little *TP63*-expression in normal murine bronchioles [34,35]. Lineage tracing experiments performed in independent laboratories have demonstrated that these cells derive from a rare population of $SOX2^+$ $p63^+$ $Krt5^{+/-}$ progenitor cells, but not from alveolar epithelial cells or BASCs [34,36,37]. Hence, studies in mouse models of lung injury have argued against an alveolar origin of bronchiolized areas in IPF and rather suggested that bronchiolization may originate from the airways.

However, it is important to mention in this context, that studies in human organoid culture systems have provided compelling evidence that, in contrast to mouse AT2 cells, human AT2 cells can give rise to $Krt5^+$ basal cells. This differentiation capacity into $Krt5^+$ basal-like cells was strictly dependent on adult human lung mesenchymal cells (AHLM) as feeder cells. The resulting $Krt5^+$ basal cells expressed canonical basal cell markers (*SOX2*,

TP63) in addition to genes typically associated with aberrant basal epithelial populations in IPF [38]. Interestingly, scRNA-Seq analysis of AHLM further revealed that during organoid culture mesenchymal subpopulations emerge that resemble such enriched in IPF lung tissue [38]. Collectively, these findings indicate that pathological mesenchymal cells in IPF generate a niche that is supportive of aberrant differentiation of human AT2 cells into KRT5$^+$ basal cells. Whether this is what happens in IPF, too, remains elusive, but it is plausible that aberrant basal cells in IPF derive from both airway and alveolar epithelial cells.

In summary, airways are drastically altered in IPF, with changes that (1) include macroscopic morphological changes visible by clinical and experimental CT imaging (airway dilation, increased airway wall thickness, honeycomb cysts), (2) manifest in physiological parameters like increased dead-space ventilation and higher FEV_1/FVC ratios, and (3) involve repopulation of the injured alveolar region with basal-like epithelial cells, which may be both airway- and alveolar-derived (Figures 1B and 2). On a cellular level, recent scRNA-Seq analyses of IPF lungs have provided even more weight to the importance of airway-like cells in IPF and will be discussed in the following chapter.

4. Recent Insights from Single Cell RNA-Sequencing (scRNA-Seq) Studies

Since the advent of single-cell RNA sequencing (scRNA-Seq), several studies in the past five years have revolutionized the concept of epithelial cell populations in IPF. In the earliest study, Xu et al. isolated Epcam$^+$/HTII-280$^+$ cells from peripheral regions of control and IPF lung and subjected that cell population to scRNA-Seq. Initially, they found that the yield of Epcam$^+$/HTII-280$^+$ cells, classically reflecting AT2 cells, drastically decreased in IPF lungs. However, more interestingly, in IPF, Epcam$^+$/HTII-280$^+$ subpopulations emerged which expressed transcripts typically associated with conducting airways and extracellular matrix-expressing cells, at the expense of genes typically associated with AT2 function [39]. Overall, the authors identified four subpopulations of Epcam$^+$/HTII-280$^+$ cells in IPF including (1) normal AT2 cells, (2) cells which expressed Goblet cell-specific markers, (3) cells which expressed basal cell-specific markers, and (4) indeterminate cells, which expressed multi-lineage markers including such for AT2, AT1, conducting airway cells and mesenchymal cells, and could thus not unambiguously be assigned to one cell type. Remarkably, the latter often co-expressed *SOX2* and *SOX9*, genes that typically define proximal airway progenitor and distal airway progenitor cells in the adult lung, respectively, thus indicating a loss of proximal-distal patterning in the IPF lung. Notably, SOX2$^+$/SOX9$^+$ progenitor cells otherwise only emerge in human lung development during the pseudoglandular stage in the distal epithelium but are already lost in the canalicular stage [40]. In addition, a more recent study suggests that surfactant processing is lost in these newly emerging epithelial cell populations, adding an important functional outcome of these changes [41]. Hence, in summary, in IPF a drastic loss of normal AT2 cells is paralleled by an increase of conducting airway characteristics in peripheral alveolar epithelial cells and an activation of aberrant differentiation programs or possibly reactivation of early lung developmental programs.

While the study above analyzed sorted Epcam$^+$/HTII-280$^+$ cells, isolated from a limited number of control and IPF lungs (n = 3), four more recent studies analyzed single cell suspensions from more specimens, without prior experimental enrichment for epithelial cells [42–45]. For visualization of the most important and consistent findings regarding epithelial cell populations in IPF/interstitial lung disease (ILD), we generated an integrative data set comprising all four studies (Figure 3A–C) using the Scanpy package (v1.8.0) [46]. To address potential batch effects, the integration was performed as described in Mayr et al. [43]. Briefly, the publicly available raw count matrices were re-processed data set wise with the same procedure. To mitigate effects of background mRNA contamination, the matrices were corrected by using the function adjustCounts() from the R library SoupX [47]. The expression matrices were normalized with scran's size factor based approach [48], log transformed via scanpy's pp.log1p() and finally scaled to unit variance and zero mean before concatenating them. A shared set of variable genes was selected by calculating gene variability patient-wise (flavor = "cell_ranger", n_top_genes = 4000) and excluding known cell cycle genes. The intersection of the variable genes across all data cohorts was used as input for principal component analysis (1311 genes). After subsetting to the epithelial cell populations, the BBKNN method [49] was used to generate a batch balanced data manifold (Munich: ILD = 7, controls n = 12; Chicago: ILD n = 9, controls n = 8; Nashville: ILD n = 20, controls n = 10; and New Haven: ILD n = 32, controls n = 22). Cell type identities from the original publication were retained and harmonized across studies. All four studies consistently confirmed the concept of an emerging diverse repertoire of epithelial cell types in ILD including IPF, most strikingly an increase in cells with features of conducting airways at the expense of classical alveolar epithelial cells (Figure 3D).

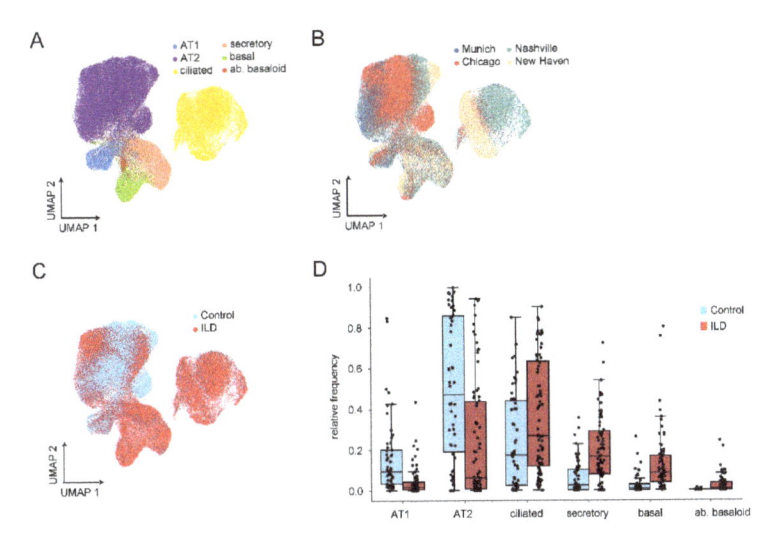

Figure 3. Single cell RNA-Sequencing has revealed drastic changes in epithelial cell populations in ILD. (**A**) Uniform Manifold Approximation and Projection (UMAP)-based dimension reduction of single cell transcriptomic data to delineate epithelial cell types, labelled by cell type. (**B**) Same UMAP visualization labelled by ILD cohort. Data used for visualization was derived from in total four datasets [42–45] of control and interstitial lung disease (ILD) samples: New Haven [45], Nashville [44], Chicago [42], and Munich [43]. (**C**) Same UMAP visualization labelled by disease. (**D**) Relative frequencies of epithelial cell populations demonstrate a consistent increase in conducting airway cell populations in ILD at the expense of alveolar type 1 (AT1) and 2 (AT2) cells. ab., aberrant.

In more detail, up to 10 distinct clusters of epithelial cells were defined in these studies. While all identified most classical epithelial cell types, i.e., AT1, AT2, basal, ciliated, and secretory cells by similar expression signatures (Figure 4), there are some differences in sub-categorization of the described cell type clusters. For instance, while Habermann et al. [44] distinguished between ciliated cells and differentiating ciliated cells, such a distinction was not made in the other studies [42,45]. Furthermore, categorization of secretory cells differs significantly between these reports. Reyfman et al. categorized club cells based on *SCGB1A1* (also termed *CC10* or *CCSP*) expression and did not report goblet cells but *MUC5B*-expressing cells within their cluster of club cells [42]. Adams et al. distinguished between club and goblet cells, but in their report *SCGB1A1* expression is a characteristic of both cell types and club and goblet cells are differentiated from each other by *SCGB3A2* and *MUC5B* expression, respectively [45]. Published and unpublished results from our lab have shown that *SCGB1A1* is expressed by a subpopulation of MUC5AC$^+$ goblet cells, too [50]; so indeed, *SCGB1A1* should rather be considered a more general marker for secretory cells than specifically for club cells. Possibly reflecting similar considerations, Habermann et al. refrained from the attempt to distinguish between club and goblet cells and instead defined several secretory cell type clusters based on expression of *SCGB1A1*, *SCGB3A2*, and *MUC5B* and combinations thereof. Collectively, these studies show that, at least based on single cell transcript analysis, there is a continuum of secretory cells with overlapping gene expression patterns, which are not easily sorted into club and goblet cells without information on cell shape, spatial distribution within the bronchial tree, and protein expression patterns. Therefore, here, we also refer to those as secretory cells, without further distinction into goblet and club cells (Figures 4 and 5). Independent of secretory cell subcategorization, all studies consistently demonstrate an increase in secretory cells including MUC5B$^+$ cells. This was equally observed in an independent scRNA-Seq study where the authors refer to SCGBB1A1$^+$ MUC5B$^+$ cells as club cells, which, as explained above, may not be entirely accurate due to the ambiguity of SCGBB1A1 as a marker in that context. Still, also this study clearly demonstrates an increase of secretory cells in IPF relative to the healthy lung [51]. Furthermore, beyond quantitative alterations in epithelial cell populations, all IPF/ILD airway subpopulations displayed many significantly upregulated genes in their expression signatures when compared to their healthy counterparts (Figure 5B).

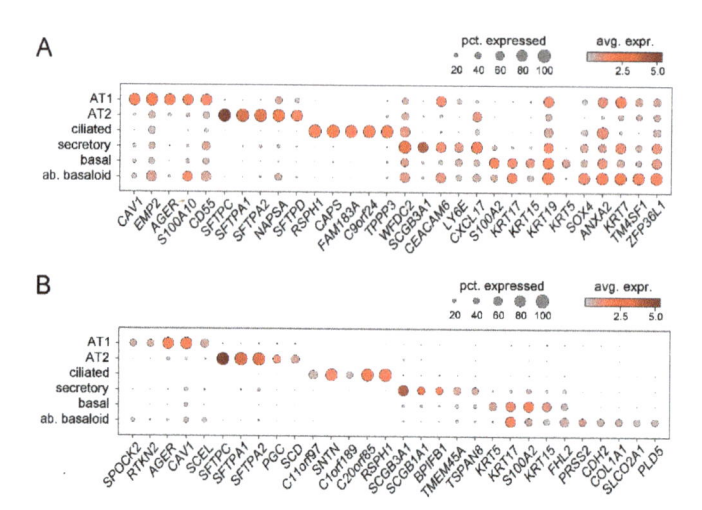

Figure 4. Cell type-specific markers for epithelial cell populations in ILD derived from scRNA-Seq data. Using the data set described in Figure 3, the top 5 specific markers for the described epithelial populations are plotted, (**A**) ranked by adjusted *p*-value or (**B**) ranked by log fold changes of relevant cell type vs. all other epithelial cell types. pct., percentage; avg. expr., average expression; ab., aberrant.

Basal cells appear to be particularly important in the context of IPF aetiology and progression for several reasons. For instance, a basal cell signature detected in the bronchioalveolar lavage transcriptome in IPF patients was predictive of mortality, strongly suggesting that basal cells play a central role in IPF progression [31]. Basal cell numbers are drastically increased in ILD (Figure 3D) and novel basal cell subpopulations and characteristics have already been demonstrated before the scRNA-Seq era. In 2015, Jonsdottir et al. reported that p63$^+$ KRT14$^+$ cells overlay fibroblastic foci in IPF (see also Figure 2B) and displayed characteristics of epithelial-to-mesenchymal transition (EMT) [52]. Shortly after, using immunofluorescence studies, Smirnova et al. quantified KRT5$^+$ and KRT14$^+$ basal cell population in healthy and IPF lungs and equally observed a drastic increase of basal cell populations in the distal IPF lung and proposed KRT14$^+$ as a marker for an aberrantly differentiating progenitor cell pool [25]. The above-mentioned scRNA-Seq studies confirm these findings, showing that *KRT14* is overexpressed in basal cells in ILD, and also a marker of aberrant basaloid cells, which will be described below [42,44,45].

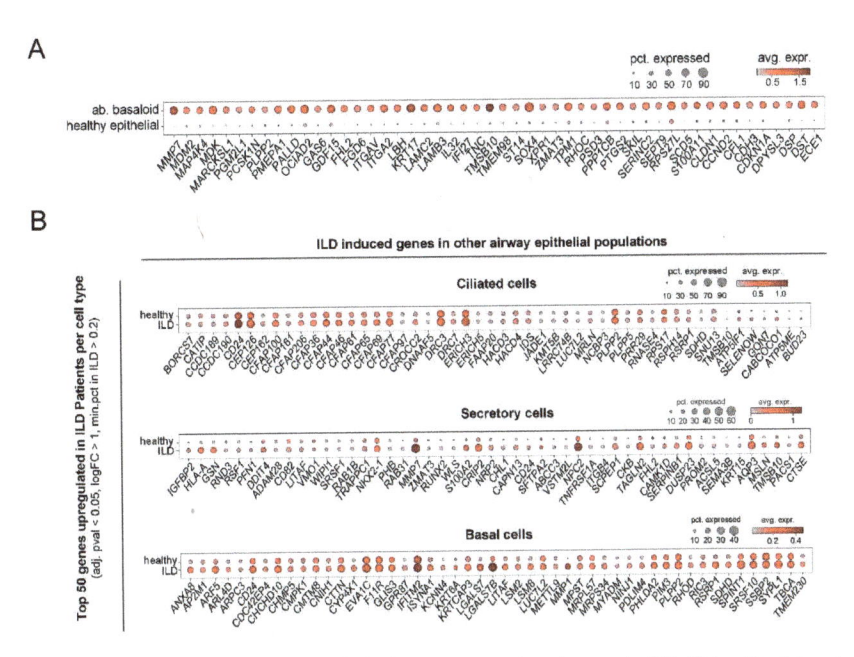

Figure 5. Epithelial cell populations show distinct expression changes in ILD. Using the data set described in Figure 3, differential gene expression analysis was performed with diffxpy (https://github.com/theislab/diffxpy, last accessed 22 December 2021) while accounting for number of transcripts per cell and patient cohort. The top 50 deregulated genes in specific subpopulations of epithelial cells are given, ranked by log2 fold change. (**A**) Top 50 genes induced in aberrant basaloid cells relative to gene expression of all other healthy epithelial cell types. (**B**) Top 50 genes increased in ILD in other airway epithelial cell populations. pct., percentage; avg. expr., average expression; ab., aberrant.

A recent scRNA-Seq study focussed on changes in basal cell plasticity in IPF and defined basal cell heterogeneity in the normal and IPF lung in greater detail [53]. According to this study, basal cells in the healthy lung can be subdivided in at least four subpopulations, namely classical multipotent basal cells (MPB), proliferating basal cells (PB), secretory-primed basal cells (SPB), and activated basal cells (AB). Based on scRNA-Seq data, surface marker screening, as well as bronchosphere assays, the authors established CD66 as a surface marker for SPBs and demonstrated an increase of CD66$^+$ KRT5$^+$ SPBs in IPF. With the importance of MUC5B and thus secretory airway cells in disease aetiology, these observations put forward modulation of basal cell priming as a novel therapeutic strategy in IPF [53].

Interestingly, Habermann et al. as well as Adams et al. identified a novel epithelial cell population with features of basal cells, which exclusively emerged in pulmonary fibrosis, namely KRT5$^-$/KRT17$^+$ epithelial cells [44], or aberrant basaloid cells [45]. These cells are comparably rare (Figure 3D) and characterized by expression of basal cell markers like *TP63*, *KRT17*, *LAMB3*, and *LAMC2* (but not *KRT5*, see Figure 4), in combination with mesenchymal markers like *COL1A1*, *VIM*, *TNC*, and *FN1*, and markers of senescence like *CDKN1A* (Figure 5A) [44,45]. Expression of *SOX9* and other markers of a distal differentiation program suggested that these cells also display characteristics of alveolar epithelial cells. Furthermore, these cells also showed the highest expression levels of *MMP7*, encoding matrix metallopeptidase 7, the probably best-validated peripheral blood biomarker for IPF (Figure 5A). Using RNA in situ hybridization, KRT17$^+$/COL1A1$^+$ basaloid cells were shown to cover fibrotic foci in IPF lungs but were not detected in non-fibrotic controls [44]. Given that these cells display characteristics of conducting and respiratory airways, the cellular origin is not clear. ScRNA-Seq-based pseudo-time analysis has raised the possibility that both transitional AT2 and *SCGB3A2*-expressing secretory cells may act as precursors for aberrant basaloid cells [43,44], a hypothesis which still requires experimental validation. Notably, studies in mouse models of lung fibrosis and injury have identified similar converging differentiation pathways, namely from club cells on the one hand and AT2 cells on the other to a population called Krt8$^+$ alveolar differentiation intermediate (ADI) cells. This cell population is highly similar to the aberrant basaloid cells in IPF [54], but of transient character in bleomycin-induced lung fibrosis: Krt8$^+$ ADI cells peak in the fibrotic phase and gradually disappear during resolution of fibrosis. Importantly, lineage tracing using Sox2- and Sftpc-Cre drivers has confirmed the dual, conducting airway and alveolar, origin of Krt8$^+$ ADI cells. Collectively, this supports a model where an intermediate cell type, transiently emerging during a normal repair process, accumulates and persists in IPF.

In summary, scRNA-Seq studies have consistently demonstrated drastic changes in epithelial subpopulations in ILD, which strongly argue for an essential role of airway epithelial cells in disease development and progression. These include: (1) A dramatic decrease of normal alveolar cell types of the respiratory zone and their replacement by diverse conducting airway cell populations (Figure 3D). (2) The emergence of a novel ILD-specific cell type reminiscent of an intermediate cell involved in normal alveolar repair, which probably derives from both proximal and distal precursors and persists in lung fibrosis (Figures 3D and 4). (3) Considerable changes in overall gene expression patterns in epithelial cell types (Figure 5).

5. Changes in Airway Function
5.1. Mucociliary Clearance

The discovery of the *MUC5B* polymorphism (see below, Section 6) has drawn a lot of attention to dysregulated mucociliary clearance as a major aetiological mechanism in IPF [29]. IPF is characterized by increased expression of *MUC5B* in the distal airways and honeycomb cysts. Increased expression is often driven by the minor allele (T) of the risk single nucleotide polymorphism (SNP) rs35705950, which is overrepresented in IPF patients. Consequently, the mucin MUC5B accumulates in airways of the distal lung where even mucous plugs can be observed within microscopic honeycomb cysts [55]. From other lung diseases, most prominently cystic fibrosis, it is very well known that overproduction of mucus impairs mucociliary clearance, leads to accumulation of particles and pathogens in the airways and increases the risk for chronic injury and inflammation. Indicating that this likely applies to lung fibrosis as well, *MUC5B* overexpression in distal airways has been shown to significantly impair mucociliary clearance and aggravate lung fibrosis in the mouse model of bleomycin-induced lung injury [56]. Importantly, in the same model, mucolytic treatment led to clearance of inflammatory cells from the lungs and counteracted the production of fibrillar collagen, providing proof-of-concept that restoring impaired mucociliary clearance may be beneficial in prevention and treatment of pulmonary fibrosis [56].

A potential key role of impaired mucociliary clearance for lung fibrogenesis is further emphasized by an independent study, where the issue of mucociliary clearance was approached from a very different angle. The E3 ubiquitin-protein ligase NEDD4-2 targets the epithelial Na$^+$ channel (ENaC, encoded by *SCNN1A*) for intracellular degradation and thus plays a key role in limiting the levels of active ENaC at the cell surface. ENaC in turn is a critical regulator of epithelial surface hydration and consequently affects mucus properties. Overexpression of *SCNN1A* and activation of ENaC increases transepithelial transport of salt and water leading to dehydration of the apical epithelial mucous layer and thus impaired mucociliary clearance [57]. NEDD4-2 levels are decreased in IPF airways.

With NEDD4-2 representing an antagonist of ENaC, conditional deletion of NEDD4-2 from airway epithelial cells in mice, as expected, increased ENaC activity and significantly impaired mucociliary clearance. A striking long-term consequence of this NEDD4-2 deficiency in murine airways, however, was the development of patchy lung fibrosis, bronchiolar remodelling, and increased MUC5B production in the peripheral airways, all features strongly reminiscent of IPF and actually reflecting IPF pathology more accurately than the most commonly used bleomycin-induced mouse model of lung fibrosis [58]. Collectively, these findings strongly indicate that mucociliary dysfunction is a major aetiological factor in IPF and, even though the minor risk allele within the *MUC5B* promoter will probably remain the most important cause, may have multiple origins including, e.g., dysregulation of epithelial surface hydration properties by NEDD4-2/ENaC.

5.2. Epithelial Barrier Dysfunction in IPF Pathogenesis

The bronchial epithelial barrier plays an important role in protecting the airways against environmental insults not only via mucociliary clearance and production of antimicrobial substances to eliminate inhaled pathogens, but also by tight junctions that maintain the cell–cell contact and regulate paracellular permeability [59]. Even if this has not been comprehensively assessed, some reports suggest that epithelial barrier function is altered during IPF pathogenesis. Zou et al., for instance, have demonstrated by immunohistochemistry (IHC) stainings for several tight junction proteins, that specifically levels of claudin-2 were elevated in IPF bronchiolar regions [60]. Others have found that levels of protein kinase D (PKD), a negative regulator of airway barrier integrity [61], were increased in IPF bronchiolar epithelium relative to normal lung tissue sections [62].

5.3. Other Changes in Airway Function

In a study designed to investigate the pathogenesis of cough in IPF, authors found increased levels of nerve growth factor and brain-derived neurotrophic factor in induced sputa of IPF patients compared to healthy control subjects [63]. These results indicated functional upregulation of sensory neurons in the proximal airways of IPF lungs.

6. Genetic Evidence Indicating Involvement of Bronchial Epithelium in IPF

IPF is a multifactorial disease where the interplay between environmental exposure and genetic susceptibility plays a central role in disease pathogenesis. Genome-wide association studies (GWAS) on large cohorts of various ethnical backgrounds have provided interesting insights into genetic susceptibility for IPF development and have linked specific genetic variants to poorer outcomes in sporadic IPF and familial pulmonary fibrosis [64]. In this context, single nucleotide polymorphisms (SNPs) conferring a higher risk for IPF were discovered in several genes reported to be expressed in airway epithelial cells, strongly suggesting a role for bronchial and bronchiolar epithelial cells in IPF aetiology [65,66]. These include mucin-5B (*MUC5B*), toll interactive protein (*TOLLIP*), desmoplakin (*DSP*), family with sequence similarity 13 member A (*FAM13A*), and A kinase anchor protein 13 (*AKAP13*). For all but *TOLLIP*, which seems comparably little expressed in airway epithelial cells, scRNA-Seq data confirms variable expression of these genes in bronchial, bronchiolar, and aberrant basaloid cells (Figure 6). While *MUC5B* and *FAM13A* are particularly expressed by secretory cells and ciliated cells, respectively, *DSP* is expressed by all bronchial and bronchiolar epithelial cell types including aberrant basaloid cells, where it is one of the top overexpressed genes relative to all other healthy epithelial cell types (Figure 5A). In contrast, except for *AKAP13*, expression of which is enriched in AT2 and aberrant basaloid cells, alveolar epithelial cells show relatively little expression of these genes (Figure 6).

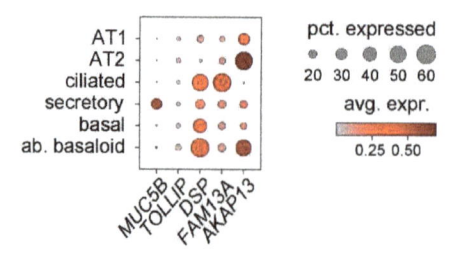

Figure 6. Expression of selected risk factor genes in epithelial cell populations. Using the data set described in Figure 3, expression of selected genes harbouring IPF risk-associated SNPs is given. Selection was based on previous reports on their expression in airway epithelium (see text for more details). pct., percentage; avg. expr., average expression; ab., aberrant.

6.1. MUC5B

A common promoter SNP in the airway gene *MUC5B* on chromosome 11, rs35705950, is the strongest risk factor for IPF, accounting for 30–35% of the overall risk to develop IPF [29,55]. *MUC5B* encodes mucin-5B, a mucin protein predominantly expressed in serous cells of submucosal glands in healthy lungs, and normally little expressed in airway surface epithelium [67]. In contrast, in IPF lungs, *MUC5B* is overexpressed in secretory cells within honeycomb cysts as well as in bronchioalveolar regions [29,30,39]. A series of elegant in vivo work has demonstrated that overexpression of *MUC5B*, both in proximal and distal airways, aggravates bleomycin-induced lung fibrosis in mice, while MUC5B-deficient mice are protected from the development of lung fibrosis. Interestingly, increased mortality was particularly observed when *MUC5B* was overexpressed in the distal murine airways [56].

6.2. TOLLIP

The gene *TOLLIP* encodes a ubiquitous protein with essential functions in the innate immune response, epithelial survival, defence against pathogens and further biological processes [68,69]. The *TOLLIP* gene is located adjacent to *MUC5B* and evidence regarding linkage disequilibrium between the *MUC5B* SNP rs35705950 and *TOLLIP* SNPs suggests that *TOLLIP* and *MUC5B* SNPs may not be passed on independently [68]. Three common variants within the *TOLLIP* locus (rs111521887, rs5743894, rs574389) have been shown to associate with higher susceptibility for IPF [66]. The minor alleles for all *TOLLIP* SNPs result in reduced expression by 20–50%, with rs111521887 and rs5743894, which are in high linkage disequilibrium, having stronger effects on expression than rs5743890 [66]. Interestingly, even though all result in reduced expression, the clinical effects of the rs111521887 and rs5743894 minor alleles are opposite to the rs5743890 minor allele: Individuals who carry the minor allele for rs111521887 and rs5743894 are more susceptible to developing IPF, while the minor allele rs5743890 is associated with less susceptibility. However, despite this initial protective effect, mortality in IPF patients with this variant is actually increased [66,68]. In the integrative scRNA-Seq data set that we examined, *TOLLIP* overall was comparably little detected (Figure 6). However, a recent study focusing on *TOLLIP* expression in the lung has demonstrated *TOLLIP* expression in AT2 cells, basal cells, and aberrant basaloid cells, but at the same time reported a global downregulation of *TOLLIP* expression in the IPF lung [70].

6.3. DSP

Linking intermediate filaments to the plasma membrane, desmoplakin, encoded by *DSP*, is a critical intracellular component of desmosomes, cell–cell adhesive junctions, which are critical for tissue integrity [71]. In the lung, *DSP* is primarily expressed in bronchi and bronchioles, with comparably little expression in alveoli [72]. The latter is also reflected by the scRNA-Seq data shown here (Figure 6). GWAS have linked at least two genetic variations in *DSP* with risk for IPF development, namely the minor alleles of rs2076295 and rs2744371 [65,72]. Among those, the minor allele of the intronic SNP rs2076295 (intron 5) is established as the strongest causal factor and is associated with an increased risk for IPF development, while the minor allele of rs2744371 confers a protective effect against IPF onset. Paradoxically, while *DSP* expression is increased in IPF lungs, the risk allele rs2076295 correlates with lower *DSP* expression. Some well-designed in vitro experiments using CRISPR/Cas9 gene editing in human bronchial epithelial cells have shown that deletion or disruption of the DNA region spanning rs2076295 as well as introduction of the minor allele (G) led to decreased expression of *DSP*, in agreement with an enhancer function of this region in intron 5 [73]. Decreased *DSP* expression in turn resulted in reduced barrier integrity, enhanced cell migration, and increased expression of markers for EMT and of ECM genes [73].

6.4. FAM13A

FAM13A encodes a so far uncharacterized protein with largely unknown function. Amino acid sequence homology suggests that FAM13A contains a Ras homologous (Rho) GTPase-activating protein (GAP) domain and hence a function in Rho GTPase signalling [74]. In the lung, *FAM13A* is primarily expressed in bronchial epithelial cells, but also by AT2 cells, and macrophages [75,76]. GWAS have identified a genetic risk variant within this gene, intronic rs2609255, that increases susceptibility for COPD and IPF with opposite risk alleles [65,77]. For IPF, this risk variant appears not to be associated with expression changes on transcript level [65]. Owing to its association with COPD and IPF disease risk, experimental studies have been performed in both disease contexts. These studies suggest that, on the one hand, FAM13A, protein levels of which are increased in COPD, may protect from cigarette smoke-induced disruption of airway integrity and neutrophilia [75], but at the same time promote β-catenin degradation, thus inhibit β-catenin signalling and associated repair processes, and increase susceptibility to emphysema [76]. On the other hand, FAM13A deficiency has been reported to exacerbate bleomycin-induced lung fibrosis in the mouse, possibly via induction of EMT-related gene expression [78]. Overall, FAM13A, even though its exact function remains unclear, appears to play an important role in airway epithelial barrier integrity and repair.

6.5. AKAP13

AKAP13, encoding A kinase anchor protein 13, is another gene with a genetic variant, rs62025270, conferring increased risk for development of IPF [79], expression of which is largely confined to the airway epithelium [80]. *AKAP13* is overexpressed in IPF where it localizes to aberrant epithelial regions [79] and functions as a Rho guanine nucleotide exchange factor regulating activation of RhoA [81], known for its involvement in profibrotic pathways.

7. Implicated Mechanisms

The precise pathogenesis of IPF is still not entirely understood, but the current knowledge on environmental and genetic risk factors strongly suggests epithelial injury-triggered reactivation of developmental pathways which, ultimately, leads to aberrant repair and regeneration resulting in drastic changes in lung structure and function. Therefore, in the following we will recapitulate these processes with a focus on what is known for the contributions of the bronchial and bronchiolar epithelium.

7.1. Types of Epithelial Injury

The airway epithelium represents the first line defence against inhaled particles, pathogens, and toxicants. Environmental and occupational triggers like cigarette smoke, wood dust, metal dust, pesticides, and herpesvirus infection are established risk factors for IPF [82,83]. Additionally, inhalation of traffic-related air pollutants has been linked to increased incidence of IPF [84]. Furthermore, gastroesophageal reflux (GER) is an overrepresented comorbidity of IPF, suggesting that microaspiration of stomach acids increases risk for IPF. Moreover, treatment of GER in IPF patients decelerates IPF disease progression and improves survival, indicating that GER also influences disease progression [82,83].

7.2. Epithelial Apoptosis

Apoptosis of alveolar epithelial cells is a well-established phenomenon in IPF and clearly reflected by the above discussed scRNA-Seq data showing a drastic decrease in normal alveolar type I and II cells in IPF relative to control lung tissue (Figure 3D). Immunofluorescent stainings of pro- and anti-apoptotic proteins in combination with terminal deoxynucleotide transferase-mediated deoxyuridine triphosphate-biotin nick end-labeling (TUNEL) stainings for DNA strand breaks have revealed that bronchiolar epithelial cells, hyperplastic epithelial cells and epithelial cells lining honeycomb cysts in the lungs of IPF patients show distinct signs of ongoing apoptosis [85–88]. While such cells in the past have often been referred to as "hyperplastic AT2 cells" [88], our recently gained more detailed understanding of the arising epithelial subpopulations in IPF, thanks to the above-described scRNA-Seq studies, strongly suggests that these cells also include epithelial cells of a bronchiolar origin like activated hyperplastic basal cells. Moreover, strengthening a potential role of apoptotic SCGBB1A1$^+$ secretory cells in IPF, a recent report has demonstrated that ablation of programmed cell death 5 (*PDCD5*) expression in these secretory cells, but not in AT2 cells protects from experimental lung fibrosis [89].

7.3. Endoplasmic Reticulum (ER) Stress as Trigger for Epithelial Apoptosis

ER stress is a well-established trigger of alveolar epithelial apoptosis in IPF [85,90], but has received less attention for bronchial or bronchiolar epithelial cells. Many types of epithelial injury linked to an increased IPF risk, as, e.g., herpesvirus infection, cigarette smoke, and particulate matter, have been shown to cause ER stress and induce the unfolded protein response (UPR), also in cultured bronchial epithelial cells [90–92]. An elegant recent study has provided an intriguing link between the *MUC5B* promoter polymorphism (see Section 6) and ER stress in secretory airway epithelial cells. Chen et al. not only demonstrated that central components of the UPR induced *MUC5B* expression in secretory airway epithelial cells in pulmonary fibrosis, but also were able to show that this induction is dependent on sequences within the promoter variant rs35705950 region which harbours the IPF risk variant. Notably, in a luciferase reporter assay, the minor risk allele T alone increased expression of *MUC5B* by almost two-fold. This study provides another piece of evidence that ER stress and induction of the UPR in bronchiolar cells likely also contributes to expression of *MUC5B*, impaired mucociliary clearance, and the development of IPF [93].

7.4. Ageing and Epithelial Senescence

IPF predominates in the elderly and is characterized by increased senescence in many cell types, presumably because of replicative exhaustion and/or repetitive injuries to the epithelium [94]. It is by now well established that epithelial cells covering fibroblast foci are positive for senescence-associated β-galactosidase activity, nuclear p16 and p21 [95–99]. In agreement, recent scRNA-Seq-based studies have demonstrated that the above-described basaloid cells as well as hyperplastic basal cell population in bronchiolized regions express genes related to growth arrest and senescence [44,45,100]. This has also been observed for the transient population of Krt8$^+$ ADI cells in mouse models of lung injury [54]. Collectively, these observations put forward an attractive hypothesis where a specific population of epithelial cells, normally committed to repair an injury of the lung mucosa followed by clearance, persists "locked in repair" in IPF [101]. Notably, senescent epithelial cells from fibrotic tissue have been shown to secrete proinflammatory and profibrotic molecules as components of their senescence-associated secretory phenotype (SASP) [97], suggesting that they may be a direct driver of disease pathogenesis.

7.5. Reactivation of Developmental Pathways

Reactivation of molecular signalling pathways such as the transforming growth factor-β (TGF-β), WNT, sonic hedgehog (SHH), and Notch pathways are critical players during the developmental stages of lung, remain largely inactive in the postnatal lung except for the maintenance of progenitor cell niches, but can become aberrantly reactivated during an injury repair response and then trigger chronic disease [102]. In the following, the induction and regulation of these developmental pathways during IPF pathogenesis is discussed with a focus in bronchial and bronchiolar epithelial cells.

7.5.1. Transforming Growth Factor-β (TGF-β) Signalling

All three TGF-β isoforms (β1, β2, β3), their receptors TGF-β receptors (TGFBR) I, II, and III, and their signalling mediators SMAD-2, -3, -4, -5, -6 and -7 are involved in embryonic lung development where they regulate branching morphogenesis and alveolarization [102]. TGF-β ligands act by binding to their cognate receptors on target cells, where they trigger intracellular signalling pathways including the canonical SMAD-mediated pathway but also non-canonical signalling pathways [103].

TGF-β is synthesized as an inactive precursor homodimer with N-terminal prodomains, which, after cleavage by the intracellular protease furin, remain non-covalently bound to the TGF-β homodimer as latency-associated peptide (LAP), collectively forming the small latent complex (SLC). Only if this complex is bound to the latent TGF-β-binding protein (LTBP), it will be secreted to the extracellular matrix as a complex called large latent complex (LLC) [104]. Hence, TGF-β is always secreted in a latent form and requires activation in situ by additional triggers.

Out of the three isoforms, TGF-β1 plays a well-recognized central role in IPF pathogenesis [105–107]. Activation of latent TGF-β1 implies the release of active TGF-β1 ligands from the ECM by proteolysis or deformation of their LAP portion. Many potential mechanisms have been observed in vitro, but for many the physiological relevance remains unclear. In vivo activation has been clearly shown for several αv integrins in the context of fibrosis, e.g., αvβ1, αvβ3, αvβ5, and αvβ6 [108]. Even though the underlying mechanisms are not fully understood, it appears that cells carrying these integrins can exert a pulling force on the LLC which "unwraps" the LAP and releases active TGF-β1 from the ECM. Other reasonably well-established activators are thrombospondin-1 (TSP1), pregnancy specific glycoproteins, and tenascin X. Additionally, activation by unspecific physico- or biochemical factors like low pH and reactive oxygen species has been described, which may also be physiologically relevant. Finally, proteolytic activation has been described for a variety of proteases, including, e.g., several matrix metalloproteinases (MMPs), calpain, plasmin, kallikrein, and cathepsin D. Interestingly, while deficiency of integrin subunits like αv, β6, and β8 in mice phenocopies the TGF-β1 knockout mouse, this has not been observed for any protease-deficient mouse so far, indicating considerable redundancy in proteolytic activation of TGF-β1 in vivo [108–110].

Bronchial epithelial cells potentially may contribute to TGF-β1-mediated mechanisms in IPF by at least three mechanisms. First, bronchial and bronchiolar epithelial cells express TGF-β1 [111,112], implying that the underlying ECM likely harbours latent TGF-β1. Second, bronchial epithelial express many of the suggested activating factors in fibrosis: Airway epithelial cells express both αvβ6 and αvβ8 integrin heterodimers, and expression of αvβ6 is dramatically increased after injury [113]. Notably, the *ITGAV* transcript for the αv integrin monomer is clearly enriched in aberrant basaloid cells relative to all other healthy epithelial cell types (Figure 5A). Second, airway and aberrant basaloid epithelial cells also have been shown to express activators of latent TGF-β1 in IPF, including MMP-8 [114], MMP-3, MMP-13, MMP14, calpain, and cathepsin D in IPF [44,45] (ipfcellatlas.com), all representing proteases previously proposed to activate latent TGF-β1 [108]. ScRNA-Seq data also demonstrates expression of the thrombospondin 1 precursor by bronchial epithelial cells [44,45] (ipfcellatlas.com). Third, bronchial epithelial cells themselves are reactive to TGF-β1 and have been shown to undergo partial epithelial-to-mesenchymal transition (pEMT) in response to TGF-β1 [115,116]. Whether EMT contributes to the myofibroblast population in IPF is controversially discussed, as conflicting results have been reported in in vivo models of pulmonary fibrosis—so far neither lineage-tracing experiments nor scRNA-Seq data have provided unambiguous evidence for a complete EMT as a source for myofibroblasts in the lung [117,118]. However, the resulting cell phenotype after pEMT is partly reminiscent of the aberrant basal-like cell phenotype observed in IPF—following pEMT, human bronchiolar epithelial cells lose epithelial morphology and polarity and upregulate mesenchymal markers like type I collagen and fibronectin. On the other hand, downregulation of expression of typical epithelial markers such as E-cadherin and up-regulation of vimentin is not evident in the scRNA-Seq data sets published so far [44,45] (ipfcellatlas.com). These discrepancies may reflect the crosstalk between variously activated profibrotic pathways and the complex cellular and ECM environment in end-stage IPF, parameters frequently not considered in studies of EMT. Clearly, further work is warranted to elucidate the role of TGF-β1 in the emergence of aberrant basaloid cells, and how this process relates to pEMT.

7.5.2. WNT Signalling Pathway

Wingless/integrase-1 (WNT) signalling pathways are fundamentally important for tissue morphogenesis including all stages of lung development [119]. The WNT ligand family comprises 19 human members which are characterized by strictly controlled spatiotemporal expression in various organs during development and tissue homeostasis and associated with a constantly growing number of human diseases by upregulation, genetic polymorphisms and mutations [120]. It is well-established that the WNT signalling pathway is reactivated in IPF [119,121] and expression of WNT ligands (WNT1, WNT3a), intracellular downstream inducers (β-catenin, GSK-3β), as well as extracellular inhibitors of canonical WNT signalling (Dickkopf proteins DKK1, DKK4 and the interacting transmembrane receptor Kremen 1) has been demonstrated in bronchial and bronchiolar epithelium in IPF [122,123]. Studies in various models of lung injury have put forward WNT signalling as a critical component for stem cell maintenance, lung regeneration, and repair [119]. WNT signalling is activated during repair after proximal lung injury and dynamically regulates submucosal gland progenitor maintenance, proliferation, and differentiation to other airway epithelial cell types [124–128]. Furthermore, in mice, expression of Wnt7b by basal cells in the proximal airways generates their own stem cell niche via induction of fibroblast growth factor 10 (Fgf10) in adjacent smooth muscle cells [129]. Airway injury induces Wnt7b in the more distal airways, generating new Fgf10-expressing mesenchymal cells and allowing for recruitment of basal cells and/or differentiation of lineage-negative progenitors into the basal progenitor cell lineage [129,130]. Collectively, these studies imply an important role of WNT signalling in aberrant bronchial and bronchiolar repair in IPF.

7.5.3. Sonic Hedgehog Signalling (SHH) Pathway

During lung development, sonic hedgehog (SHH) is expressed in the respiratory epithelium in a gradient with higher levels in the branching tips, presumably providing polarization during branching morphogenesis in the embryonic and pseudoglandular stage. Furthermore, SHH is essential for the coordination of epithelial-mesenchymal compartment growth, also during the alveolarization phase [131,132]. Bolaños et al. systematically assessed expression of SHH signalling pathway components in control lung tissue and IPF and found that expression of all SHH signalling components was induced or drastically increased in IPF. They observed expression of the ligand SHH exclusively in bronchial, bronchiolar, and alveolar epithelial cells, but expression of the receptors transmembrane receptor Patched-1 and the G-protein coupled receptor Smoothened mainly in fibroblasts and inflammatory cells. While the SHH signalling transcription factor glioma-associated oncogene homolog (*GLI*) 1 was expressed ubiquitously, including in fibroblasts, nuclear GLI2 was confined to distal epithelial cells [133]. Furthermore, the authors could show that recombinant SHH increased proliferation, expression of ECM components, and migration of primary human lung fibroblasts and at the same time inhibited fibroblast apoptosis [133]. These results indicate that SHH generated by distal, bronchiolar and alveolar, epithelial cells activates fibroblasts, which indicates an important profibrotic contribution of epithelial-derived SHH in IPF pathogenesis. Interestingly, a more recent study provided evidence that a profibrotic feed-forward mechanism may exist in this context: Gli^+ mesenchymal stromal cells promote differentiation of airway progenitors into aberrant metaplastic $Krt5^+$ basal cells by antagonizing activation of the bone morphogenetic protein (BMP) pathway [134]. Overall, this suggests that upregulation of epithelial SHH may be an early event in IPF pathogenesis and trigger reciprocal epithelial-mesenchymal interactions that propagate lung fibrogenesis.

7.5.4. Notch Signalling Pathway

In lung development, Notch signalling determines ciliated versus secretory cell fate in conducting airways [135,136]. Following bleomycin injury or influenza infection in mice, Notch signalling has been shown to activate proliferation and migration of a $KRT5^+$ progenitor cell lineage in the context of repair after injury while blockade of Notch signalling induced an alveolar cell type faith. Importantly, active Notch signalling was detected in IPF honeycomb cysts [130], indicating a role for Notch signalling in aberrant epithelial repair and honeycomb cyst formation. Interestingly, overexpression of Notch can also induce EMT [137]; so, Notch signalling may not only promote aberrant cyst formation, but also contribute to the emergence of the above- described aberrant basaloid cells. In mice, Dlk1-mediated temporal regulation of Notch signalling is required for differentiation of AT2 to AT1 cells during repair [138]. Interestingly, deletion of Dlk1 in AT2 cells led to the accumulation of an intermediate cell population. We may speculate that a similar Notch-dependent mechanism might drive the appearance of aberrant basaloid cells in IPF.

In summary, bronchial and bronchiolar epithelial cells including airway-cell derived disease-specific lineages contribute to the reactivation of developmental pathways in IPF, including central pathways like the TGF-β1, WNT, SHH, and Notch signalling pathways. The collective evidence clearly demonstrates that, via autocrine and paracrine mechanisms, conducting airway epithelial-derived factors induce and modulate developmental programmes in IPF and drive major pathological outcomes in this disease like excessive ECM deposition and honeycomb cyst formation.

7.6. Epigenetic Mechanisms

Epigenetics traditionally comprises DNA methylation and histone modification, molecular alterations in chromatin which serve as marks for transcriptional activation or repression without affecting the DNA sequence per se. Epigenetic regulation mechanisms are typically persistent, can be inherited, and have the potential to translate environmental exposures into regulation of gene transcription at the level of chromatin structure [139,140]. This applies particularly to the airway mucosa, which represents a direct interface between environment and human body [141,142]. As IPF development seems to be orchestrated by genetic predisposition and environmental risk factors, epigenetic mechanisms may provide important mechanistic links and novel targets for therapy. Indeed, a number of studies have established that epigenetic signatures are changed in IPF, including DNA methylation and expression of DNA methyl transferases [143,144] as well as single histone modification marks [140] and expression of histone modifying enzymes [145]. To the best of our knowledge, genome-wide histone modification studies in IPF are lacking to date.

Our knowledge on epigenetic marks in IPF and their cell type-specific contribution to disease pathogenesis and progression is still very limited. However, it is well-known that IPF risk factors like cigarette smoke or particulate matter, for instance, induce epigenetic alterations in bronchial epithelial cells [146–148], indicating that such changes may be frequent in IPF. Furthermore, increased expression and activity of histone deacetylases in IPF has been localized to myofibroblasts, but also to aberrant basal cells in IPF [145]. Clearly, the role of epigenetic changes in airway epithelial cells requires more attention and detailed mechanistic studies, and such investigations may ultimately provide interesting novel therapeutic intervention opportunities for early therapy.

7.7. Non-Coding RNAs

Non-coding RNA (ncRNA), i.e., RNA which is not translated to proteins, constitutes approximately 98% of the total transcribed RNA in humans [149]. NcRNAs include housekeeping RNAs, such as ribosomal, spliceosomal, or transfer RNA, expression of which is constitutive, but also regulatory RNAs, such as long noncoding RNAs (lncRNA) or microRNAs (miRNA), which are expressed in a cell type- and tissue-specific manner and often altered in disease. LncRNA molecules are arbitrarily defined as >200 nucleotides in length and can regulate gene expression by transcriptional interference, chromatin remodelling, promoter inactivation, activation and transport of accessory and transcription factors, epigenetic silencing, and as precursors for small interfering RNAs [150,151]. In contrast, miRNAs are short, approximately 22 nucleotides long, RNA molecules which suppress protein translation by non-perfect complementary binding to regions in the 3'UTR of their target mRNAs.

Even though our knowledge on function and regulation of lncRNAs in general is still very limited, several studies support the concept that lncRNAs contribute to profibrotic cellular mechanisms in IPF [152,153]. While some studies in this context focussed on the function of specific lncRNAs in lung fibroblasts [154], other recent reports highlight altered lncRNA expression and function in bronchial epithelial cells. For instance, increased expression of lncRNA *MEG3* was observed in atypical KRT5+ p63+ basal cells in IPF relative to normal donor lung tissue. In vitro studies showed that *MEG3* induced basal cell gene transcription (*KRT14, TP63*) in bronchial cell lines, but also fundamental events of EMT, including increased cellular migration and downregulation of *CDH1* (E-cadherin) [155]. *MEG3* may thus cause or at least contribute to the emergence of the aberrant basal-like cell populations in IPF described above (see Section 4). In contrast, loss of the terminal differentiation-induced lncRNA (TINCR), a lncRNA normally expressed in the bronchial epithelium, but decreased in IPF, has been described to, among others, induce basal cell markers and ECM genes [156,157], reminiscent of gene expression signatures of aberrant basal and basaloid cells in IPF [42,44,45]. Studies in mouse models of lung fibrosis and primary human cells have proposed additional lncRNAs as regulators of EMT in bronchial epithelial cells, but localization in the IPF lung has, to the best of our knowledge, not yet been demonstrated. These include lncRNAs uc.77 and 2700086A05Rik [158] and lncRNA H19 [159]. Collectively, these studies support the concept of bronchial epithelial cell-specific lncRNA expression as an emerging driver in IPF pathogenesis.

To date, few studies have addressed the function of airway epithelial miRNAs in IPF pathogenesis. A pioneering study has globally assessed expression of miRNAs in bronchoscopy-assisted bronchial brushes from fibrotic airways of bronchiolitis obliterans syndrome (BOS) and found that miR-323a-3p was drastically downregulated (>18-fold) in airways of BOS patients relative to control lung transplant patients. The authors also examined miR-323a-3p expression in isolated AT2 cells from IPF lung explants and from fibrotic mouse lungs after bleomycin injury and observed significant downregulation, indicating general downregulation in lung epithelium during fibrogenesis [160]. Furthermore, miR-323a-3p mimics and miR-323a-3p antagomirs suppressed and exacerbated lung fibrogenesis, respectively, in the bleomycin mouse model. In vitro studies suggested that miR-323a-3p directly targets central mediators of TGF-α and TGF-β signalling as well as caspase 3, thereby attenuating key profibrotic mechanisms and epithelial cell apoptosis [160]. Given that miRNA therapeutics are coming of age and, in the case of the lung, can be easily delivered to the epithelium by inhalation, more such studies are warranted to identify further epithelial-specific miRNA-based profibrotic mechanisms.

8. Summary, Conclusions, and Emerging Questions

The last decade has transformed our understanding of IPF pathogenesis and set forth multiple evidence that strongly argues for a critical role of conducting airway epithelial cell populations in IPF aetiology and disease development (summarized in Figure 7). The discovery of the *MUC5B* promoter polymorphism as the strongest causative factor for IPF onset drew attention from the alveolar department to bronchial and bronchiolar cell contributions to lung fibrogenesis. IPF airways are drastically distorted, and alveolar areas are repopulated by airway-like epithelial cells in a process termed bronchiolization. In agreement, several recent scRNA-Seq analyses of IPF lungs have consistently revealed drastic alterations in epithelial subpopulations including the replacement of alveolar epithelial cells by various airway-like cells that are either directly distal airway-derived or the result of alveolar epithelial cell transdifferentiation or a combination of both. Emerging new evidence suggests that specific mesenchymal niche environments in the IPF patient may promote plasticity of the alveolar epithelium that leads to full transdifferentiation towards airway-like states [38]. Another line of evidence shows that persistent alveolar repair generates intermediate cells, which display features of senescence and p53 activation. In mice, inducing senescence in AT2 cells and thereby shifting them to a state that resembles injury-induced alveolar differentiation intermediates [54,161] and the aberrant basaloid cells [42,44,45] leads to progressive pulmonary fibrosis as seen in IPF patients [162]. Future work needs to leverage histopathological disease grade staging to further clarify the cellular origins of these intermediate cell populations and the natural evolution of epithelial metaplasia and bronchiolization in IPF disease progression.

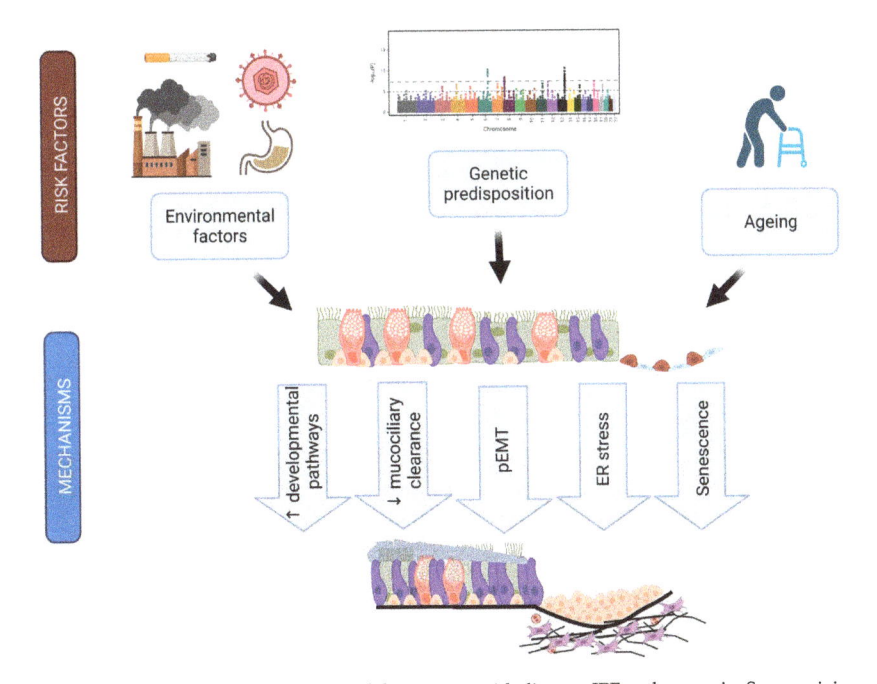

Figure 7. Hypothetical contributions of the airway epithelium to IPF pathogenesis. Summarizing scheme linking established environmental and genetic risk factors via the bronchial and bronchiolar epithelium to IPF-specific disease mechanisms and outcomes like bronchiolization and interstitial scarring. Figure was created with biorender.com.

Critical airway functions like mucociliary clearance and epithelial barrier integrity are also affected in IPF. Genetic risk factors beyond the *MUC5B* promoter polymorphism, in particular the *DSP* and *FAM13A* risk SNPs, argue for airway epithelial cells as central culprits in disease onset. Finally, evidence is accumulating that bronchial epithelial cells directly trigger central profibrotic mechanisms like the reactivation of multiple developmental programmes in an aberrant injury response.

The balance between epithelial proliferation, trans-differentiation, apoptosis and cellular senescence is drastically disturbed in IPF airway epithelial cells. Impaired mucociliary clearance may be a key disease-initiating feature in this context. However, we still understand very little about the mechanisms that trigger the balance to tip from normal alveolar repair towards this aberrant, airway epithelial cell-driven repair process leading to the emergence of epithelial metaplasia and aberrant basaloid cells in the lung periphery. Similarly, the sequence of events that ultimately lead to IPF development remains ill-defined. For instance, is bronchiolization an epiphenomenon and characteristic of end-stage disease, or may pEMT of airway epithelial cells actually precede activation of fibroblasts? What are key mechanisms that can be safely and effectively employed to target profibrotic epithelial-mesenchymal cross-talk and regenerate normal stem cell niches? In particular epigenetic mechanisms, the role of epithelial non-coding RNAs, how these affect profibrotic and disease-perpetuating mechanisms, and whether they can be targeted for therapy remains a largely unexplored area. Additionally, the contributions of immune cells to the described processes remain little understood. Evidently, more mechanistic studies are needed to decipher these processes in molecular detail. It is becoming increasingly clear that, for this aim, we need to develop novel animal lung fibrosis models, which recapitulate impaired mucociliary function and environmental exposure. The above-described mouse model derived by conditional deletion of NEDD4-2 from airway epithelial cells represents a great opportunity to study in more detail the mechanisms that trigger fibrosis as a result of impaired mucociliary clearance. The good news about airway epithelial cells as emerging central culprits in IPF pathogenesis is that, finally, targeting airway epithelial cells is a more straightforward task than targeting fibroblasts, because, given that fibrotic areas are ventilated, the inhalatory route would deliver the drug directly and specifically onto the aberrant epithelium.

Author Contributions: Writing—review and editing, A.C., M.M., M.A., H.B.S., C.A.S.-W.; supervision, C.A.S.-W.; funding acquisition, H.B.S., C.A.S.-W. All authors have read and agreed to the published version of the manuscript.

Funding: Work in the authors' laboratories is supported by the Helmholtz Association, the German Center for Lung Research (DZL), the Deutsche Forschungsgemeinschaft (DFG) within the Research Training Group GRK2338 (grant to C.A.S.-W.), the Federal Institute for Risk Assessment (Bundesinstitut für Risikobewertung, BfR) (#1328-570, grant to C.A.S.-W.), the European Union's Horizon 2020 research and innovation program (grant agreement 874656, to H.B.S.) and the Chan Zuckerberg Initiative (CZF2019-002438, to H.B.S.).

Institutional Review Board Statement: For previously unpublished stainings given in Figure 2B, the study was conducted in accordance with the Declaration of Helsinki, and approved by the Ethics Committee of the Ludwig-Maximilians University of Munich, Germany (Ethic vote #333-10, #382-10). For all other data extracted from previous work, please refer to the original publications.

Informed Consent Statement: Informed consent was obtained from all subjects involved in the study.

Data Availability Statement: Count tables of the Munich single-cell cohort as well as custom preprocessing code can be accessed at https://github.com/theislab/2020_Mayr (last accessed 22 December 2021). Raw count tables for additional cohorts were retrieved from the Gene Expression Omnibus database by the accession numbers as provided in the original publications (Chicago cohort GSE122960; Nashville cohort GSE135893; New Haven cohort GSE136831).

Acknowledgments: We gratefully acknowledge the provision of human biomaterial and clinical data from the CPC-M bioArchive and its partners at the Asklepios Biobank Gauting, the Klinikum der Universität München and the Ludwig-Maximilians-Universität München.

Conflicts of Interest: The authors declare no conflict of interest. The funders had no role in the design of the study; in the collection, analyses, or interpretation of data; in the writing of the manuscript, or in the decision to publish the results.

References

1. Richeldi, L.; Du Bois, R.M.; Raghu, G.; Azuma, A.; Brown, K.K.; Costabel, U.; Cottin, V.; Flaherty, K.R.; Hansell, D.M.; Inoue, Y.; et al. Efficacy and safety of nintedanib in idiopathic pulmonary fibrosis. *N. Engl. J. Med.* **2014**, *370*, 2071–2082. [CrossRef] [PubMed]
2. King, T.E., Jr.; Bradford, W.Z.; Castro-Bernardini, S.; Fagan, E.A.; Glaspole, I.; Glassberg, M.K.; Gorina, E.; Hopkins, P.M.; Kardatzke, D.; Lancaster, L.; et al. A Phase 3 Trial of pirfenidone in patients with idiopathic pulmonary fibrosis. *N. Engl. J. Med.* **2014**, *370*, 2083–2092. [CrossRef]
3. Lederer, D.J.; Martinez, F.J. Idiopathic Pulmonary Fibrosis. *N. Engl. J. Med.* **2018**, *379*, 797–798. [CrossRef] [PubMed]
4. Crystal, R.G.; Randell, S.H.; Engelhardt, J.F.; Voynow, J.; Sunday, M.E. Airway epithelial cells: Current concepts and challenges. *Proc. Am. Thorac. Soc.* **2008**, *5*, 772–777. [CrossRef]
5. Rock, J.R.; Randell, S.H.; Hogan, B.L.M. Airway basal stem cells: A perspective on their roles in epithelial homeostasis and remodeling. *Dis. Model. Mech.* **2010**, *3*, 545–556. [CrossRef] [PubMed]
6. Rock, J.R.; Onaitis, M.W.; Rawlins, E.L.; Lu, Y.; Clark, C.P.; Xue, Y.; Randell, S.H.; Hogan, B.L.M. Basal cells as stem cells of the mouse trachea and human airway epithelium. *Proc. Natl. Acad. Sci. USA* **2009**, *106*, 12771–12775. [CrossRef]
7. Barkauskas, C.E.; Cronce, M.J.; Rackley, C.R.; Bowie, E.J.; Keene, D.R.; Stripp, B.R.; Randell, S.H.; Noble, P.W.; Hogan, B.L.M. Type 2 alveolar cells are stem cells in adult lung. *J. Clin. Investig.* **2013**, *123*, 3025–3036. [CrossRef]
8. Liu, Q.; Liu, K.; Cui, G.; Huang, X.; Yao, S.; Guo, W.; Qin, Z.; Li, Y.; Yang, R.; Pu, W.; et al. Lung regeneration by multipotent stem cells residing at the bronchioalveolar-duct junction. *Nat. Genet.* **2019**, *51*, 728–738. [CrossRef]
9. McLellan, T.; George, P.M.; Ford, P.; De Backer, J.; Van Holsbeke, C.; Mignot, B.; Screaton, N.J.; Ruggiero, A.; Thillai, M. Idiopathic pulmonary fibrosis: Airway volume measurement identifies progressive disease on computed tomography scans. *ERJ Open Res.* **2020**, *6*, 00290-2019. [CrossRef]
10. Tanabe, N.; McDonough, J.E.; Vasilescu, D.M.; Ikezoe, K.; Verleden, S.E.; Xu, F.; Wuyts, W.A.; Vanaudenaerde, B.M.; Colby, T.V.; Hogg, J.C. Pathology of idiopathic pulmonary fibrosis assessed by a combination of microcomputed tomography, histology, and immunohistochemistry. *Am. J. Pathol.* **2020**, *190*, 2427–2435. [CrossRef]
11. McDonough, J.E.; Verleden, S.E.; Verschakelen, J.; Wuyts, W.; Vanaudenaerde, B.M. The structural origin of honeycomb cysts in IPF. *Am. J. Respir. Crit. Care Med.* **2018**, *197*, A6388.
12. Ikezoe, K.; Hackett, T.-L.; Peterson, S.; Prins, D.; Hague, C.J.; Murphy, D.; LeDoux, S.; Chu, F.; Xu, F.; Cooper, J.D.; et al. Small Airway Reduction and Fibrosis Is an Early Pathologic Feature of Idiopathic Pulmonary Fibrosis. *Am. J. Respir. Crit. Care Med.* **2021**, *204*, 1048–1059. [CrossRef] [PubMed]
13. Pastre, J.; Plantier, L.; Planes, C.; Borie, R.; Nunes, H.; Delclaux, C.; Israël-Biet, D. Different KCO and VA combinations exist for the same DLCO value in patients with diffuse parenchymal lung diseases. *BMC Pulm. Med.* **2015**, *15*, 100. [CrossRef]
14. Plantier, L.; Cazes, A.; Dinh-Xuan, A.-T.; Bancal, C.; Marchand-Adam, S.; Crestani, B. Physiology of the lung in idiopathic pulmonary fibrosis. *Eur. Respir. Rev. Off. J. Eur. Respir. Soc.* **2018**, *27*, 170062. [CrossRef] [PubMed]
15. Brand, P.; Kohlha, M.; Meyer, T.; Selzer, T.; Heyder, J.; Häussinger, K.; Ha¨ußinger, K. Aerosol-derived airway morphometry and aerosol bolus dispersion in patients with lung fibrosis and lung emphysema. *Chest* **1999**, *116*, 543–548. [CrossRef] [PubMed]
16. Plantier, L.; Debray, M.-P.; Estellat, C.; Flamant, M.; Roy, C.; Bancal, C.; Borie, R.; Israel-Biet, D.; Mal, H.; Crestani, B.; et al. Increased volume of conducting airways in idiopathic pulmonary fibrosis is independent of disease severity: A volumetric capnography study. *J. Breath Res.* **2016**, *10*, 16005. [CrossRef] [PubMed]
17. Westcott, J.L.; Cole, S.R. Traction bronchiectasis in end-stage pulmonary fibrosis. *Radiology* **1986**, *161*, 665–669. [CrossRef]
18. Hino, T.; Lee, K.S.; Han, J.; Hata, A.; Ishigami, K.; Hatabu, H. Spectrum of pulmonary fibrosis from interstitial lung abnormality to usual interstitial pneumonia: Importance of identification and quantification of traction bronchiectasis in patient management. *Korean J. Radiol.* **2021**, *22*, 811–828. [CrossRef]
19. Walsh, S.L.F.; Wells, A.U.; Sverzellati, N.; Devaraj, A.; von der Thusen, J.; Yousem, S.A.; Colby, T.V.; Nicholson, A.G.; Hansell, D.M. Relationship between fibroblastic foci profusion and high resolution CT morphology in fibrotic lung disease. *BMC Med.* **2015**, *13*, 1–8. [CrossRef]
20. Piciucchi, S.; Tomassetti, S.; Ravaglia, C.; Gurioli, C.; Gurioli, C.; Dubini, A.; Carloni, A.; Chilosi, M.; Colby, T.V.; Poletti, V. From "traction bronchiectasis" to honeycombing in idiopathic pulmonary fibrosis: A spectrum of bronchiolar remodeling also in radiology? *BMC Pulm. Med.* **2016**, *16*, 1–4. [CrossRef]
21. Verleden, S.; Tanabe, N.; McDonough, J.; Vasilescu, D.M.; Xu, F.; A Wuyts, W.; Piloni, D.; De Sadeleer, L.; Willems, S.; Mai, C.; et al. Small airways pathology in idiopathic pulmonary fibrosis: A retrospective cohort study. *Lancet Respir. Med.* **2020**, *8*, 573–584. [CrossRef]
22. Miller, E.R.; Putman, R.K.; Diaz, A.A.; Xu, H.; Estépar, R.S.J.; Araki, T.; Nishino, M.; De Frías, S.P.; Hida, T.; Ross, J.; et al. Increased airway wall thickness in interstitial lung abnormalities and idiopathic pulmonary fibrosis. *Ann. Am. Thorac. Soc.* **2019**, *16*, 447–454. [CrossRef]

23. Chilosi, M.; Poletti, V.; Murer, B.; Lestani, M.; Cancellieri, A.; Montagna, L.; Piccoli, P.; Cangi, G.; Doglioni, C. Abnormal re-epithelialization and lung remodeling in idiopathic pulmonary fibrosis: The role of deltaN-P63. *Lab. Investig.* **2002**, *82*, 1335–1345. [CrossRef] [PubMed]
24. Chilosi, M.; Zamò, A.; Doglioni, C.; Reghellin, D.; Lestani, M.; Montagna, L.; Pedron, S.; Ennas, M.G.; Cancellieri, A.; Murer, B.; et al. Migratory marker expression in fibroblast foci of idiopathic pulmonary fibrosis. *Respir. Res.* **2006**, *7*, 95. [CrossRef]
25. Smirnova, N.F.; Schamberger, A.C.; Nayakanti, S.; Hatz, R.; Behr, J.; Eickelberg, O. Detection and quantification of epithelial progenitor cell populations in human healthy and IPF lungs. *Respir. Res.* **2016**, *17*, 1–11. [CrossRef]
26. Strickland, N.H.; Hughes, J.M.B.; Hart, D.A.; Myers, M.J.; Lavender, J.P. Cause of regional ventilation-perfusion mismatching in patients with idiopathic pulmonary fibrosis: A combined CT and scintigraphic study. *Am. J. Roentgenol.* **1993**, *161*, 719–725. [CrossRef]
27. Hansell, D.M.; Bankier, A.A.; MacMahon, H.; McLoud, T.C.; Müller, N.L.; Remy, J. Fleischner society: Glossary of terms for thoracic imaging. *Radiology* **2008**, *246*, 697–722. [CrossRef]
28. Akira, M. Radiographic differentiation of advanced fibrocystic lung diseases. *Ann. Am. Thorac. Soc.* **2017**, *14*, 432–440. [CrossRef]
29. Evans, C.M.; Fingerlin, T.E.; Schwarz, M.I.; Lynch, D.; Kurche, J.; Warg, L.; Yang, I.V.; Schwartz, D.A. Idiopathic pulmonary fibrosis: A genetic disease that involves mucociliary dysfunction of the peripheral airways. *Physiol. Rev.* **2016**, *96*, 1567–1591. [CrossRef] [PubMed]
30. Seibold, M.A.; Smith, R.W.; Urbanek, C.; Groshong, S.D.; Cosgrove, G.P.; Brown, K.K.; Schwarz, M.I.; Schwartz, D.A.; Reynolds, S.D. The idiopathic pulmonary fibrosis honeycomb cyst contains a mucocilary pseudostratified epithelium. *PLoS ONE* **2013**, *8*, e58658. [CrossRef] [PubMed]
31. Prasse, A.; Binder, H.; Schupp, J.; Kayser, G.; Bargagli, E.; Jaeger, B.; Hess, M.; Rittinghausen, S.; Vuga, L.; Lynn, H.; et al. BAL cell gene expression is indicative of outcome and airway basal cell involvement in idiopathic pulmonary fibrosis. *Am. J. Respir. Crit. Care Med.* **2019**, *199*, 622–630. [CrossRef] [PubMed]
32. Salwig, I.; Spitznagel, B.; Vazquez-Armendariz, A.I.; Khalooghi, K.; Guenther, S.; Herold, S.; Szibor, M.; Braun, T. Bronchioalveolar stem cells are a main source for regeneration of distal lung epithelia in vivo. *EMBO J.* **2019**, *38*. [CrossRef] [PubMed]
33. Plantier, L.; Crestani, B.; E Wert, S.; Dehoux, M.; Zweytick, B.; Guenther, A.; A Whitsett, J. Ectopic respiratory epithelial cell differentiation in bronchiolised distal airspaces in idiopathic pulmonary fibrosis. *Thorax* **2011**, *66*, 651–657. [CrossRef] [PubMed]
34. Kumar, P.A.; Hu, Y.; Yamamoto, Y.; Hoe, N.B.; Wei, T.S.; Mu, D.; Sun, Y.; Joo, L.S.; Dagher, R.; Zielonka, E.M.; et al. Distal airway stem cells yield alveoli in vitro and during lung regeneration following H1N1 influenza infection. *Cell* **2011**, *147*, 525–538. [CrossRef]
35. Zuo, W.; Zhang, T.; Wu, D.Z.; Guan, S.P.; Liew, A.-A.; Yamamoto, Y.; Wang, X.; Lim, S.J.; Vincent, M.; Lessard, M.; et al. p63(+)Krt5(+) distal airway stem cells are essential for lung regeneration. *Nature* **2014**, *517*, 616–620. [CrossRef]
36. Xi, Y.; Kim, T.; Brumwell, A.N.; Driver, I.; Wei, Y.; Tan, V.; Jackson, J.R.; Xu, J.; Lee, D.-K.; Gotts, J.E.; et al. Local lung hypoxia determines epithelial fate decisions during alveolar regeneration. *Nat. Cell Biol.* **2017**, *19*, 904–914. [CrossRef]
37. Ray, S.; Chiba, N.; Yao, C.; Guan, X.; McConnell, A.M.; Brockway, B.; Que, L.; McQualter, J.L.; Stripp, B.R. Rare SOX2$^+$ airway progenitor cells generate KRT5$^+$ cells that repopulate damaged alveolar parenchyma following influenza virus infection. *Stem Cell Rep.* **2016**, *7*, 817–825. [CrossRef]
38. Kathiriya, J.J.; Wang, C.; Zhou, M.; Brumwell, A.; Cassandras, M.; Le Saux, C.J.; Cohen, M.; Alysandratos, K.-D.; Wang, B.; Wolters, P.; et al. Human alveolar type 2 epithelium transdifferentiates into metaplastic KRT5(+) basal cells. *Nature* **2021**, *24*, 10–23. [CrossRef]
39. Xu, Y.; Mizuno, T.; Sridharan, A.; Du, Y.; Guo, M.; Tang, J.; Wikenheiser-Brokamp, K.A.; Perl, A.-K.T.; Funari, V.A.; Gokey, J.; et al. Single-cell RNA sequencing identifies diverse roles of epithelial cells in idiopathic pulmonary fibrosis. *JCI Insight* **2016**, *1*, e90558. [CrossRef]
40. Danopoulos, S.; Alonso, I.; Thornton, M.E.; Grubbs, B.H.; Bellusci, S.; Warburton, D.; Al Alam, D. Human lung branching morphogenesis is orchestrated by the spatiotemporal distribution of ACTA2, SOX2, and SOX. *Am. J. Physiol. Cell. Mol. Physiol.* **2018**, *314*, L144–L149. [CrossRef]
41. Wasnick, R.M.; Shalashova, I.; Wilhelm, J.; Khadim, A.; Schmidt, N.; Hackstein, H.; Hecker, A.; Hoetzenecker, K.; Seeger, W.; Bellusci, S.; et al. Differential lysotracker uptake defines two populations of distal epithelial cells in idiopathic pulmonary fibrosis. *Cells* **2022**, *11*, 235. [CrossRef]
42. Reyfman, P.A.; Walter, J.M.; Joshi, N.; Anekalla, K.R.; McQuattie-Pimentel, A.C.; Chiu, S.; Fernandez, R.; Akbarpour, M.; Chen, C.-I.; Ren, Z.; et al. Single-cell transcriptomic analysis of human lung provides insights into the pathobiology of pulmonary fibrosis. *Am. J. Respir. Crit. Care Med.* **2019**, *199*, 1517–1536. [CrossRef]
43. Mayr, C.H.; Simon, L.M.; Leuschner, G.; Ansari, M.; Schniering, J.; E Geyer, P.; Angelidis, I.; Strunz, M.; Singh, P.; Kneidinger, N.; et al. Integrative analysis of cell state changes in lung fibrosis with peripheral protein biomarkers. *EMBO Mol. Med.* **2021**, *13*, e12871. [CrossRef]
44. Habermann, A.C.; Gutierrez, A.J.; Bui, L.T.; Yahn, S.L.; Winters, N.I.; Calvi, C.L.; Peter, L.; Chung, M.-I.; Taylor, C.J.; Jetter, C.; et al. Single-cell RNA sequencing reveals profibrotic roles of distinct epithelial and mesenchymal lineages in pulmonary fibrosis. *Sci. Adv.* **2020**, *6*, eaba1972. [CrossRef]

45. Adams, T.S.; Schupp, J.C.; Poli, S.; Ayaub, E.A.; Neumark, N.; Ahangari, F.; Chu, S.G.; Raby, B.A.; DeIuliis, G.; Januszyk, M.; et al. Single-cell RNA-seq reveals ectopic and aberrant lung-resident cell populations in idiopathic pulmonary fibrosis. *Sci. Adv.* **2020**, *6*, eaba1983. [CrossRef]
46. Wolf, F.A.; Angerer, P.; Theis, F.J. SCANPY: Large-scale single-cell gene expression data analysis. *Genome Biol.* **2018**, *19*, 1–5. [CrossRef] [PubMed]
47. Young, M.D.; Behjati, S. SoupX removes ambient RNA contamination from droplet-based single-cell RNA sequencing data. *GigaScience* **2020**, *9*, giaa151. [CrossRef]
48. Lun, A.T.; McCarthy, D.; Marioni, J. A step-by-step workflow for low-level analysis of single-cell RNA-seq data with Bioconductor. *F1000Research* **2016**, *5*, 2122. [CrossRef] [PubMed]
49. Polański, K.; Young, M.D.; Miao, Z.; Meyer, K.B.; A Teichmann, S.; Park, J.-E. BBKNN: Fast batch alignment of single cell transcriptomes. *Bioinformatics* **2019**, *36*, 964–965. [CrossRef]
50. Schamberger, A.C.; Staab-Weijnitz, C.; Mise-Racek, N.; Eickelberg, O. Cigarette smoke alters primary human bronchial epithelial cell differentiation at the air-liquid interface. *Sci. Rep.* **2015**, *5*, 8163. [CrossRef] [PubMed]
51. Zuo, W.-L.; Rostami, M.R.; Leblanc, M.; Kaner, R.J.; O'Beirne, S.L.; Mezey, J.G.; Leopold, P.L.; Quast, K.; Visvanathan, S.; Fine, J.S.; et al. Dysregulation of club cell biology in idiopathic pulmonary fibrosis. *PLoS ONE* **2020**, *15*, e0237529. [CrossRef] [PubMed]
52. Jonsdottir, H.R.; Arason, A.J.; Palsson, R.; Franzdottir, S.R.; Gudbjartsson, T.; Isaksson, H.J.; Gudmundsson, G.; Gudjonsson, T.; Magnusson, M.K. Basal cells of the human airways acquire mesenchymal traits in idiopathic pulmonary fibrosis and in culture. *Lab. Investig.* **2015**, *95*, 1418–1428. [CrossRef] [PubMed]
53. Carraro, G.; Mulay, A.; Yao, C.; Mizuno, T.; Konda, B.; Petrov, M.; Lafkas, D.; Arron, J.R.; Hogaboam, C.M.; Chen, P.; et al. Single cell reconstruction of human basal cell diversity in normal and idiopathic pulmonary fibrosis lungs. *Am. J. Respir. Crit. Care Med.* **2020**, *202*, 1540–1550. [CrossRef] [PubMed]
54. Strunz, M.; Simon, L.M.; Ansari, M.; Kathiriya, J.J.; Angelidis, I.; Mayr, C.H.; Tsidiridis, G.; Lange, M.; Mattner, L.F.; Yee, M.; et al. Alveolar regeneration through a Krt8+ transitional stem cell state that persists in human lung fibrosis. *Nat. Commun.* **2020**, *11*, 1–20. [CrossRef] [PubMed]
55. Seibold, M.A.; Anastasia, L.; Wise, L.; Speer, M.C.; Steele, M.P.; Brown, K.K.; Loyd, J.E.; Fingerlin, T.E.; Zhang, W.; Gudmundsson, G.; et al. A common MUC5B promoter polymorphism and pulmonary fibrosis. *N. Engl. J. Med.* **2011**, *364*, 1503–1512. [CrossRef] [PubMed]
56. Hancock, L.A.; Hennessy, C.E.; Solomon, G.M.; Dobrinskikh, E.; Estrella, A.; Hara, N.; Hill, D.B.; Kissner, W.J.; Markovetz, M.R.; Villalon, D.E.G.; et al. Muc5b overexpression causes mucociliary dysfunction and enhances lung fibrosis in mice. *Nat. Commun.* **2018**, *9*, 5363. [CrossRef] [PubMed]
57. Mall, M.; Grubb, B.R.; Harkema, J.R.; O'Neal, W.K.; Boucher, R.C. Increased airway epithelial Na+ absorption produces cystic fibrosis-like lung disease in mice. *Nat. Med.* **2004**, *10*, 487–493. [CrossRef] [PubMed]
58. Duerr, J.; Leitz, D.H.W.; Szczygiel, M.; Dvornikov, D.; Fraumann, S.G.; Kreutz, C.; Zadora, P.K.; Agircan, A.S.; Konietzke, P.; Engelmann, T.A.; et al. Conditional deletion of Nedd4-2 in lung epithelial cells causes progressive pulmonary fibrosis in adult mice. *Nat. Commun.* **2020**, *11*, 1–18. [CrossRef] [PubMed]
59. Ganesan, S.; Comstock, A.T.; Sajjan, U.S. Barrier function of airway tract epithelium. *Tissue Barriers* **2013**, *1*, e24997. [CrossRef] [PubMed]
60. Zou, J.; Li, Y.; Yu, J.; Dong, L.; Husain, A.N.; Shen, L.; Weber, C.R. Idiopathic pulmonary fibrosis is associated with tight junction protein alterations. *Biochim. Et Biophys. Acta (BBA)-Biomembr.* **2020**, *1862*, 183205. [CrossRef] [PubMed]
61. Gan, H.; Wang, G.; Hao, Q.; Wang, Q.J.; Tang, H. Protein kinase D promotes airway epithelial barrier dysfunction and permeability through down-regulation of claudin-1. *J. Biol. Chem.* **2013**, *288*, 37343–37354. [CrossRef] [PubMed]
62. Gan, H.; McKenzie, R.; Hao, Q.; Idell, S.; Tang, H. Protein kinase d is increased and activated in lung epithelial cells and macrophages in idiopathic pulmonary fibrosis. *PLoS ONE* **2014**, *9*, e101983. [CrossRef] [PubMed]
63. Hope-Gill, B.D.M.; Hilldrup, S.; Davies, C.; Newton, R.P.; Harrison, N.K. A study of the cough reflex in idiopathic pulmonary fibrosis. *Am. J. Respir. Crit. Care Med.* **2003**, *168*, 995–1002. [CrossRef] [PubMed]
64. Kaur, A.; Mathai, S.K.; Schwartz, D.A. Genetics in idiopathic pulmonary fibrosis pathogenesis, prognosis, and treatment. *Front. Med.* **2017**, *4*, 154. [CrossRef] [PubMed]
65. Fingerlin, T.E.; Murphy, E.; Zhang, W.; Peljto, A.L.; Brown, K.K.; Steele, M.P.; Loyd, J.E.; Cosgrove, G.P.; Lynch, D.; Groshong, S. Genome-wide association study identifies multiple susceptibility loci for pulmonary fibrosis. *Nat. Genet.* **2013**, *45*, 613–620. [CrossRef] [PubMed]
66. Noth, I.; Zhang, Y.; Ma, S.-F.; Flores, C.; Barber, M.; Huang, Y.; Broderick, S.M.; Wade, M.S.; Hysi, P.; Scuirba, J.; et al. Genetic variants associated with idiopathic pulmonary fibrosis susceptibility and mortality: A genome-wide association study. *Lancet Respir. Med.* **2013**, *1*, 309–317. [CrossRef]
67. Chen, Y.; Zhao, Y.H.; Di, Y.-P.; Wu, R. Characterization of human mucin 5b gene expression in airway epithelium and the genomic clone of the amino-terminal and 5′-flanking region. *Am. J. Respir. Cell Mol. Biol.* **2001**, *25*, 542–553. [CrossRef] [PubMed]
68. Li, X.; Goobie, G.C.; Gregory, A.D.; Kass, D.J.; Zhang, Y. Toll-Interacting Protein in Pulmonary Diseases. Abiding by the Goldilocks Principle. *Am. J. Respir. Cell Mol. Biol.* **2021**, *64*, 536–546. [CrossRef] [PubMed]
69. Michalski, J.E.; A Schwartz, D.A. Genetic risk factors for idiopathic pulmonary fibrosis: Insights into immunopathogenesis. *J. Inflamm. Res.* **2021**, *13*, 1305–1318. [CrossRef] [PubMed]

70. Li, X.; Kim, S.E.; Chen, T.; Wang, J.; Yang, X.; Tabib, T.; Tan, J.; Guo, B.; Fung, S.; Zhao, J.; et al. Toll interacting protein protects bronchial epithelial cells from bleomycin-induced apoptosis. *FASEB J.* **2020**, *34*, 9884–9898. [CrossRef] [PubMed]
71. Delva, E.; Tucker, D.K.; Kowalczyk, A.P. The desmosome. *Cold Spring Harb. Perspect. Biol.* **2009**, *1*, a002543. [CrossRef] [PubMed]
72. Mathai, S.K.; Pedersen, B.S.; Smith, K.; Russell, P.; Schwarz, M.I.; Brown, K.K.; Steele, M.P.; Loyd, J.; Crapo, J.D.; Silverman, E.K.; et al. Desmoplakin Variants Are Associated with Idiopathic Pulmonary Fibrosis. *Am. J. Respir. Crit. Care Med.* **2016**, *193*, 1151–1160. [CrossRef] [PubMed]
73. Hao, Y.; Bates, S.; Mou, H.; Yun, J.H.; Pham, B.; Liu, J.; Qiu, W.; Guo, F.; Morrow, J.D.; Hersh, C.P.; et al. Genome-wide association study: Functional variant rs2076295 regulates desmoplakin expression in airway epithelial cells. *Am. J. Respir. Crit. Care Med.* **2020**, *202*, 1225–1236. [CrossRef] [PubMed]
74. Corvol, H.; Hodges, C.A.; Drumm, M.L.; Guillot, L. Moving beyond genetics: Is FAM13A a major biological contributor in lung physiology and chronic lung diseases? *J. Med. Genet.* **2014**, *51*, 646–649. [CrossRef] [PubMed]
75. Chen, Q.; de Vries, M.; Nwozor, K.O.; Noordhoek, J.A.; Brandsma, C.-A.; Boezen, H.M.; Heijink, I.H. A protective role of fam13a in human airway epithelial cells upon exposure to cigarette smoke extract. *Front. Physiol.* **2021**, *12*. [CrossRef] [PubMed]
76. Jiang, Z.; Lao, T.; Qiu, W.; Polverino, F.; Gupta, K.; Guo, F.; Mancini, J.D.; Naing, Z.Z.C.; Cho, M.H.; Castaldi, P.J.; et al. A chronic obstructive pulmonary disease susceptibility gene, fam13a, regulates protein stability of β-catenin. *Am. J. Respir. Crit. Care Med.* **2016**, *194*, 185–197. [CrossRef] [PubMed]
77. Hobbs, B.D.; de Jong, K.; Lamontagne, M.; Bossé, M.L.Y.; Shrine, N.; Artigas, M.S.; Wain, L.V.; Hall, I.; Jackson, V.E.; Wyss, A.B.; et al. Genetic loci associated with chronic obstructive pulmonary disease overlap with loci for lung function and pulmonary fibrosis. *Nat. Genet.* **2017**, *49*, 426–432. [CrossRef] [PubMed]
78. Rahardini, E.P.; Ikeda, K.; Nugroho, D.B.; Hirata, K.-I.; Emoto, N. loss of family with sequence similarity 13, member a exacerbates pulmonary fibrosis potentially by promoting epithelial to mesenchymal transition. *Kobe J. Med. Sci.* **2020**, *65*, E100–E109. [PubMed]
79. Allen, R.J.; Porte, J.; Braybrooke, R.; Flores, C.; E Fingerlin, T.; Oldham, J.M.; Guillen-Guio, B.; Ma, S.-F.; Okamoto, T.; E John, A.; et al. Genetic variants associated with susceptibility to idiopathic pulmonary fibrosis in people of European ancestry: A genome-wide association study. *Lancet Respir. Med.* **2017**, *5*, 869–880. [CrossRef]
80. Organ, L.; Porte, J.; John, A.; Jenkins, G. Investigating the role of AKAP13 on epithelial cell TGFß activation. *Eur. Respir. J.* **2019**, *54*, PA2429.
81. Diviani, D.; Soderling, J.; Scott, J.D. AKAP-Lbc anchors protein kinase A and nucleates Galpha 12-selective Rho-mediated stress fiber formation. *J. Biol. Chem.* **2001**, *276*, 44247–44257. [CrossRef] [PubMed]
82. Park, Y.; Ahn, C.; Kim, T.-H. Occupational and environmental risk factors of idiopathic pulmonary fibrosis: A systematic review and meta-analyses. *Sci. Rep.* **2021**, *11*, 1–10. [CrossRef] [PubMed]
83. Wolters, P.J.; Collard, H.R.; Jones, K.D. Pathogenesis of Idiopathic Pulmonary Fibrosis. *Annu. Rev. Pathol. Mech. Dis.* **2014**, *9*, 157–179. [CrossRef] [PubMed]
84. Conti, S.; Harari, S.; Caminati, A.; Zanobetti, A.; Schwartz, J.D.; Bertazzi, P.A.; Cesana, G.; Madotto, F. The association between air pollution and the incidence of idiopathic pulmonary fibrosis in Northern Italy. *Eur. Respir. J.* **2018**, *51*, 1700397. [CrossRef] [PubMed]
85. Korfei, M.; Ruppert, C.; Mahavadi, P.; Henneke, I.; Markart, P.; Koch, M.; Lang, G.; Fink, L.; Bohle, R.-M.; Seeger, W.; et al. Epithelial endoplasmic reticulum stress and apoptosis in sporadic idiopathic pulmonary fibrosis. *Am. J. Respir. Crit. Care Med.* **2008**, *178*, 838–846. [CrossRef] [PubMed]
86. Kuwano, K.; Kunitake, R.; Kawasaki, M.; Nomoto, Y.; Hagimoto, N.; Nakanishi, Y.; Hara, N. P21Waf1/Cip1/Sdi1 and p53 expression in association with DNA strand breaks in idiopathic pulmonary fibrosis. *Am. J. Respir. Crit. Care Med.* **1996**, *154*, 477–483. [CrossRef] [PubMed]
87. Maher, T.M.; Evans, I.C.; Bottoms, S.E.; Mercer, P.F.; Thorley, A.J.; Nicholson, A.G.; Laurent, G.J.; Tetley, T.D.; Chambers, R.C.; McAnulty, R.J. Diminished prostaglandin E₂ contributes to the apoptosis paradox in idiopathic pulmonary fibrosis. *Am. J. Respir. Crit. Care Med.* **2010**, *182*, 73–82. [CrossRef] [PubMed]
88. Plataki, M.; Koutsopoulos, A.V.; Darivianaki, K.; Delides, G.; Siafakas, N.M.; Bouros, D. Expression of apoptotic and antiapoptotic markers in epithelial cells in idiopathic pulmonary fibrosis. *Chest* **2005**, *127*, 266–274. [CrossRef] [PubMed]
89. Park, S.-Y.; Hong, J.Y.; Lee, S.Y.; Lee, S.-H.; Kim, M.J.; Kim, S.Y.; Kim, K.W.; Shim, H.S.; Park, M.S.; Lee, C.G.; et al. Club cell-specific role of programmed cell death 5 in pulmonary fibrosis. *Nat. Commun.* **2021**, *12*, 1–13. [CrossRef] [PubMed]
90. Lawson, W.E.; Crossno, P.F.; Polosukhin, V.V.; Roldan, J.; Cheng, D.-S.; Lane, K.B.; Blackwell, T.R.; Xu, C.; Markin, C.; Ware, L.B.; et al. Endoplasmic reticulum stress in alveolar epithelial cells is prominent in IPF: Association with altered surfactant protein processing and herpesvirus infection. *Am. J. Physiol. Cell. Mol. Physiol.* **2008**, *294*, L1119–L1126. [CrossRef] [PubMed]
91. Johnston, B.P.; McCormick, C. Herpesviruses and the unfolded protein response. *Viruses* **2019**, *12*, 17. [CrossRef]
92. Tanjore, H.; Lawson, W.E.; Blackwell, T.S. Endoplasmic reticulum stress as a pro-fibrotic stimulus. *Biochim. Et. Biophys. Acta BBA-Mol. Basis Dis.* **2012**, *1832*, 940–947. [CrossRef] [PubMed]
93. Chen, G.; Ribeiro, C.M.P.; Sun, L.; Okuda, K.; Kato, T.; Glimore, R.C.; Martino, M.B.; Dang, H.; Abzhanove, A.; Lin, J.M.; et al. XBP1S regulates MUC5B in a promoter variant-dependent pathway in idiopathic pulmonary fibrosis airway epithelia. *Am. J. Respir. Crit. Care Med.* **2019**, *200*, 220–234. [CrossRef] [PubMed]

94. Selman, M.; Pardo, A. Revealing the pathogenic and aging-related mechanisms of the enigmatic idiopathic pulmonary fibrosis. an integral model. *Am. J. Respir. Crit. Care Med.* **2014**, *189*, 1161–1172. [CrossRef] [PubMed]
95. Araya, J.; Kojima, J.; Takasaka, N.; Ito, S.; Fuji, S.; Hara, H.; Yanagisawa, H.; Kobayashim, K.; Tsurushige, C.; Kawaishi, M.; et al. Insufficient autophagy in idiopathic pulmonary fibrosis. *Am. J. Physiol. Lung Cell. Mol. Physiol.* **2013**, *304*, L56–L69. [CrossRef] [PubMed]
96. Hecker, L.; Logsdon, N.J.; Kurundkar, D.; Kurundkar, A.; Bernard, K.; Hock, T.; Meldrum, E.; Sanders, Y.Y.; Thannickal, V.J. Reversal of persistent fibrosis in aging by targeting Nox4-Nrf2 redox imbalance. *Sci. Transl. Med.* **2014**, *6*, 231ra47. [CrossRef] [PubMed]
97. Lehmann, M.; Mutze, K.; Korfei, M.; Klee, S.; Wagner, D.; Costa, R.; Schiller, H.; Günther, A.; Königshoff, M. LSC-2017-Senolytic drugs target alveolar epithelial cell function and attenuate experimental lung fibrosis ex vivo. *Eur. Respir. J.* **2017**, *50*, PA3471. [CrossRef]
98. Minagawa, S.; Araya, J.; Numata, T.; Nojiri, S.; Hara, H.; Yumino, Y.; Kawaishi, M.; Odaka, M.; Morikawa, T.; Nishimura, S.L.; et al. Accelerated epithelial cell senescence in IPF and the inhibitory role of SIRT6 in TGF-beta-induced senescence of human bronchial epithelial cells. *Am. J. Physiol. Lung Cell. Mol. Physiol.* **2011**, *300*, L391–L401. [CrossRef] [PubMed]
99. Schafer, M.J.; White, T.A.; Iijima, K.; Haak, A.J.; Ligresti, G.; Atkinson, E.J.; Oberg, A.L.; Birch, J.; Salmonowicz, H.; Zhu, Y.; et al. Cellular senescence mediates fibrotic pulmonary disease. *Nat. Commun.* **2017**, *8*, 14532. [CrossRef]
100. DePianto, D.J.; Heiden, J.A.V.; Morshead, K.B.; Sun, K.-H.; Modrusan, Z.; Teng, G.; Wolters, P.J.; Arron, J.R. Molecular mapping of interstitial lung disease reveals a phenotypically distinct senescent basal epithelial cell population. *JCI Insight* **2021**, *6*. [CrossRef]
101. Meiners, S.; Lehmann, M. Senescent cells in IPF: Locked in repair? *Front. Med.* **2020**, *7*, 606330. [CrossRef] [PubMed]
102. Chanda, D.; Otoupalova, E.; Smith, S.R.; Volckaert, T.; De Langhe, S.P.; Thannickal, V.J. Developmental pathways in the pathogenesis of lung fibrosis. *Mol. Asp. Med.* **2018**, *65*, 56–69. [CrossRef] [PubMed]
103. Massague, J. TGFbeta signalling in context. *Nat. Rev. Mol. Cell Biol.* **2012**, *13*, 616–630. [CrossRef] [PubMed]
104. Shi, M.; Zhu, J.; Wang, R.; Chen, X.; Mi, L.; Walz, T.; Springer, T.A. Latent TGF-beta structure and activation. *Nature* **2011**, *474*, 343–349. [CrossRef] [PubMed]
105. Ask, K.; Bonniaud, P.; Maass, K.; Eickelberg, O.; Margetts, P.J.; Warburton, D.; Groffen, J.; Gauldie, J.; Kolb, M. Progressive pulmonary fibrosis is mediated by TGF-beta isoform 1 but not TGF-beta. *Int. J. Biochem. Cell Biol.* **2008**, *40*, 484–495. [PubMed]
106. Fernandez, I.E.; Eickelberg, O. The impact of TGF-beta on lung fibrosis: From targeting to biomarkers. *Proc. Am. Thorac. Soc.* **2012**, *9*, 111–116. [CrossRef] [PubMed]
107. Xaubet, A.; Marin-Arguedas, A.; Lario, S.; Ancochea, J.; Morell, F.; Ruiz-Manzano, J.; Rodriguez-Becerra, E.; Rodriguez-Arias, J.M.; Sanz, S.; Campistol, J.M.; et al. Transforming growth factor-beta1 gene polymorphisms are associated with disease progression in idiopathic pulmonary fibrosis. *Am. J. Respir. Crit. Care Med.* **2003**, *168*, 431–435. [CrossRef] [PubMed]
108. Lodyga, M.; Hinz, B. TGF-beta1-A truly transforming growth factor in fibrosis and immunity. *Semin. Cell Dev. Biol.* **2020**, *101*, 123–139. [CrossRef] [PubMed]
109. Jenkins, G. The role of proteases in transforming growth factor-beta activation. *Int. J. Biochem. Cell Biol.* **2008**, *40*, 1068–1078. [PubMed]
110. Robertson, I.B.; Rifkin, D.B. Regulation of the Bioavailability of TGF-beta and TGF-beta-Related Proteins. *Cold Spring Harb. Perspect. Biol.* **2016**, *8*, a021907. [CrossRef] [PubMed]
111. Coker, R.K.; Laurent, G.J.; Shahzeidi, S.; Hernandez-Rodriguez, N.A.; Pantelidis, P.; du Bois, R.M.; Jeffery, P.K.; McAnulty, R.J. Diverse cellular TGF-beta 1 and TGF-beta 3 gene expression in normal human and murine lung. *Eur. Respir. J.* **1996**, *9*, 2501–2507. [CrossRef] [PubMed]
112. Kang, Y.; Prentice, M.A.; Mariano, J.M.; Davarya, S.; Linnoila, R.I.; Moody, T.W.; Wakefield, L.M.; Jakowlew, S.B. Transforming growth factor-beta 1 and its receptors in human lung cancer and mouse lung carcinogenesis. *Exp. Lung Res.* **2000**, *26*, 685–707. [CrossRef] [PubMed]
113. Sheppard, D. Functions of pulmonary epithelial integrins: From development to disease. *Physiol. Rev.* **2003**, *83*, 673–686. [CrossRef] [PubMed]
114. Craig, V.J.; Polverino, F.; Laucho-Contreras, M.E.; Shi, Y.; Liu, Y.; Osorio, J.C.; Tesfaigzi, Y.; Pinto-Plata, V.; Gochuico, B.R.; Rosas, I.O.; et al. Mononuclear phagocytes and airway epithelial cells: Novel sources of matrix metalloproteinase-8 (MMP-8) in patients with idiopathic pulmonary fibrosis. *PLoS ONE* **2014**, *9*, e97485. [CrossRef] [PubMed]
115. Câmara, J.; Jarai, G. Epithelial-mesenchymal transition in primary human bronchial epithelial cells is Smad-dependent and enhanced by fibronectin and TNF-α. *Fibrogenesis Tissue Repair* **2010**, *3*, 2. [CrossRef] [PubMed]
116. Hackett, T.-L.; Warner, S.M.; Stefanowicz, D.; Shaheen, F.; Pechkovsky, D.V.; Murray, L.A.; Argentieri, R.; Kicic, A.; Sick, S.M.; Bai, T.R.; et al. Induction of epithelial-mesenchymal transition in primary airway epithelial cells from patients with asthma by transforming growth factor-beta. *Am. J. Respir. Crit. Care Med.* **2009**, *180*, 122–133. [CrossRef] [PubMed]
117. Gabasa, M.; Duch, P.; Jorba, I.; Giménez, A.; Lugo, R.; Pavelescu, I.; Rodriguez-Pascual, F.; Molina, M.M.; Xaubet, A.; Pereda, J.; et al. Epithelial contribution to the profibrotic stiff microenvironment and myofibroblast population in lung fibrosis. *Mol. Biol. Cell* **2017**, *28*, 3741–3755. [CrossRef] [PubMed]
118. LeBleu, V.S.; Neilson, E.G. Origin and functional heterogeneity of fibroblasts. *FASEB J.* **2020**, *34*, 3519–3536. [CrossRef] [PubMed]
119. Aros, C.J.; Pantoja, C.J.; Gomperts, B.N. Wnt signaling in lung development, regeneration, and disease progression. *Commun. Biol.* **2021**, *4*, 1–13. [CrossRef]

120. Herr, P.; Hausmann, G.; Basler, K. WNT secretion and signalling in human disease. *Trends Mol. Med.* **2012**, *18*, 483–493. [CrossRef]
121. Baarsma, H.A.; Königshoff, M. 'WNT-er is coming': WNT signalling in chronic lung diseases. *Thorax* **2017**, *72*, 746–759. [CrossRef] [PubMed]
122. Königshoff, M.; Balsara, N.; Pfaff, E.-M.; Kramer, M.; Chrobak, I.; Seeger, W.; Eickelberg, O. Functional wnt signaling is increased in idiopathic pulmonary fibrosis. *PLoS ONE* **2008**, *3*, e2142. [CrossRef] [PubMed]
123. Pfaff, E.-M.; Becker, S.; Gunther, A.; Konigshoff, M. Dickkopf proteins influence lung epithelial cell proliferation in idiopathic pulmonary fibrosis. *Eur. Respir. J.* **2010**, *37*, 79–87. [CrossRef] [PubMed]
124. Aros, C.J.; Paul, M.; Pantoja, C.J.; Bisht, B.; Meneses, K.; Vijayaraj, P.; Sandlin, J.M.; France, B.; Tse, J.A.; Chen, M.W.; et al. High-throughput drug screening identifies a potent wnt inhibitor that promotes airway basal stem cell homeostasis. *Cell Rep.* **2020**, *30*, 2055–2064.e5. [CrossRef] [PubMed]
125. Aros, C.J.; Vijayaraj, P.; Pantoja, C.J.; Bisht, B.; Meneses, L.K.; Sandlin, J.M.; Tse, J.A.; Chen, M.W.; Purkayastha, A.; Shia, D.W.; et al. Distinct spatiotemporally dynamic wnt-secreting niches regulate proximal airway regeneration and aging. *Cell Stem Cell* **2020**, *27*, 413–429. [CrossRef] [PubMed]
126. Lynch, T.J.; Anderson, P.J.; Rotti, P.G.; Tyler, S.R.; Crooke, A.K.; Choi, S.H.; Montoro, D.T.; Montoro, C.L.; Silverman, C.L.; Shahin, W.; et al. Submucosal gland myoepithelial cells are reserve stem cells that can regenerate mouse tracheal epithelium. *Cell Stem Cell* **2018**, *22*, 779. [CrossRef] [PubMed]
127. Lynch, T.J.; Anderson, P.J.; Xie, W.; Crooke, A.K.; Liu, X.; Tyler, S.R.; Luo, M.; Kusner, D.M.; Zhang, Y.; Neff, T.; et al. Wnt signaling regulates airway epithelial stem cells in adult murine submucosal glands. *Stem Cells* **2016**, *34*, 2758–2771. [CrossRef] [PubMed]
128. Haas, M.; Vázquez, G.J.L.; Sun, D.I.; Tran, H.T.; Brislinger, M.; Tasca, A.; Shomroni, O.; Vleminckx, K.; Walentek, P. DeltaN-Tp63 mediates wnt/beta-catenin-induced inhibition of differentiation in basal stem cells of mucociliary epithelia. *Cell Rep.* **2019**, *28*, 3338–3352. [CrossRef] [PubMed]
129. Volckaert, T.; Yuan, T.; Chao, C.-M.; Bell, H.; Sitaula, A.; Szimmtenings, L.; El Agha, E.; Chanda, D.; Majka, S.; Bellusci, S.; et al. Fgf10-hippo epithelial-mesenchymal crosstalk maintains and recruits lung basal stem cells. *Dev. Cell* **2017**, *43*, 48–59. [CrossRef] [PubMed]
130. Vaughan, A.E.; Brumwell, A.N.; Xi, Y.; Gotts, J.E.; Brownfield, D.G.; Treutlein, B.; Tan, K.; Tan, V.; Liu, F.C.; Looney, M.R.; et al. Lineage-negative progenitors mobilize to regenerate lung epithelium after major injury. *Nature* **2015**, *517*, 621–625. [CrossRef] [PubMed]
131. Kugler, M.C.; Joyner, A.L.; Loomis, C.A.; Munger, J.S. Sonic hedgehog signaling in the lung. From development to disease. *Am. J. Respir. Cell Mol. Biol.* **2015**, *52*, 1–13. [CrossRef] [PubMed]
132. Kugler, M.C.; Loomis, C.A.; Zhao, Z.; Cushman, J.C.; Liu, L.; Munger, J.S. Sonic hedgehog signaling regulates myofibroblast function during alveolar septum formation in murine postnatal lung. *Am. J. Respir. Cell Mol. Biol.* **2017**, *57*, 280–293. [CrossRef] [PubMed]
133. Bolanos, A.L.; Milla, C.M.; Liram, J.C.; Ramírez, R.; Checa, M.; Barrera, L.; García-Alvarez, J.; Carbajal, V.; Becerril, C.; Gaxiola, M. Role of Sonic Hedgehog in idiopathic pulmonary fibrosis. *Am. J. Physiol. Lung Cell. Mol. Physiol.* **2012**, *303*, 978–990. [CrossRef] [PubMed]
134. Cassandras, M.; Wang, C.; Kathiriya, J.; Tsukui, T.; Matatia, P.; Matthay, M.; Wolters, P.; Molofsky, A.; Sheppard, D.; Chapman, H.; et al. Gli1+ mesenchymal stromal cells form a pathological niche to promote airway progenitor metaplasia in the fibrotic lung. *Nat. Cell Biol.* **2020**, *22*, 1295–1306. [CrossRef] [PubMed]
135. Morimoto, M.; Liu, Z.; Cheng, H.-T.; Winters, N.; Bader, D.; Kopan, R. Canonical Notch signaling in the developing lung is required for determination of arterial smooth muscle cells and selection of Clara versus ciliated cell fate. *J. Cell Sci.* **2010**, *123*, 213–224. [CrossRef] [PubMed]
136. Tsao, P.-N.; Vasconcelos, M.; Izvolsky, K.I.; Qian, J.; Lu, J.; Cardoso, W.V. Notch signaling controls the balance of ciliated and secretory cell fates in developing airways. *Development* **2009**, *136*, 2297–2307. [CrossRef] [PubMed]
137. Aoyagi-Ikeda, K.; Maeno, T.; Hiroki Matsui, H.; Ueno, M.; Hara, K.; Aoki, Y.; Aoki, F.; Shimizu, T.; Doi, H.; Kawai-Kowase, K.; et al. Notch induces myofibroblast differentiation of alveolar epithelial cells via transforming growth factor-{beta}-Smad3 pathway. *Am. J. Respir. Cell Mol. Biol.* **2011**, *45*, 136–144.
138. Finn, J.; Sottoriva, K.; Pajcini, K.V.; Kitajewski, J.K.; Chen, C.; Zhang, W.; Malik, A.B.; Liu, Y. Dlk1-mediated temporal regulation of notch signaling is required for differentiation of alveolar type ii to type i cells during repair. *Cell Rep.* **2019**, *26*, 2942–2954. [CrossRef]
139. Portela, A.; Esteller, M. Epigenetic modifications and human disease. *Nat. Biotechnol.* **2010**, *28*, 1057–1068. [CrossRef] [PubMed]
140. Yang, I.V.; Schwartz, D.A. Epigenetics of idiopathic pulmonary fibrosis. *Transl. Res. J. Lab. Clin. Med.* **2015**, *165*, 48–60. [CrossRef]
141. Alhamwe, B.A.; Miethe, S.; Von Strandmann, E.P.; Potaczek, D.P.; Garn, H. Epigenetic regulation of airway epithelium immune functions in asthma. *Front. Immunol.* **2020**, *11*, 1747. [CrossRef] [PubMed]
142. Acevedo, N.; Alashkar Alhamwe, B.; Caraballo, L.; Ding, M.; Ferrante, A.; Garn, H.; Garssen, J.; Hii, C.S.; Irvine, J.; Llinás-Caballero, K.; et al. Perinatal and early-life nutrition, epigenetics, and allergy. *Nutrients* **2021**, *13*, 724. [CrossRef] [PubMed]
143. Sanders, Y.Y.; Ambalavanan, N.; Halloran, B.; Zhang, X.; Liu, H.; Crossman, D.K.; Bray, M.; Zhang, K.; Thannickal, V.J.; Hagood, J.S. Altered DNA methylation profile in idiopathic pulmonary fibrosis. *Am. J. Respir. Crit. Care Med.* **2012**, *186*, 525–535. [CrossRef] [PubMed]

144. Yang, I.V.; Pedersen, B.S.; Rabinovich, E.; Hennessy, C.E.; Davidson, E.J.; Murphy, E.; Guardela, B.J.; Tedrow, J.R.; Zhang, Y.; Singh, M.K.; et al. Relationship of DNA methylation and gene expression in idiopathic pulmonary fibrosis. *Am. J. Respir. Crit. Care Med.* **2014**, *190*, 1263–1272. [CrossRef] [PubMed]
145. Korfei, M.; Skwarna, S.; Henneke, I.; MacKenzie, B.; Klymenko, O.; Saito, S.; Ruppert, C.; von der Beck, D.; Mahavadi, P.; Klepetko, W.; et al. Aberrant expression and activity of histone deacetylases in sporadic idiopathic pulmonary fibrosis. *Thorax* **2015**, *70*, 1022–1032. [CrossRef] [PubMed]
146. Leclercq, B.; Platel, A.; Antherieu, S.; Alleman, L.; Hardy, E.; Perdrix, E.; Grova, N.; Riffault, V.; Appenzeller, B.; Happillon, M.; et al. Genetic and epigenetic alterations in normal and sensitive COPD-diseased human bronchial epithelial cells repeatedly exposed to air pollution-derived $PM_{2.5}$. *Environ. Pollut.* **2017**, *230*, 163–177. [CrossRef] [PubMed]
147. Real, A.D.; Santurtún, A.; Zarrabeitia, M.T. Epigenetic related changes on air quality. *Environ. Res.* **2021**, *197*, 111155. [CrossRef] [PubMed]
148. Vaz, M.; Hwang, S.Y.; Kagiampakis, I.; Phallen, J.; Patil, A.; O'Hagan, H.M.; Murphy, L.; Zahnow, C.A.; Gabrielson, E.; Velculescu, V.E.; et al. Chronic cigarette smoke-induced epigenomic changes precede sensitization of bronchial epithelial cells to single-step transformation by KRAS mutations. *Cancer Cell* **2017**, *32*, 360–376. [CrossRef] [PubMed]
149. Mattick, J.S. Non-coding RNAs: The architects of eukaryotic complexity. *EMBO Rep.* **2001**, *2*, 986–991. [CrossRef] [PubMed]
150. Ponting, C.P.; Oliver, P.L.; Reik, W. Evolution and functions of long noncoding RNAs. *Cell* **2009**, *136*, 629–641. [CrossRef] [PubMed]
151. Ulitsky, I. Interactions between short and long noncoding RNAs. *FEBS Lett.* **2018**, *592*, 2874–2883. [CrossRef] [PubMed]
152. Hadjicharalambous, M.R.; Lindsay, M.A. Idiopathic pulmonary fibrosis: Pathogenesis and the emerging role of long non-coding RNAs. *Int. J. Mol. Sci.* **2020**, *21*, 524. [CrossRef] [PubMed]
153. Omote, N.; Sauler, M. Non-coding RNAs as regulators of cellular senescence in idiopathic pulmonary fibrosis and chronic obstructive pulmonary disease. *Front. Med.* **2020**, *7*, 603047. [CrossRef] [PubMed]
154. Savary, G.; Savary, G.; Dewaeles, E.; Diazzi, S.; Buscot, M.; Nottet, N.; Fassy, J.; Courcot, E.; Henaoui, I.-S.; Lemaire, J.; et al. The long noncoding RNA DNM3OS is a reservoir of fibromirs with major functions in lung fibroblast response to TGF-beta and pulmonary fibrosis. *Am. J. Respir. Crit. Care Med.* **2019**, *200*, 184–198. [CrossRef] [PubMed]
155. Gokey, J.; Snowball, J.; Sridharan, A.; Speth, J.P.; Black, K.E.; Hariri, L.P.; Perl, A.-K.T.; Xu, Y.; Whitsett, J.A. MEG3 is increased in idiopathic pulmonary fibrosis and regulates epithelial cell differentiation. *JCI Insight* **2018**, *3*, e122490. [CrossRef] [PubMed]
156. Omote, N.; Sakamoto, K.; Li, Q.; Schupp, J.C.; Adams, T.; Ahangari, F.; Chioccioli, M.; DeIuliis, G.; Hashimoto, N.; Hasegawa, Y.; et al. Long noncoding RNA TINCR is a novel regulator of human bronchial epithelial cell differentiation state. *Physiol. Rep.* **2021**, *9*, e14727. [CrossRef] [PubMed]
157. Omote, N.; Sakamoto, K.; Li, Q.; Schupp, J.; Adams, T.; Ahangari, F.; Chioccioli, M.; Xylourgidis, N.; Deiuliis, G.; Hashimoto, N.; et al. TINCR, a long intergenic noncoding RNA decreased in IPF, is a novel regulator of airway epithelial cell differentiation. *Am. J. Respir. Crit. Care Med.* **2019**, *199*, A5406. [CrossRef]
158. Sun, H.; Chen, J.; Qian, W.; Kang, J.; Wang, J.; Jiang, L.; Qiao, L.; Chen, W.; Zhang, J. Integrated long non-coding RNA analyses identify novel regulators of epithelial-mesenchymal transition in the mouse model of pulmonary fibrosis. *J. Cell. Mol. Med.* **2016**, *20*, 1234–1246. [CrossRef] [PubMed]
159. Wang, X.; Cheng, Z.; Dai, L.; Jiang, T.; Jia, L.; Jing, X.; An, L.; Wang, H.; Liu, M. Knockdown of long noncoding RNA H19 represses the progress of pulmonary fibrosis through the transforming growth factor beta/smad3 pathway by regulating microRNA 140. *Mol. Cell. Biol.* **2019**, *39*, e00143-19. [CrossRef] [PubMed]
160. Ge, L.; Habiel, D.M.; Hansbro, P.; Kim, R.Y.; Gharib, S.A.; Edelman, J.D.; Koenigshoff, M.; Parimon, T.; Brauer, R.; Huang, Y.; et al. miR-323a-3p regulates lung fibrosis by targeting multiple profibrotic pathways. *JCI Insight* **2016**, *1*, e90301. [CrossRef] [PubMed]
161. Kobayashi, Y.; Tata, A.; Konkimalla, A.; Katsura, H.; Lee, R.F.; Ou, J.; Banovich, N.E.; Kropski, J.A.; Tata, P.R. Persistence of a regeneration-associated, transitional alveolar epithelial cell state in pulmonary fibrosis. *Nat. Cell Biol.* **2020**, *22*, 934–946. [CrossRef] [PubMed]
162. Yao, C.; Guan, X.; Carraro, G.; Parimon, T.; Liu, X.; Huang, G.; Mulay, A.; Soukiasian, H.J.; David, G.; Weigt, S.S.; et al. Senescence of Alveolar Type 2 Cells Drives Progressive Pulmonary Fibrosis. *Am. J. Respir. Crit. Care Med.* **2021**, *203*, 707–717. [CrossRef] [PubMed]

Review

EGFR Signaling in Lung Fibrosis

Fabian Schramm [1,†], Liliana Schaefer [2] and Malgorzata Wygrecka [1,*,†]

[1] Center for Infection and Genomics of the Lung (CIGL), Universities of Giessen and Marburg, 35392 Giessen, Germany; fabian.schramm@med.uni-giessen.de
[2] Institute of Pharmacology and Toxicology, Goethe University Frankfurt, 60590 Frankfurt, Germany; schaefer@med.uni-frankfurt.de
* Correspondence: malgorzata.wygrecka@innere.med.uni-giessen.de
† Member of the German Center for Lung Research.

Abstract: In this review article, we will first provide a brief overview of the ErbB receptor–ligand system and its importance in developmental and physiological processes. We will then review the literature regarding the role of ErbB receptors and their ligands in the maladaptive remodeling of lung tissue, with special emphasis on idiopathic pulmonary fibrosis (IPF). Here we will focus on the pathways and cellular processes contributing to epithelial–mesenchymal miscommunication seen in this pathology. We will also provide an overview of the in vivo studies addressing the efficacy of different ErbB signaling inhibitors in experimental models of lung injury and highlight how such studies may contribute to our understanding of ErbB biology in the lung. Finally, we will discuss what we learned from clinical applications of the ErbB1 signaling inhibitors in cancer in order to advance clinical trials in IPF.

Keywords: epidermal growth factor; epidermal growth factor receptor; ErbB-signaling; pulmonary fibrosis; idiopathic pulmonary fibrosis; lung fibrosis; tyrosine kinase inhibitor; TGF-α; TGF-β; amphiregulin; neuregulin 1

1. Introduction

The epidermal growth factor (EGF) receptor (EGFR), belongs to the family of the ErbB tyrosine kinase receptors [1,2]. EGFR is also known as ErbB1 or HER1. Other members of this family are ErbB2 (HER2) [3], ErbB3 (HER3) [4] and ErbB4 (HER4) [5]. Following ligand binding, ErbB receptors form homo- or heterodimers that are autophosphorylated on tyrosine residues by intrinsic tyrosine kinase activity and mediate signal transduction to the nucleus [6]. Several ErbB ligands have been identified thus far, including EGF [7,8], transforming growth factor-α (TGF-α) [9], amphiregulin (AREG) [10], heparin-binding EGF-like growth factor (HB-EGF) [11], betacellulin (BC) [12], epiregulin (EREG) [13], epigen (EPG) [14] and neuregulins (NRGs) [15]. All ErbB ligands exist as membrane-anchored precursors that are released in an active form by enzymatic cleavage to the extracellular milieu. Matrix metalloproteinases (MMPs) and A disintegrin and metalloproteinases (ADAMs) were found to be responsible for the shedding of ErbB ligands [16–18]. The main sheddases of ErbB ligands are ADAM-10 and -17. ADAM-10 was reported to release EGF and BC [18], whereas ADAM-17 to cleave TGF-α, AREG, HB-EGF and EREG. In addition, MMP-3 was described to release HB-EGF from rat ventral prostate epithelial cells [17].

EGF is a prototype member of the ErbB ligand family. This polypeptide was originally identified in the submaxillary glands of mice and the urine of humans. EGF was discovered by Stanley Cohen while working with Rita Levi-Montalcini on nerve growth factors. For these discoveries, Stanley Cohen and Rita Levi-Montalcini were awarded the Nobel Prize in Physiology or Medicine in 1986 [19]. EGF, TGF-α, AREG and EPG only interact with ErbB1, while EREG, BC and HB-EGF bind to ErbB1 and ErbB4. A heterogeneous group of ligands called neuregulins (NRG) interacts with ErbB3 and ErbB4 [15] (Figure 1). The NRG family is composed of NRG1 isoforms, NRG2 (also known as neural- and thymus-derived activator for ErbB kinases (NTAK)) [11,20], NRG3 [21] and NRG4 [22]. The different NRG1 isoforms can be categorized into three smaller groups: type I NRG1, which includes heregulins (HRGs) [23], neu differentiation factor (NDF) [24,25] and acetylcholine receptor-inducing activity (ARIA) [26]; type II NRG1, which contains the glial growth factors (GGFs) [24] and type III NRG1, which comprises the sensory and motor neuron-derived factor (SMDF) [27]. While NRG1 and NRG2 bind to ErbB3 and ErbB4, NRG3 and NRG4 only interact with ErbB4 [15] (see Figure 1).

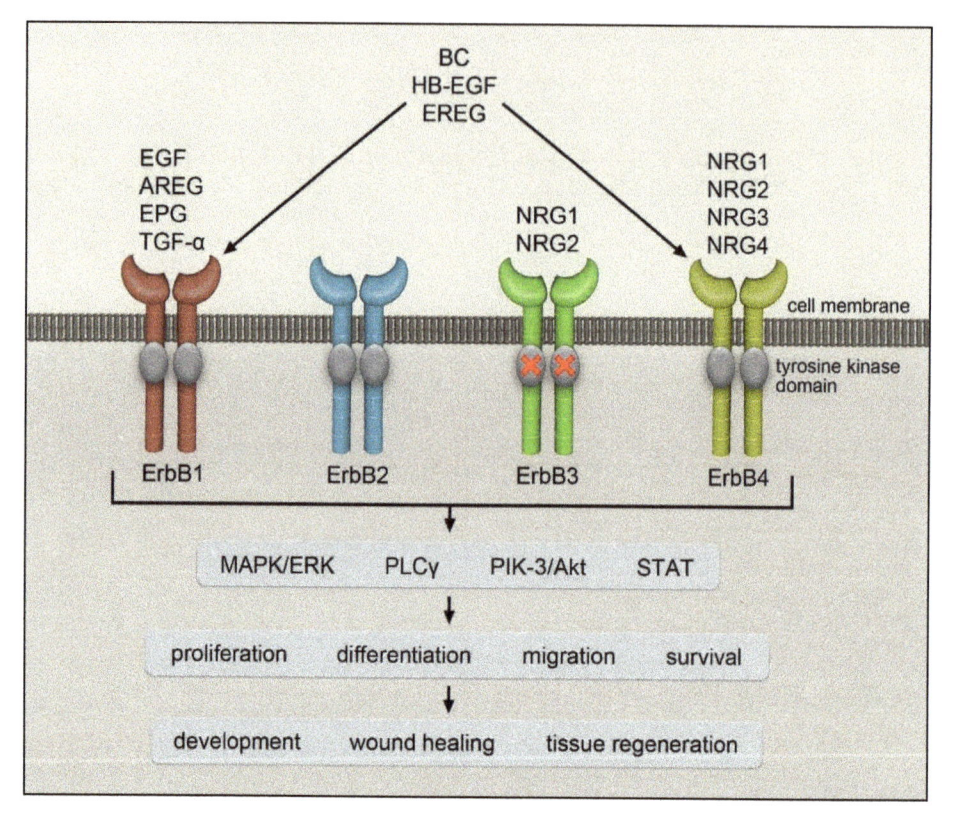

Figure 1. ErbB receptors and their ligands. ErbB2 has no known ligand, while ErbB3 lacks intrinsic kinase activity (indicated by a cross). Following ligand binding, the receptors activate several downstream signaling pathways thereby regulating cell growth, proliferation, and survival. These processes play an important role in development, wound healing and tissue regeneration. EGF, epidermal growth factor; TGFα, transforming growth factor-α; EPG, epigen; AREG, amphiregulin; EREG, epiregulin; BC, betacellulin; HB-EGF, heparin-binding EGF-like growth factor; NRG1-4, neuregulin 1-4; STAT, signal transducer and activator of transcription; MAPK/ERK, mitogen-activated protein kinase/extracellular signal-regulated kinase; PIK3/Akt, phosphoinositide 3-kinase/protein kinase B; PLCγ, phospholipase Cγ.

So far, there is no known ligand for the ErbB2 receptor [28], however, ErbB2 is a preferred partner when forming heterodimers with other ErbB receptors [29]. For instance, binding of EGF to ErbB1 may induce phosphorylation of ErbB2 [30] and thus marked amplification of a signal. Furthermore, binding of NRG1 or NRG2 to ErbB3, which lacks intrinsic catalytic activity, can trigger ErbB3 phosphorylation by the kinase-active partner ErbB2 and thus transduction of a potent mitogenic signal [31].

Upon ligand binding, ErbB receptors trigger phosphorylation of diverse effector proteins and activation of multiple downstream signaling pathways. There is a number of excellent reviews describing downstream signaling pathways initiated by ErbB receptors for those interested in this topic [8,15]. Here, only some of the major ErbB downstream signaling pathways are listed. These include: mitogen-activated protein kinase (MAPK)/extracellular signal-regulated kinase (ERK) pathway [32], phosphoinositide 3-kinase (PIK3)/protein kinase B (Akt) pathway [33], phospholipase Cγ (PLCγ) pathway [34], or signal transducers and activators of transcription (STAT) pathway [8]. Activation of the ErbB receptors regulates cell growth, proliferation, and survival and it is associated with a number of biological processes such as organ development, tissue regeneration, and wound healing [35]. The importance of the ErbB-mediated signaling for organogenesis is underscored by the studies showing that inhibition of ErbB1 impairs the development of epithelia in almost every organ including the heart [36], skin [37], lung, brain, kidney and liver [38,39], leading to mouse death shortly after birth [37,39]. Deficiency in single ErbB ligands results in similar pathological changes as the lack of the receptors themselves [40,41].

Besides its role in many developmental and physiological processes, overactivation of ErbB signaling has been widely described in many forms of cancer, including glioblastoma [42] and lung [43], breast and ovarian cancer [44–46]. These findings led to the development of ErbB signaling inhibitors for the treatment of the aforementioned pathologies [47,48]. Emerging interest in the ErbB signaling and its function during carcinogenesis brought attention to the role of the ErbB receptors and their ligands in other hyperproliferative diseases including lung fibrosis [49].

In this review, we will focus on the ErbB signaling in lung fibrosis, with special emphasis on idiopathic pulmonary fibrosis (IPF). We will discuss the implications of the ErbB signaling in processes that are hallmarks of the maladaptive remodeling of lung tissue. Lastly, we will critically discuss recent advances and future perspectives in targeting the ErbB signaling for lung fibrosis therapy.

2. Idiopathic Pulmonary Fibrosis

Idiopathic pulmonary fibrosis (IPF) is one of the most common forms of diffuse parenchymal lung diseases and is characterized by excessive deposition of extracellular matrix proteins in the lung [50]. IPF is an age-related disease, and with the human population aging worldwide, the economic burden of IPF is expected to constantly increase in the future. The pathomechanism of IPF remains elusive, with preferred concepts of disease pathobiology involving recurrent microinjuries to a genetically predisposed alveolar epithelium, followed by an abnormal activation of mesenchymal cells ((myo)fibroblasts), their expansion and massive accumulation of collagens in the lung. Aggregates of active (myo)fibroblasts, so-called fibroblastic foci, are typical histological features of IPF [50]. Fibroblastic foci are often covered by aberrant basaloid cells [51] and MUC5B-producing airway secretory cells [52]. Repopulation of alveoli by abnormal airway epithelial cells is associated with the formation of honeycomb cysts, which are indicators of advanced fibrosis and poor prognosis [50]. Active involvement of airway epithelial cells in the pathogenesis of IPF is reinforced by the fact that the gain-of-function *MUC5B* promoter variant rs35705950 is the dominant risk factor for disease development [53]. Although, it is not entirely clear how increased expression of MUC5B contributes to IPF pathobiology, the study by Hancock et al. [52] linked MUC5B overexpression to impaired mucociliary clearance accompanied by progressive lung tissue scarring.

Increased expression of several cytokine/growth factors have been considered to drive profibrotic processes in the lung, including transforming growth factor-β1 (TGF-β1), platelet-derived growth factor-BB (PDGF-BB), connective tissue growth factor (CTGF), vascular endothelial growth factor (VEGF), and tumor necrosis factor-α (TNF-α). These mediators contribute to lung tissue scarring by deregulating activation, survival, proliferation, and differentiation of a variety of cells, including mesenchymal and epithelial cells [54,55].

For instance, TGF-β1, which is stored in the ECM in a latent form and activated by cell contractile forces, drives the conversion of fibroblasts to matrix-producing myofibroblasts. Excessive deposition of ECM and its stiffening lower the threshold for TGF-β1 activation thereby creating a self-amplifying loop that promotes the expansion of myofibroblasts and fibrosis development [56]. These processes may be enhanced by factors such as interleukin (IL)-6, IL-1β, or TNF-α, which potentiate TGF-β1 expression and activation of the TGF-β1 signaling pathway [57,58]. All these changes are aggravated by the resistance of IPF (myo)fibroblasts to apoptosis [59].

Despite the approval of pirfenidone [60] and nintedanib [61], IPF has a very poor prognosis with a life expectancy of 3–5 years once diagnosed [54]. Thus, lung transplantation still remains the only treatment option that markedly improves the quality of life and survival of IPF patients [50]. Both pirfenidone and nintedanib delay disease progression by exerting pleiotropic effects, which range from the inhibition of inflammatory processes to the blockage of fibroblast proliferation and ECM production. Although the pirfenidone mode of action remains elusive, several studies demonstrated the direct impact of this drug on the Hedgehog and TGF-β signaling pathways [60,62]. In contrast to pirfenidone, nintedanib is a tyrosine kinase inhibitor (TKI) of PDGF, VEGF, and fibroblast growth factor (FGF) receptors. In addition, it also inhibits a narrow range of other targets at pharmacologically-relevant doses including the Src family and Flt-3 kinases. Ligands of PDGF, VEGF, and FGF receptors are known to have potent profibrotic effects [61]. While the approval of pirfenidone and nintedanib was a milestone in the care of IPF, there is still a high and unmet clinical need in this patient group. A multi-targeted approach, potentially with combination therapies and the identification of subsets of IPF patients who may respond more favorably to specific agents, are likely to dominate future clinical studies.

Targeting ErbB receptors and their ligands may serve as a potential therapeutic option for IPF, in particular, that different elements of the ErbB signaling can be pharmacologically targeted. However, a complex ligand–receptor network and the involvement of the ErbB signaling in the tissue regenerative process may encounter some unexpected surprises, thus further studies critically evaluating the role of ErbB receptors and their ligands in adaptive versus maladaptive remodeling of lung tissue are urgently needed.

3. ErbB Receptor–Ligand System in Lung Fibrosis

ErbB receptors and their ligands are expressed in a large variety of human tissues including the epithelial cells of the lung [63]. Under physiological conditions, ErbB1–4 are expressed in bronchial epithelial and alveolar type II (ATII) cells [64,65], whereas ErbB ligands, such as TGF-α, AREG, and HB-EGF, are expressed in bronchial epithelial cells [65]. Furthermore, TGF-α, AREG, HB-EGF, BTC, and EGF are produced in serous acinar cells from submucosal glands beneath the respiratory epithelium [64]. In cell culture, naïve lung fibroblasts were found to express TGF-α, HB-EGF, HRG and AREG but not BTC [66].

Increased expression of various ErbB ligands is associated with fibrosis development in multiple organs, including, lung, liver, or pancreas. For example, overexpression of HB-EGF and AREG causes pancreatic fibrosis [67,68], while high levels of AREG alone are sufficient to trigger liver fibrosis [69]. Furthermore, increased expression of EPG results in the fibrosis of the nerve system, and overexpression of TGF-α is associated with fibrosis of the lung [70]. Interestingly, deficiency of HB-EGF is linked to liver fibrosis [71], thus pointing towards a dual and organ-specific role of the ErbB receptor–ligand system in the tissue scarring processes. Below, we provide evidence for a dual ("good" versus "bad") role of ErbB receptors and their ligands in lung fibrosis and, in particular, in IPF.

3.1. ErbB1/EGFR Receptor

Besides being overexpressed in many types of cancer, ErbB1 is also upregulated in lung epithelial cells from patients with different forms of pulmonary fibrosis [72]. In IPF, abundant ErbB1 immunostaining was found in the hyperplastic alveolar epithelium surrounding areas of fibrosis and inflammation. In addition, increased ErbB1 protein levels were reported in IPF fibroblastic foci and in fibroblasts isolated from IPF lungs [73]. Furthermore, IPF lung fibroblast (LF)-derived culture supernatants were found to stimulate expression of ErbB1 in donor LF in an FGF-dependent manner [73]. In addition, a negative correlation between ErbB1 mRNA levels and the indicators of IPF progression, such as forced vital capacity (FVC) and diffusion capacity of the lung for carbon monoxide (DLCO) [72], was reported.

After the introduction of ErbB1 TKI to cancer therapy, the discussion on their repurposing and usage in the treatment of other hyperproliferative diseases, including lung fibrosis, began. Quickly, first studies demonstrated that tyrphostin AG1478 reduces proliferation of LF and attenuates pulmonary fibrosis caused by intratracheal instillation of vanadium pentoxide in rats [74]. Another ErbB1 TKI, gefitinib, suppressed proliferation of LF and diminished pulmonary fibrosis in the bleomycin-treated mice [75,76]. In contrast, Suzuki et al. [77] demonstrated that gefitinib aggravates bleomycin-induced lung fibrosis in mice by reducing the regenerative potential of alveolar epithelial cells. Although the reasons for these contradictory findings are unknown, differences in mouse strains, dosages, intervals and mode of drug application could have played a role.

Development of acute lung injury and ILD in non-small cell lung cancer (NSCLC) patients receiving gefitinib demonstrates possible deleterious effects of the ErbB1 signaling inhibition [78,79]. Interestingly, similar harmful effects were also observed in NSCLC patients treated with another ErbB1 TKI, erlotinib [80,81]. The incidence of ILD in TKI-treated NSCLC patients is ~1% worldwide [82]. In the Japanese population, it is significantly higher at ~2%. Despite this observation, the *EGFR* polymorphism leading to the genetic susceptibility to the treatment with ErbB1 TKI in the Japanese was not observed [82]. Pre-existing lung disorders, such as interstitial pneumonia or pulmonary fibrosis, male sex and history of smoking, were identified as risk factors for the development of gefitinib-associated ILD [83,84]. Considering the chemical and pharmacological similarities between gefitinib and erlotinib, the same risk factors may apply to the erlotinib-trigger ILD. In addition, radio- and chemotherapy, both used to treat cancer, seem to aggravate ErbB1 TKI-induced ILD [85]. Currently, it is not known what mechanisms lead to the development of ILD in NSCLS patients receiving gefitinib or erlotinib. However, it is increasingly recognized that the border between adaptive and maladaptive repair of the lung tissue is thin and the clue to success is maintaining the balance between all the factors involved [86].

3.2. Transforming Growth Factor-α

Among all ErbB1 ligands, TGF-α is the one with a well-described function in pulmonary fibrosis. TGF-α was found to be overexpressed in ATII cells, endothelial cells and fibroblasts in the lungs of IPF patients [87]. In addition, its levels were reported to be increased in IPF bronchoalveolar lavage fluid (BALF) [88]. The profibrotic potential of TGF-α was demonstrated in several studies, in which lung-specific overexpression of TGF-α in mice was conducted. For example, chronic production of TGF-α in surfactant protein-C (SP-C)-expressing cells disrupted alveolar and vascular development and caused pulmonary fibrosis and pulmonary hypertension in mice [85]. Similarly, chronic conditional expression of TGF-α driven by the doxycycline-regulatable Clara cell secretory protein (dox-CCSP) promoter triggered progressive vascular adventitial, peribronchial, interstitial, and pleural fibrosis, which was independent of inflammation and TGF-β activation [89]. Further studies demonstrated transcriptional similarities between dox-CCSP-TGF-α-induced lung fibrosis and IPF, thus pointing towards an essential role of the ErbB1–TGF-α axis in the development of IPF. In the rat bleomycin model, increased immunoreactivity for TGF-α and ErbB1 was observed in macrophages, alveolar septal cells and respiratory epithelial cells. Both proteins were predominantly detected in foci of cellular proliferation and in areas of intra-alveolar fibrosis [90]. Accordingly, TGF-α-deficient mice showed reduced hydroxyproline levels and partially preserved lung structure following bleomycin application as compared to wild-type littermates [91]. Interestingly, overexpression of TGF-α under the control of SP-C promoter protected mice against acute lung injury was caused by inhalation of polytetrafluoroethylene (PTFE; teflon) fumes. Histological hallmarks of this model are pulmonary hemorrhage and inflammation. Indeed, SP-C-TGFα-transgenic mice exhibited reduced levels of IL-6 and macrophage inflammatory protein 2 in lung homogenates and decreased total protein levels and neutrophil numbers in BALF as compared to non-transgenic controls. Altogether, these findings demonstrate the etiology-dependent role of TGF-α in lung pathologies.

In line with these observations, ErbB1 TKI, gefitinib, partially reduced collagen levels and improved lung compliance, tissue and airway elastance, and airway resistance in mice overexpressing TGF-α under tetracycline-inducible CCSP (rtTA-CCSP) promoter [89]. These changes were supported by the decreased expression of several genes associated with lung parenchymal and vascular remodeling. It is worth mentioning here that gefitinib neither induced chronic lung injury nor exacerbated pulmonary fibrosis, thus supporting further studies to determine the role of ErbB1 in human lung fibrotic diseases [85,92]. Furthermore, the same group demonstrated that blockage of the ErbB1 downstream signaling mediator, PI3K, by the PX-866 pan-inhibitor reduced total lung collagen content and improved pulmonary mechanics in rtTA-CCSP-TGF-α overexpressing mice [93]. These results were recapitulated when another ErbB1 signaling pathway, MAPK/ERK, was targeted. Administration of an allosteric MEK inhibitor, ARRY-142886, prevented the progression of established lung fibrosis in rtTA-CCSP-TGF-α overexpressing mice [94]. To sum up, a growing body of evidence suggests that TGF-α-driven activation of the ErbB1 signaling pathways may play an important role in the development of lung fibrosis and that TGF-α might be amenable to targeted therapy.

3.3. Amphiregulin

Amphiregulin, another ErbB1 ligand, was discussed in the context of maladaptive remodeling of the liver and lung. In this respect, AREG-deficient mice were found to be protected against liver fibrosis induced by chronic administration of carbon tetrachloride (CCl_4) [69]. To decipher the underlying molecular mechanism, several studies focused on the link between AREG and a master regulator of fibrogenesis, TGF-β1. Zhou et al. [95] reported that stimulation of fibroblasts with TGF-β1 elevates AREG production, which in turn increases cell proliferation and the expression of profibrotic genes, such as α-smooth muscle actin, collagen 1-α1/α2, fibronectin and tenascin. These effects were reversed by the treatment of TGF-β1-stimulated fibroblasts with AREG siRNA or ErbB1 inhibitors, AG1478 or gefitinib [95]. Consistent with these in vitro findings, AREG expression was markedly increased in the lungs of dox-CC10-TGF-β1 overexpressing mice and administration of AREG siRNA or AG1478 reduced collagen content and attenuated lung fibrosis in these animals. Besides AREG, the increased expression of other ErbB1 ligands, such as EREG and HB-EGF following exposure of fibroblasts to TGF-β1, was reported [96,97]. Andrianifahanana et al. [97] documented that TGFβ-induced AREG, EREG, and HB-EGF production requires the integration of an autocrine signal from a PDGF receptor and engages a positive feedback loop through ErbB1. The same authors demonstrated the pathological relevance of PDGFR-ErbB1 cooperation in the bleomycin model of lung fibrosis. Namely, they observed that simultaneous application of imatinib (a PDGF receptor inhibitor) and lapatinib (an ErbB1/2 inhibitor) is more effective than either treatment alone. Although, there is no evidence that pirfenidone and nintedanib directly interfere with the ErbB1, their ability to inhibit TGFβ and VEGF/PDGF/FGF receptors, respectively, might influence the overall ErbB1 activity in lung fibrosis. Accordingly, Shochet et al. reported that ErbB1 expression in donor LF triggered by IPF LF-culture media depends on FGF and can be reversed by nintedanib [73]. Interconnections of ErbB1 with other signaling pathways have to be considered when designing future IPF therapies.

The complexity of AREG cellular effects is underscored by the recent publication by Stancil et al., who showed the role of the AREG–ErbB1 axis in the jamming–unjamming of airway epithelial cells in IPF. Jamming transition describes a process of epithelial cell transformation from migratory (unjammed) to non-migratory (jammed) status in the absence of wounding or cell-type changes. This transition is believed to play an important role during embryogenesis, in processes such as axis elongation and tissue development [98–100]. It was also associated with the pathogenesis of carcinomas [101] and asthma [102]. Stancil et al. [103] demonstrated in vitro that the unjammed phase is extended in distal airway epithelial cells of IPF patients and is associated with increased activity of the ErbB-YAP (Yes-Associated Protein) signaling pathway. YAP is a transcriptional co-activator, which was found to regulate epithelial progenitor cell proliferation in the lung [104] and epithelial–mesenchymal transition in lung cancer cells following exposure to TGF-β [105]. These findings are supported by the increased levels of AREG in IPF distal airway epithelial cells and its ability to induce jammed to unjammed transition in controlling distal airway epithelial cells in vitro [103]. Interestingly, the AREG-triggered extended unjammed phase of distal airway epithelial cells correlated with activation of the fibroblasts lying underneath [103], thus providing ample evidence for the contribution of airways epithelial cells repopulating distal parts of IPF lungs to the disease progression. The association between the AREG-driven prolonged unjammed status of distal airway epithelial cells and the gain-of-function *MUC5B* promotor variant underscores this assumption.

Besides its "bad" role in lung fibrosis, AREG was also found to contribute to the restoration of tissue homeostasis after acute lung injury driven by infection. Minutti et al. [106] showed that macrophage-derived AREG promotes TGF-β1 activation and subsequent differentiation of pericytes into collagen-producing myofibroblasts leading to restoration of vascular integrity in injured tissue and wound healing. Thus, not only TGF-β1 may regulate AREG expression but vice versa AREG can control the levels of active TGF-β1. It seems that the first scenario operates in fibrosis and the second under inflammatory conditions. Thus, the function of AREG may depend on its source, concentration and cellular and molecular landscape of the surrounding area. Although further research is needed to decipher the function of AREG in acute versus chronic pathological conditions, it becomes clear that identification of dynamics and causal flows in complex AREG signaling networks is crucial for its use as a therapeutic target. This assumption is supported by the study demonstrating attenuation of bleomycin-induced lung fibrosis upon AREG application during the late inflammatory phase [107]. This observation is in sharp contrast to the lung fibrosis reports mentioned above but it may be explained by the findings of Minutti et al. [106], namely, the AREG effects on blood vessel regeneration and thus epithelial cell survival in acute lung injury [95]. Overall, it seems that AREG properties may depend on the genetic background and the immune system condition, thus preselecting the potential responders prior to the treatment may raise the possibility of the success of an anti-AREG therapy in IPF.

3.4. ErbB2 and ErbB3 Receptors and Their Ligands

Another ErbB receptor that was linked to pulmonary fibrosis is ErbB2. Besides being an important oncogene in breast and ovarian cancer [44], ErbB2 was found to be involved in epithelial cell recovery upon acute lung injury. While ErbB2 was detected on the basolateral side of airway epithelial cells, HRG-α was only found in the apical membrane of these cells and in the overlying mucus film [108]. When epithelial integrity is disrupted, HRG-α translocates to Erb2 and enables a rapid response to injury. Thus, the Erb2-HRG-α systems sense changes in the extracellular environment and ensure restoration of barrier function that may be critical for survival. As there is no known ligand for ErbB2, this receptor is able to transduce intracellular signaling only upon forming a complex with other ErbB receptors. In pulmonary epithelial cells, ErbB2 is the preferred binding partner for ErbB3. Besides being engaged in the HRG-α-triggered intracellular signaling, the ErbB2–ErbB3 complex also responds to NRG1. Using a dominant-negative mutant of ErbB3 expressed under the SP-C promotor, Nethery et al. [109] demonstrated that SP-C-ErbB3 transgenic mice exhibit reduce collagen levels in the lung and better survival following bleomycin administration. The effect was associated with the inability of NRG1 to signal *via* the nonfunctional ErbB2–ErbB3 complex. These findings are corroborated by Faress et al. [110], who reported preserved lung structure and diminished lung collagen content upon administration of an anti-ErbB2 antibody (2C4) to bleomycin-treated mice.

The important role of ErbB2 in bronchial epithelial cell differentiation and proliferation was shown by Vermeer et al. [66]. These authors demonstrated that treatment of airway epithelial cells with an anti-ErbB2 antibody, trastuzumab, induces their de-differentiation associated with an increase in the numbers of non-ciliated and metaplastic, flat cells. By contrast, the exposure of the cells to HRG-α preserved normal differentiation of airway epithelial cells. Most interestingly, co-culturing of airway epithelial cells with fibroblasts potentiated epithelial cell differentiation comparable to that achieved following treatment with HRG-α, pointing towards the ability of fibroblasts to produce ErbB ligands. Indeed, further studies demonstrated that normal human LF express TGF-α, HB-EGF, EREG, AREG, and HRG-α [66]. These observations were in line with the clinical case report describing reversible changes in airway epithelial cell differentiation of a breast cancer patient that coincided with the initiation and discontinuation of a trastuzumab therapy [66].

The ErbB3–NRG1-α axis was also discussed in the context of alveolar bronchiolization seen in the lungs of IPF patients. In these patients, NRG1-α was detected in epithelial cells lining honeycombing areas, as well as in normal submucosal glands [111]. In addition, elevated levels of this molecule were measured in IPF BALF [112]. Given the ability of NRG1-α to regulate airway mucus cell differentiation and MUC5B expression, it is worth speculating about its pivotal role in airway epithelial cell reprogramming and thus honeycomb cyst formation in IPF [113].

Taken together, it seems that ErbB2–ErbB3 activation is essential for the differentiation of airway epithelial cells and their integrity. Overactivation of this receptor complex system may induce abnormal behavior of airway epithelial cells thereby contributing to the honeycomb cyst formation and fibrosis progression. Because of the risks associated with the ErbB2–ErbB3 complex inhibition, close patient monitoring and patient categorization have to be taken into account when considering an anti-ErbB2–ErbB3 therapy in IPF.

4. Conclusions

A growing body of evidence suggests the pivotal role of the ErbB-ligand system in irreversible lung tissue scarring (Figure 2). The ErbB receptors and ligands were found to be overexpressed in IPF lungs and a number of preclinical studies demonstrated their pro-fibrotic properties in the loss-of-function and gain-of-function approaches. In addition, the therapeutic application of ErbB receptor/ligand inhibitors was often associated with favorable outcomes in lung fibrosis models (see Table 1). However, in view of the multi-functionality of the ErbB receptor–ligand system and its role in tissue regeneration, concern remains. Identification of dynamics and causal flows in the ligand–ErbB signaling network in acute versus chronic lung injury will be a prerequisite to maximize the chance of success of anti-ErbB/ligand agents in the clinical trials for IPF.

In addition, a lesson has to be also drawn from the remarkable progress in understanding the ErbB biology in cancer. It is now clear that the results of clinical trials can only be improved by taking into account a number of important issues. First, the effects of the targeted therapy may be weakened because of differences in etiology and heterogeneity. Furthermore, stratification of the patients according to a predominant disease mechanism have to be considered. Molecular endotyping should be integrated into the protocols of clinical trials. This strategy may promote the prudent use of novel targeted therapies. Finally, identification of the factors that can predict drug response or resistance will play a fundamental role to tailor individual ErbB-based therapy regimens.

in vitro

- ErbB1 activation induces survival and proliferation of LF
- LF express TGF-α, HB-EGF, EREG, AREG and HRG-α
- TGF-β potentiates expression of AREG, EREG and HB-EGF in LF
- AREG increases proliferation of LF and expression of profibrotic genes in these cells
- AREG induces jammed to unjammed transition in distal airway epithelial cells contributing to their abnormal behaviour
- HRG-α-ErbB2 axis is involved in restoration of airway epithelial cell integrity following mechanical injury
- ErbB2 regulates airway epithelial cell differentiation
- Macrophage-derived AREG stimulates TGF-β expression in pericytes thereby driving their differentiation to myofibroblasts

in vivo

- Expression of TGF-α, AREG, and ErbB1 is elevated in fibrotic lungs
- Overexpression of TGF-α under control of CCSP or SP-C promoter causes lung fibrosis in mice
- TGF-α deficient mice are protected against bleomycin - induced lung fibrosis
- Tyrphostin attenuates pulmonary fibrosis caused by intratracheal instillation of vanadium pentoxide in rats
- Gefitinib and lapatinib diminish bleomycin - triggered lung fibrosis in mice
- Gefitinib, PI3K inhibitor (PX-866), or MEK inhibitor (ARRY-142886) reduce lung fibrosis in mice overexpressing TGF-α under control of CCSP
- Mice overexpressing dominant negative mutant of ErbB3 under control of SP-C promotor exhibit reduced lung fibrosis following bleomycin administration
- Anti-ErbB2 antibody (2C4) decreases bleomycin - induced lung fibrosis in mice
- **AREG application attenuates bleomycin - triggered lung fibrosis in mice**
- **Overexpression of TGF-α under control of SP-C promoter protects mice against acute lung injury caused by inhalation of polytetrafluoroethylene (teflon)**

In IPF

- ErbB1 is expressed in hyperplastic alveolar epithelium and fibroblast foci in IPF lungs
- TGF-α is produced by ATII cells, endothelial cells and fibroblasts in IPF lungs
- AREG expression is eleavted in distal airway epithelial cells in IPF lungs
- NRG1-α is detected in epithelial cells lining honeycombing areas in IPF lungs
- TGF-α and NRG1 levels are increased in IPF BALF
- ErbB1 mRNA levels negatively correlate with FCV adn DL$_{CO}$ of IPF patients
- **Gefitinib and erlotinib cause ILD in NSCLC patients**

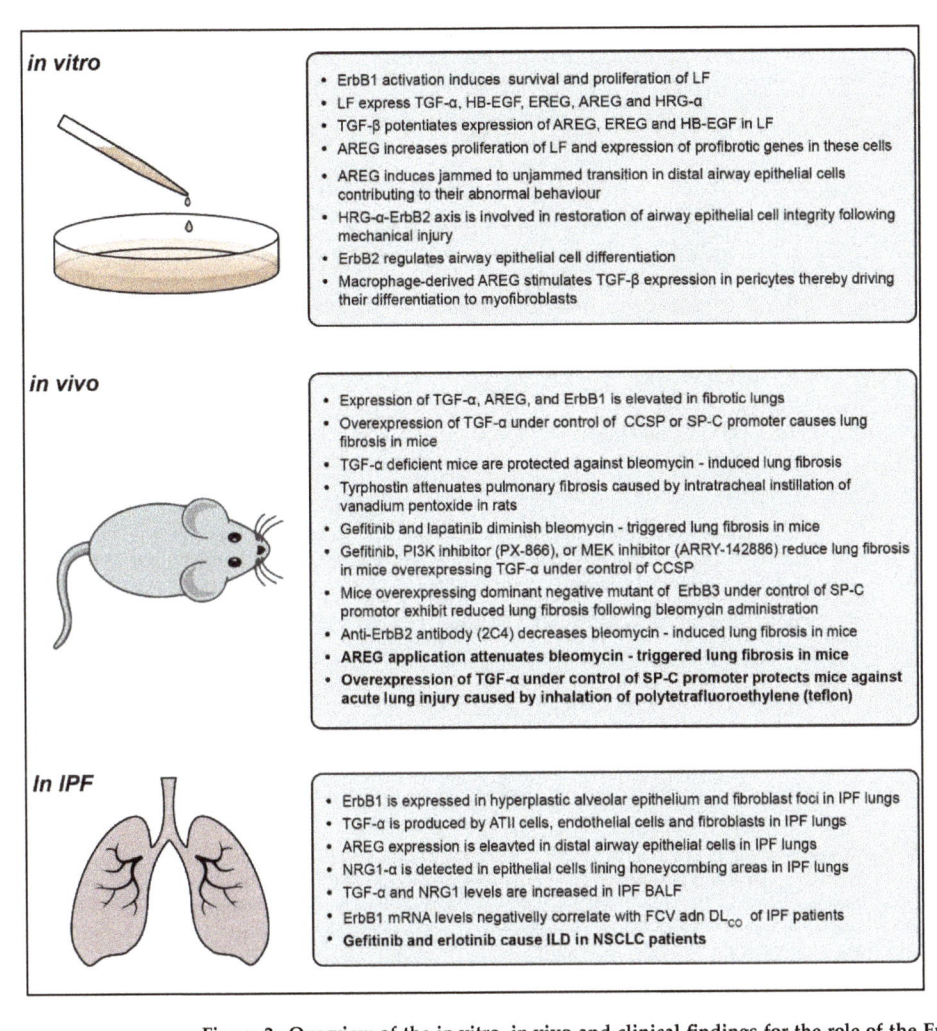

Figure 2. Overview of the in vitro, in vivo and clinical findings for the role of the ErbB/ligand system in lung fibrosis. LF, lung fibroblasts; TGFα, transforming growth factor-α; HB-EGF, heparin-binding epidermal growth factor-like growth factor; EREG, epiregulin; *AREG*, amphiregulin; HRG-α, heregulins; TGF-β, transforming growth factor-β; CCSP, Clara cell secretory protein; SP-C, surfactant protein-C; PI3K, phosphoinositide 3-kinase; MEK, mitogen-activated protein kinase kinase; IPF, idiopathic pulmonary fibrosis; ATII cells, alveolar type II cells; NRG1α, neuregulin-1α; BALF, bronchoalveolar lavage fluid; FVC, forced vital capacity; DL$_{CO}$, diffusion capacity of the lung for carbon monoxide; ILD, interstitial lung disease; NSCLC, non-small-cell lung cancer.

Table 1. Anti-ErbB/ligand approaches in preclinical models of lung fibrosis.

Targeted Molecule	Inhibitor/Antibody	Animal Model	Outcome	Reference
ErbB1	AG1478	Vanadium pentoxide	Favorable	Rice et al., 1999 [73]
ErbB1	Gefitinib	Bleomycin	Favorable	Ishii et al., 2006 [75]; Wang et al., 2010 [74]
ErbB1	Gefitinib	Bleomycin	Harmful	Suzuki et al., 2003 [76]
ErbB1	Gefitinib	rtTA-CCSP [4]-TGF-α [5]	Favorable	Hardie et al. 2004 [88]
PI3K [1]	PX-866	rtTA-CCSP-TGF-α	Favorable	Hardie et al., 2010 [92]
MEK [2]	ARRY-142886	rtTA-CCSP-TGF-α	Favorable	Madala et al., 2012 [93]
AREG [3]	AREG siRNA	dox-CC10 [6]-TGF-β1 [7]	Favorable	Zhou et al., 2012 [94]
ErbB1	AG1478	dox-CC10-TGF-β1	Favorable	Zhou et al., 2012 [94]
ErbB1/2	Lapatinib	Bleomycin	Favorable	Andrianifahanana et al., 2013 [96]
ErbB2	anti-ErbB2 antibody (2C4)	Bleomycin	Favorable	Faress et al., 2007 [109]

[1] PI3K, phosphoinositide 3-kinase; [2] MEK, mitogen-activated protein kinase; [3] AREG, amphiregulin; [4] rtTA-CCSP, tetracycline-inducible Clara cell secretory protein; [5] TGF-α, transforming growth factor α; [6] dox-CC10, doxycycline-regulatable Clara cell 10-kDa protein; [7] TGF-β, transforming growth factor β1.

Author Contributions: Conceptualization, F.S.; original draft preparation, F.S. and M.W.; review and editing, F.S., L.S. and M.W.; discussions and suggestions, M.W. All authors have read and agreed to the published version of the manuscript.

Funding: M.W. acknowledges financial support from the German Center for Lung Research (82 DZL 005A1).

Institutional Review Board Statement: Not applicable.

Informed Consent Statement: Not applicable.

Data Availability Statement: Not applicable.

Conflicts of Interest: The authors declare no conflict of interest.

References

1. Cohen, S.; Carpenter, G.; King, L. Epidermal growth factor-receptor-protein kinase interactions. Co-purification of receptor and epidermal growth factor-enhanced phosphorylation activity. *J. Biol. Chem.* **1980**, *255*, 4834–4842. [CrossRef]
2. Ullrich, A.; Coussens, L.; Hayflick, J.S.; Dull, T.J.; Gray, A.; Tam, A.W.; Lee, J.; Yarden, Y.; Libermann, T.A.; Schlessinger, J. Human epidermal growth factor receptor cDNA sequence and aberrant expression of the amplified gene in A431 epidermoid carcinoma cells. *Nature* **1984**, *309*, 418–425. [CrossRef] [PubMed]
3. Yamamoto, T.; Ikawa, S.; Akiyama, T.; Semba, K.; Nomura, N.; Miyajima, N.; Saito, T.; Toyoshima, K. Similarity of protein encoded by the human c-erb-B-2 gene to epidermal growth factor receptor. *Nature* **1986**, *319*, 230–234. [CrossRef] [PubMed]
4. Kraus, M.H.; Issing, W.; Miki, T.; Popescu, N.C.; Aaronson, S.A. Isolation and characterization of ERBB3, a third member of the ERBB/epidermal growth factor receptor family: Evidence for overexpression in a subset of human mammary tumors. *Proc. Natl. Acad. Sci. USA* **1989**, *86*, 9193–9197. [CrossRef]
5. Plowman, G.D.; Culouscou, J.M.; Whitney, G.S.; Green, J.M.; Carlton, G.W.; Foy, L.; Neubauer, M.G.; Shoyab, M. Ligand-specific activation of HER4/p180erbB4, a fourth member of the epidermal growth factor receptor family. *Proc. Natl. Acad. Sci. USA* **1993**, *90*, 1746–1750. [CrossRef] [PubMed]
6. Yarden, Y.; Schlessinger, J. Self-phosphorylation of epidermal growth factor receptor: Evidence for a model of intermolecular allosteric activation. *Biochemistry* **1987**, *26*, 1434–1442. [CrossRef] [PubMed]
7. Cohen, S. Isolation of a Mouse Submaxillary Gland Protein Accelerating Incisor Eruption and Eyelid Opening in the New-born Animal. *J. Biol. Chem.* **1962**, *237*, 1555–1562. [CrossRef]
8. Jones, S.; Rappoport, J.Z. Interdependent epidermal growth factor receptor signalling and trafficking. *Int. J. Biochem. Cell Biol.* **2014**, *51*, 23–28. [CrossRef]
9. Marquardt, H.; Hunkapiller, M.W.; Hood, L.E.; Todaro, G.J. Rat transforming growth factor type 1: Structure and relation to epidermal growth factor. *Science* **1984**, *223*, 1079–1082. [CrossRef]
10. Shoyab, M.; Plowman, G.D.; McDonald, V.L.; Bradley, J.G.; Todaro, G.J. Structure and function of human amphiregulin: A member of the epidermal growth factor family. *Science* **1989**, *243 Pt 1*, 1074–1076. [CrossRef]
11. Higashiyama, S.; Abraham, J.A.; Miller, J.; Fiddes, J.C.; Klagsbrun, M. A heparin-binding growth factor secreted by macrophage-like cells that is related to EGF. *Science* **1991**, *251*, 936–939. [CrossRef] [PubMed]

12. Shing, Y.; Christofori, G.; Hanahan, D.; Ono, Y.; Sasada, R.; Igarashi, K.; Folkman, J. Betacellulin: A mitogen from pancreatic beta cell tumors. *Science* **1993**, *259*, 1604–1607. [CrossRef] [PubMed]
13. Komurasaki, T.; Toyoda, H.; Uchida, D.; Morimoto, S. Epiregulin binds to epidermal growth factor receptor and ErbB-4 and induces tyrosine phosphorylation of epidermal growth factor receptor, ErbB-2, ErbB-3 and ErbB-4. *Oncogene* **1997**, *15*, 2841–2848. [CrossRef] [PubMed]
14. Strachan, L.; Murison, J.G.; Prestidge, R.L.; Sleeman, M.A.; Watson, J.D.; Kumble, K.D. Cloning and biological activity of epigen, a novel member of the epidermal growth factor superfamily. *J. Biol. Chem.* **2001**, *276*, 18265–18271. [CrossRef] [PubMed]
15. Yarden, Y.; Sliwkowski, M.X. Untangling the ErbB signalling network. Nature reviews. *Mol. Cell Biol.* **2001**, *2*, 127–137.
16. Harris, R. EGF receptor ligands. *Exp. Cell Res.* **2003**, *284*, 2–13. [CrossRef]
17. Suzuki, M.; Raab, G.; Moses, M.A.; Fernandez, C.A.; Klagsbrun, M. Matrix metalloproteinase-3 releases active heparin-binding EGF-like growth factor by cleavage at a specific juxtamembrane site. *J. Biol. Chem.* **1997**, *272*, 31730–31737. [CrossRef]
18. Sahin, U.; Weskamp, G.; Kelly, K.; Zhou, H.-M.; Higashiyama, S.; Peschon, J.; Hartmann, D.; Saftig, P.; Blobel, C.P. Distinct roles for ADAM10 and ADAM17 in ectodomain shedding of six EGFR ligands. *J. Cell Biol.* **2004**, *164*, 769–779. [CrossRef]
19. NobelPrize.org. Available online: https://www.nobelprize.org/prizes/medicine/1986/summary/ (accessed on 22 January 2022).
20. Chang, H.; Riese, D.J.; Gilbert, W.; Stern, D.F.; McMahan, U.J. Ligands for ErbB-family receptors encoded by a neuregulin-like gene. *Nature* **1997**, *387*, 509–512. [CrossRef]
21. Zhang, D.; Sliwkowski, M.X.; Mark, M.; Frantz, G.; Akita, R.; Sun, Y.; Hillan, K.; Crowley, C.; Brush, J.; Godowski, P.J. Neuregulin-3 (NRG3): A novel neural tissue-enriched protein that binds and activates ErbB4. *Proc. Natl. Acad. Sci. USA* **1997**, *94*, 9562–9567. [CrossRef]
22. Harari, D.; Tzahar, E.; Romano, J.; Shelly, M.; Pierce, J.H.; Andrews, G.C.; Yarden, Y. Neuregulin-4: A novel growth factor that acts through the ErbB-4 receptor tyrosine kinase. *Oncogene* **1999**, *18*, 2681–2689. [CrossRef] [PubMed]
23. Holmes, W.E.; Sliwkowski, M.X.; Akita, R.W.; Henzel, W.J.; Lee, J.; Park, J.W.; Yansura, D.; Abadi, N.; Raab, H.; Lewis, G.D. Identification of heregulin, a specific activator of p185erbB2. *Science* **1992**, *256*, 1205–1210. [CrossRef] [PubMed]
24. Wen, D.; Peles, E.; Cupples, R.; Suggs, S.V.; Bacus, S.S.; Luo, Y.; Trail, G.; Hu, S.; Silbiger, S.M.; Levy, R.B.; et al. Neu differentiation factor: A transmembrane glycoprotein containing an EGF domain and an immunoglobulin homology unit. *Cell* **1992**, *69*, 559–572. [CrossRef]
25. Peles, E.; Bacus, S.S.; Koski, R.A.; Lu, H.S.; Wen, D.; Ogden, S.G.; Levy, R.B.; Yarden, Y. Isolation of the NeuHER-2 stimulatory ligand: A 44 kd glycoprotein that induces differentiation of mammary tumor cells. *Cell* **1992**, *69*, 205–216. [CrossRef]
26. Falls, D. ARIA, a protein that stimulates acetylcholine receptor synthesis, is a member of the neu ligand family. *Cell* **1993**, *72*, 801–813. [CrossRef]
27. Ho, W.H.; Armanini, M.P.; Nuijens, A.; Phillips, H.S.; Osheroff, P.L. Sensory and motor neuron-derived factor. A novel heregulin variant highly expressed in sensory and motor neurons. *J. Biol. Chem.* **1995**, *270*, 14523–14532. [CrossRef]
28. Klapper, L.N.; Glathe, S.; Vaisman, N.; Hynes, N.E.; Andrews, G.C.; Sela, M.; Yarden, Y. The ErbB-2/HER2 oncoprotein of human carcinomas may function solely as a shared coreceptor for multiple stroma-derived growth factors. *Proc. Natl. Acad. Sci. USA* **1999**, *96*, 4995–5000. [CrossRef]
29. Tzahar, E.; Levkowitz, G.; Karunagaran, D.; Yi, L.; Peles, E.; Lavi, S.; Chang, D.; Liu, N.; Yayon, A.; Wen, D. ErbB-3 and ErbB-4 function as the respective low and high affinity receptors of all Neu differentiation factor/heregulin isoforms. *J. Biol. Chem.* **1994**, *269*, 25226–25233. [CrossRef]
30. King, C.R.; Borrello, I.; Bellot, F.; Comoglio, P.; Schlessinger, J. Egf binding to its receptor triggers a rapid tyrosine phosphorylation of the erbB-2 protein in the mammary tumor cell line SK-BR-3. *EMBO J.* **1988**, *7*, 1647–1651. [CrossRef]
31. Sliwkowski, M.X.; Schaefer, G.; Akita, R.W.; Lofgren, J.A.; Fitzpatrick, V.D.; Nuijens, A.; Fendly, B.M.; Cerione, R.A.; Vandlen, R.L.; Carraway, K.L. Coexpression of erbB2 and erbB3 proteins reconstitutes a high affinity receptor for heregulin. *J. Biol. Chem.* **1994**, *269*, 14661–14665. [CrossRef]
32. Batzer, A.G.; Rotin, D.; Ureña, J.M.; Skolnik, E.Y.; Schlessinger, J. Hierarchy of binding sites for Grb2 and Shc on the epidermal growth factor receptor. *Mol. Cell. Biol.* **1994**, *14*, 5192–5201. [PubMed]
33. Rodrigues, G.A.; Falasca, M.; Zhang, Z.; Ong, S.H.; Schlessinger, J. A novel positive feedback loop mediated by the docking protein Gab1 and phosphatidylinositol 3-kinase in epidermal growth factor receptor signaling. *Mol. Cell. Biol.* **2000**, *20*, 1448–1459. [CrossRef]
34. Margolis, B.; Rhee, S.G.; Felder, S.; Mervic, M.; Lyall, R.; Levitzki, A.; Ullrich, A.; Zilberstein, A.; Schlessinger, J. EGF induces tyrosine phosphorylation of phospholipase C-II: A potential mechanism for EGF receptor signaling. *Cell* **1989**, *57*, 1101–1107. [CrossRef]
35. Zeng, F.; Harris, R.C. Epidermal growth factor, from gene organization to bedside. *Semin. Cell Dev. Biol.* **2014**, *28*, 2–11. [CrossRef] [PubMed]
36. Chen, B.; Bronson, R.T.; Klaman, L.D.; Hampton, T.G.; Wang, J.F.; Green, P.J.; Magnuson, T.; Douglas, P.S.; Morgan, J.P.; Neel, B.G. Mice mutant for Egfr and Shp2 have defective cardiac semilunar valvulogenesis. *Nat. Genet.* **2000**, *24*, 296–299. [CrossRef] [PubMed]
37. Sibilia, M.; Wagner, B.; Hoebertz, A.; Elliott, C.; Marino, S.; Jochum, W.; Wagner, E.F. Mice humanised for the EGF receptor display hypomorphic phenotypes in skin, bone and heart. *Development* **2003**, *130*, 4515–4525. [CrossRef] [PubMed]

38. Threadgill, D.W.; Dlugosz, A.A.; Hansen, L.A.; Tennenbaum, T.; Lichti, U.; Yee, D.; LaMantia, C.; Mourton, T.; Herrup, K.; Harris, R.C. Targeted disruption of mouse EGF receptor: Effect of genetic background on mutant phenotype. *Science* **1995**, *269*, 230–234. [CrossRef] [PubMed]
39. Miettinen, P.J.; Berger, J.E.; Meneses, J.; Phung, Y.; Pedersen, R.A.; Werb, Z.; Derynck, R. Epithelial immaturity and multiorgan failure in mice lacking epidermal growth factor receptor. *Nature* **1995**, *376*, 337–341. [CrossRef] [PubMed]
40. Luetteke, N.C.; Qiu, T.H.; Peiffer, R.L.; Oliver, P.; Smithies, O.; Lee, D.C. TGFα deficiency results in hair follicle and eye abnormalities in targeted and waved-1 mice. *Cell* **1993**, *73*, 263–278. [CrossRef]
41. Luetteke, N.C.; Qiu, T.H.; Fenton, S.E.; Troyer, K.L.; Riedel, R.F.; Chang, A.; Lee, D.C. Targeted inactivation of the EGF and amphiregulin genes reveals distinct roles for EGF receptor ligands in mouse mammary gland development. *Development* **1999**, *126*, 2739–2750. [CrossRef]
42. Ekstrand, A.J.; Sugawa, N.; James, C.D.; Collins, V.P. Amplified and rearranged epidermal growth factor receptor genes in human glioblastomas reveal deletions of sequences encoding portions of the N- and/or C-terminal tails. *Proc. Natl. Acad. Sci. USA* **1992**, *89*, 4309–4313. [CrossRef] [PubMed]
43. Yun, C.-H.; Boggon, T.J.; Li, Y.; Woo, M.S.; Greulich, H.; Meyerson, M.; Eck, M.J. Structures of lung cancer-derived EGFR mutants and inhibitor complexes: Mechanism of activation and insights into differential inhibitor sensitivity. *Cancer Cell* **2007**, *11*, 217–227. [CrossRef] [PubMed]
44. Slamon, D.J.; Godolphin, W.; Jones, L.A.; Holt, J.A.; Wong, S.G.; Keith, D.E.; Levin, W.J.; Stuart, S.G.; Udove, J.; Ullrich, A. Studies of the HER-2/neu proto-oncogene in human breast and ovarian cancer. *Science* **1989**, *244*, 707–712. [CrossRef] [PubMed]
45. Hynes, N. The biology of erbB-2/nue/HER-2 and its role in cancer. *Biochim. Biophys. Acta (BBA)-Rev. Cancer* **1994**, *1198*, 165–184. [CrossRef]
46. Stancovski, I.; Sela, M.; Yarden, Y. Molecular and clinical aspects of the Neu/ErbB-2 receptor tyrosine kinase. *Cancer Treat. Res.* **1994**, *71*, 161–191.
47. Fukuoka, M.; Yano, S.; Giaccone, G.; Tamura, T.; Nakagawa, K.; Douillard, J.-Y.; Nishiwaki, Y.; Vansteenkiste, J.; Kudoh, S.; Rischin, D.; et al. Multi-institutional randomized phase II trial of gefitinib for previously treated patients with advanced non-small-cell lung cancer (The IDEAL 1 Trial) corrected. *J. Clin. Oncol. Off. J. Am. Soc. Clin. Oncol.* **2003**, *21*, 2237–2246. [CrossRef] [PubMed]
48. Kris, M.G.; Natale, R.B.; Herbst, R.S.; Lynch, T.J.; Prager, D.; Belani, C.P.; Schiller, J.H.; Kelly, K.; Spiridonidis, H.; Sandler, A.; et al. Efficacy of gefitinib, an inhibitor of the epidermal growth factor receptor tyrosine kinase, in symptomatic patients with non-small cell lung cancer: A randomized trial. *JAMA* **2003**, *290*, 2149–2158. [CrossRef] [PubMed]
49. Coward, W.R.; Saini, G.; Jenkins, G. The pathogenesis of idiopathic pulmonary fibrosis. *Ther. Adv. Respir. Dis.* **2010**, *4*, 367–388. [CrossRef]
50. Travis, W.D.; Costabel, U.; Hansell, D.M.; King, T.E.; Lynch, D.A.; Nicholson, A.G.; Ryerson, C.J.; Ryu, J.H.; Selman, M.; Wells, A.U.; et al. An official American Thoracic Society/European Respiratory Society statement: Update of the international multidisciplinary classification of the idiopathic interstitial pneumonias. *Am. J. Respir. Crit. Care Med.* **2013**, *188*, 733–748. [CrossRef]
51. Adams, T.S.; Schupp, J.C.; Poli, S.; Ayaub, E.A.; Neumark, N.; Ahangari, F.; Chu, S.G.; Raby, B.A.; DeIuliis, G.; Januszyk, M.; et al. Single-cell RNA-seq reveals ectopic and aberrant lung-resident cell populations in idiopathic pulmonary fibrosis. *Sci. Adv.* **2020**, *6*, eaba1983. [CrossRef]
52. Hancock, L.A.; Hennessy, C.E.; Solomon, G.M.; Dobrinskikh, E.; Estrella, A.; Hara, N.; Hill, D.B.; Kissner, W.J.; Markovetz, M.R.; Grove Villalon, D.E.; et al. Muc5b overexpression causes mucociliary dysfunction and enhances lung fibrosis in mice. *Nat. Commun.* **2018**, *9*, 5363. [CrossRef] [PubMed]
53. Seibold, M.A.; Wise, A.L.; Speer, M.C.; Steele, M.P.; Brown, K.K.; Loyd, J.E.; Fingerlin, T.E.; Zhang, W.; Gudmundsson, G.; Groshong, S.D.; et al. A common MUC5B promoter polymorphism and pulmonary fibrosis. *N. Engl. J. Med.* **2011**, *364*, 1503–1512. [CrossRef] [PubMed]
54. King, T.E.; Pardo, A.; Selman, M. Idiopathic pulmonary fibrosis. *Lancet* **2011**, *378*, 1949–1961. [CrossRef]
55. Selman, M.; King, T.E.; Pardo, A. Idiopathic pulmonary fibrosis: Prevailing and evolving hypotheses about its pathogenesis and implications for therapy. *Ann. Intern. Med.* **2001**, *134*, 136–151. [CrossRef] [PubMed]
56. Hinz, B. Mechanical aspects of lung fibrosis: A spotlight on the myofibroblast. *Proc. Am. Thorac. Soc.* **2012**, *9*, 137–147. [CrossRef] [PubMed]
57. Epstein Shochet, G.; Bardenstein-Wald, B.; Brook, E.; Shitrit, D. Transforming growth factor beta (TGF-β) pathway activation by IPF fibroblast-derived soluble factors is mediated by IL-6 trans-signaling. *Eur. Respir.* **2020**, *56*, 3352.
58. Epstein Shochet, G.; Brook, E.; Bardenstein-Wald, B.; Shitrit, D. TGF-β pathway activation by idiopathic pulmonary fibrosis (IPF) fibroblast derived soluble factors is mediated by IL-6 trans-signaling. *Respir. Res.* **2020**, *21*, 56. [CrossRef]
59. Kulasekaran, P.; Scavone, C.A.; Rogers, D.S.; Arenberg, D.A.; Thannickal, V.J.; Horowitz, J.C. Endothelin-1 and transforming growth factor-beta1 independently induce fibroblast resistance to apoptosis via AKT activation. *Am. J. Respir. Cell Mol. Biol.* **2009**, *41*, 484–493. [CrossRef] [PubMed]
60. Noble, P.W.; Albera, C.; Bradford, W.Z.; Costabel, U.; Du Bois, R.M.; Fagan, E.A.; Fishman, R.S.; Glaspole, I.; Glassberg, M.K.; Lancaster, L.; et al. Pirfenidone for idiopathic pulmonary fibrosis: Analysis of pooled data from three multinational phase 3 trials. *Eur. Respir. J.* **2016**, *47*, 243–253. [CrossRef] [PubMed]

61. Richeldi, L.; Du Bois, R.M.; Raghu, G.; Azuma, A.; Brown, K.K.; Costabel, U.; Cottin, V.; Flaherty, K.R.; Hansell, D.M.; Inoue, Y.; et al. Efficacy and safety of nintedanib in idiopathic pulmonary fibrosis. *N. Engl. J. Med.* **2014**, *370*, 2071–2082. [CrossRef]
62. Didiasova, M.; Singh, R.; Wilhelm, J.; Kwapiszewska, G.; Wujak, L.; Zakrzewicz, D.; Schaefer, L.; Markart, P.; Seeger, W.; Lauth, M.; et al. Pirfenidone exerts antifibrotic effects through inhibition of GLI transcription factors. *FASEB J. Off. Publ. Fed. Am. Soc. Exp. Biol.* **2017**, *31*, 1916–1928. [CrossRef]
63. Kajikawa, K.; Yasui, W.; Sumiyoshi, H.; Yoshida, K.; Nakayama, H.; Ayhan, A.; Yokozaki, H.; Ito, H.; Tahara, E. Expression of epidermal growth factor in human tissues. Immunohistochemical and biochemical analysis. *Vichows Arch. A Pathol Anat* **1991**, *418*, 27–32. [CrossRef]
64. Polosa, R.; Prosperini, G.; Leir, S.H.; Holgate, S.T.; Lackie, P.M.; Davies, D.E. Expression of c-erbB receptors and ligands in human bronchial mucosa. *Am. J. Respir. Cell Mol. Biol.* **1999**, *20*, 914–923. [CrossRef]
65. Aida, S.; Tamai, S.; Sekiguchi, S.; Shimizu, N. Distribution of epidermal growth factor and epidermal growth factor receptor in human lung: Immunohistochemical and immunoelectron-microscopic studies. *Respir. Int. Rev. Thorac. Dis.* **1994**, *61*, 161–166. [CrossRef]
66. Vermeer, P.D.; Panko, L.; Karp, P.; Lee, J.H.; Zabner, J. Differentiation of human airway epithelia is dependent on erbB2. *Am. J. Physiol.-Lung Cell. Mol. Physiol.* **2006**, *291*, L175–L180. [CrossRef]
67. Wagner, M.; Weber, C.K.; Bressau, F.; Greten, F.R.; Stagge, V.; Ebert, M.; Leach, S.D.; Adler, G.; Schmid, R.M. Transgenic overexpression of amphiregulin induces a mitogenic response selectively in pancreatic duct cells. *Gastroenterology* **2002**, *122*, 1898–1912. [CrossRef]
68. Means, A.L.; Ray, K.C.; Singh, A.B.; Washington, M.K.; Whitehead, R.H.; Harris, R.C.; Wright, C.V.E.; Coffey, R.J.; Leach, S.D. Overexpression of heparin-binding EGF-like growth factor in mouse pancreas results in fibrosis and epithelial metaplasia. *Gastroenterology* **2003**, *124*, 1020–1036. [CrossRef]
69. Perugorria, M.J.; Latasa, M.U.; Nicou, A.; Cartagena-Lirola, H.; Castillo, J.; Goñi, S.; Vespasiani-Gentilucci, U.; Zagami, M.G.; Lotersztajn, S.; Prieto, J.; et al. The epidermal growth factor receptor ligand amphiregulin participates in the development of mouse liver fibrosis. *Hepatology* **2008**, *48*, 1251–1261. [CrossRef]
70. Dahlhoff, M.; Emrich, D.; Wolf, E.; Schneider, M.R. Increased activation of the epidermal growth factor receptor in transgenic mice overexpressing epigen causes peripheral neuropathy. *Biochim. Biophys. Acta* **2013**, *1832*, 2068–2076. [CrossRef]
71. Takemura, T.; Yoshida, Y.; Kiso, S.; Kizu, T.; Furuta, K.; Ezaki, H.; Hamano, M.; Egawa, M.; Chatani, N.; Kamada, Y.; et al. Conditional loss of heparin-binding EGF-like growth factor results in enhanced liver fibrosis after bile duct ligation in mice. *Biochem. Biophys. Res. Commun.* **2013**, *437*, 185–191. [CrossRef]
72. Tzouvelekis, A.; Ntolios, P.; Karameris, A.; Vilaras, G.; Boglou, P.; Koulelidis, A.; Archontogeorgis, K.; Kaltsas, K.; Zacharis, G.; Sarikloglou, E.; et al. Increased expression of epidermal growth factor receptor (EGF-R) in patients with different forms of lung fibrosis. *BioMed Res. Int.* **2013**, *2013*, 654354. [CrossRef] [PubMed]
73. Epstein Shochet, G.; Brook, E.; Eyal, O.; Edelstein, E.; Shitrit, D. Epidermal growth factor receptor paracrine upregulation in idiopathic pulmonary fibrosis fibroblasts is blocked by nintedanib. *Am. J. Physiol.-Lung Cell. Mol. Physiol.* **2019**, *316*, L1025–L1034. [CrossRef] [PubMed]
74. Rice, A.B.; Moomaw, C.R.; Morgan, D.L.; Bonner, J.C. Specific Inhibitors of Platelet-Derived Growth Factor or Epidermal Growth Factor Receptor Tyrosine Kinase Reduce Pulmonary Fibrosis in Rats. *Am. J. Pathol.* **1999**, *155*, 213–221. [CrossRef]
75. Wang, P.; Tian, Q.; Liang, Z.; Yang, Z.; Xu, S.; Sun, J.; Chen, L. Gefitinib attenuates murine pulmonary fibrosis induced by bleomycin. *Chin. Med. J.* **2010**, *123*, 2259–2264. [PubMed]
76. Ishii, Y.; Fujimoto, S.; Fukuda, T. Gefitinib prevents bleomycin-induced lung fibrosis in mice. *Am. J. Respir. Crit. Care Med.* **2006**, *174*, 550–556. [CrossRef] [PubMed]
77. Suzuki, H.; Aoshiba, K.; Yokohori, N.; Nagai, A. Epidermal growth factor receptor tyrosine kinase inhibition augments a murine model of pulmonary fibrosis. *Cancer Res.* **2003**, *63*, 5054–5059. [PubMed]
78. Inomata, S.; Takahashi, H.; Nagata, M.; Yamada, G.; Shiratori, M.; Tanaka, H.; Satoh, M.; Saitoh, T.; Sato, T.; Abe, S. Acute lung injury as an adverse event of gefitinib. *Anti-Cancer Drugs* **2004**, *15*, 461–467. [CrossRef] [PubMed]
79. Inoue, A.; Saijo, Y.; Maemondo, M.; Gomi, K.; Tokue, Y.; Kimura, Y.; Ebina, M.; Kikuchi, T.; Moriya, T.; Nukiwa, T. Severe acute interstitial pneumonia and gefitinib. *Lancet* **2003**, *361*, 137–139. [CrossRef]
80. Ten Heine, R.; van den Bosch, R.T.A.; Schaefer-Prokop, C.M.; Lankheet, N.A.G.; Beijnen, J.H.; Staaks, G.H.A.; van der Westerlaken, M.M.; Malingré, M.M.; van den Brand, J.J.G. Fatal interstitial lung disease associated with high erlotinib and metabolite levels. A case report and a review of the literature. *Lung Cancer* **2012**, *75*, 391–397. [CrossRef]
81. Ren, S.; Li, Y.; Li, W.; Zhao, Z.; Jin, C.; Zhang, D. Fatal asymmetric interstitial lung disease after erlotinib for lung cancer. *Respir. Int. Rev. Thorac. Dis.* **2012**, *84*, 431–435. [CrossRef]
82. Cohen, M.H.; Williams, G.A.; Sridhara, R.; Chen, G.; Pazdur, R. FDA drug approval summary: Gefitinib (ZD1839) (Iressa) tablets. *Oncologist* **2003**, *8*, 303–306. [CrossRef] [PubMed]
83. Akamatsu, H.; Inoue, A.; Mitsudomi, T.; Kobayashi, K.; Nakagawa, K.; Mori, K.; Nukiwa, T.; Nakanishi, Y.; Yamamoto, N. Interstitial lung disease associated with gefitinib in Japanese patients with EGFR-mutated non-small-cell lung cancer: Combined analysis of two Phase III trials (NEJ 002 and WJTOG 3405). *Jpn. J. Clin. Oncol.* **2013**, *43*, 664–668. [CrossRef] [PubMed]

84. Ando, M.; Okamoto, I.; Yamamoto, N.; Takeda, K.; Tamura, K.; Seto, T.; Ariyoshi, Y.; Fukuoka, M. Predictive factors for interstitial lung disease, antitumor response, and survival in non-small-cell lung cancer patients treated with gefitinib. *J. Clin. Oncol. Off. J. Am. Soc. Clin. Oncol.* **2006**, *24*, 2549–2556. [CrossRef]
85. Hardie, W.D.; Davidson, C.; Ikegami, M.; Leikauf, G.D.; Le Cras, T.D.; Prestridge, A.; Whitsett, J.A.; Korfhagen, T.R. EGF receptor tyrosine kinase inhibitors diminish transforming growth factor-alpha-induced pulmonary fibrosis. *Am. J. Physiol.-Lung Cell. Mol. Physiol.* **2008**, *294*, L1217–L1725. [CrossRef] [PubMed]
86. Li, C.; Wei, R.; Jones-Hall, Y.L.; Vittal, R.; Zhang, M.; Liu, W. Epidermal growth factor receptor (EGFR) pathway genes and interstitial lung disease: An association study. *Sci. Rep.* **2014**, *4*, 4893. [CrossRef]
87. Baughman, R.P.; Lower, E.E.; Miller, M.A.; Bejarano, P.A.; Heffelfinger, S.C. Overexpression of transforming growth factor-alpha and epidermal growth factor-receptor in idiopathic pulmonary fibrosis. *Sarcoidosis Vasc. Diffus. Lung Dis. Off. J. WASOG* **1999**, *16*, 57–61.
88. Madtes, D.K.; Rubenfeld, G.; Klima, L.D.; Milberg, J.A.; Steinberg, K.P.; Martin, T.R.; Raghu, G.; Hudson, L.D.; Clark, J.G. Elevated transforming growth factor-alpha levels in bronchoalveolar lavage fluid of patients with acute respiratory distress syndrome. *Am. J. Respir. Crit. Care Med.* **1998**, *158*, 424–430. [CrossRef] [PubMed]
89. Hardie, W.D.; Le Cras, T.D.; Jiang, K.; Tichelaar, J.W.; Azhar, M.; Korfhagen, T.R. Conditional expression of transforming growth factor-alpha in adult mouse lung causes pulmonary fibrosis. *Am. J. Physiol.-Lung Cell. Mol. Physiol.* **2004**, *286*, L741–L749. [CrossRef] [PubMed]
90. Madtes, D.K.; Busby, H.K.; Strandjord, T.P.; Clark, J.G. Expression of transforming growth factor-alpha and epidermal growth factor receptor is increased following bleomycin-induced lung injury in rats. *Am. J. Respir. Cell Mol. Biol.* **1994**, *11*, 540–551. [CrossRef]
91. Madtes, D.K.; Elston, A.L.; Hackman, R.C.; Dunn, A.R.; Clark, J.G. Transforming growth factor-alpha deficiency reduces pulmonary fibrosis in transgenic mice. *Am. J. Respir. Cell Mol. Biol.* **1999**, *20*, 924–934. [CrossRef]
92. Hardie, W.D.; Korfhagen, T.R.; Sartor, M.A.; Prestridge, A.; Medvedovic, M.; Le Cras, T.D.; Ikegami, M.; Wesselkamper, S.C.; Davidson, C.; Dietsch, M.; et al. Genomic profile of matrix and vasculature remodeling in TGF-alpha induced pulmonary fibrosis. *Am. J. Respir. Cell Mol. Biol.* **2007**, *37*, 309–321. [CrossRef] [PubMed]
93. Hardie, W.D.; Hagood, J.S.; Dave, V.; Perl, A.-K.T.; Whitsett, J.A.; Korfhagen, T.R.; Glasser, S. Signaling pathways in the epithelial origins of pulmonary fibrosis. *Cell Cycle* **2010**, *9*, 2769–2776. [CrossRef] [PubMed]
94. Madala, S.K.; Schmidt, S.; Davidson, C.; Ikegami, M.; Wert, S.; Hardie, W.D. MEK-ERK pathway modulation ameliorates pulmonary fibrosis associated with epidermal growth factor receptor activation. *Am. J. Respir. Cell Mol. Biol.* **2012**, *46*, 380–388. [CrossRef]
95. Zhou, Y.; Lee, J.-Y.; Lee, C.-M.; Cho, W.-K.; Kang, M.-J.; Koff, J.L.; Yoon, P.-O.; Chae, J.; Park, H.-O.; Elias, J.A.; et al. Amphiregulin, an epidermal growth factor receptor ligand, plays an essential role in the pathogenesis of transforming growth factor-β-induced pulmonary fibrosis. *J. Biol. Chem.* **2012**, *287*, 41991–42000. [CrossRef]
96. Andrianifahanana, M.; Wilkes, M.C.; Repellin, C.E.; Edens, M.; Kottom, T.J.; Rahimi, R.A.; Leof, E.B. ERBB receptor activation is required for profibrotic responses to transforming growth factor beta. *Cancer Res.* **2010**, *70*, 7421–7430. [CrossRef] [PubMed]
97. Andrianifahanana, M.; Wilkes, M.C.; Gupta, S.K.; Rahimi, R.A.; Repellin, C.E.; Edens, M.; Wittenberger, J.; Yin, X.; Maidl, E.; Becker, J.; et al. Profibrotic TGFβ responses require the cooperative action of PDGF and ErbB receptor tyrosine kinases. *FASEB J. Off. Publ. Fed. Am. Soc. Exp. Biol.* **2013**, *27*, 4444–4454. [CrossRef]
98. Mongera, A.; Rowghanian, P.; Gustafson, H.J.; Shelton, E.; Kealhofer, D.A.; Carn, E.K.; Serwane, F.; Lucio, A.A.; Giammona, J.; Campàs, O. A fluid-to-solid jamming transition underlies vertebrate body axis elongation. *Nature* **2018**, *561*, 401–405. [CrossRef]
99. Atia, L.; Fredberg, J.J.; Gov, N.S.; Pegoraro, A.F. Are cell jamming and unjamming essential in tissue development? *Cells Dev.* **2021**, *4*, 203727. [CrossRef]
100. Bi, D.; Lopez, J.H.; Schwarz, J.M.; Manning, M.L. A density-independent glass transition in biological tissues. *Nat. Phys.* **2015**, *11*, 1074–1079. [CrossRef]
101. Palamidessi, A.; Malinverno, C.; Frittoli, E.; Corallino, S.; Barbieri, E.; Sigismund, S.; Beznoussenko, G.V.; Martini, E.; Garre, M.; Ferrara, L.; et al. Unjamming overcomes kinetic and proliferation arrest in terminally differentiated cells and promotes collective motility of carcinoma. *Nat. Mater.* **2019**, *18*, 1252–1263. [CrossRef]
102. Park, J.-A.; Atia, L.; Mitchel, J.A.; Fredberg, J.J.; Butler, J.P. Collective migration and cell jamming in asthma, cancer and development. *J. Cell Sci.* **2016**, *129*, 3375–3383. [CrossRef] [PubMed]
103. Stancil, I.T.; Michalski, J.E.; Davis-Hall, D.; Chu, H.W.; Park, J.-A.; Magin, C.M.; Yang, I.V.; Smith, B.J.; Dobrinskikh, E.; Schwartz, D.A. Pulmonary fibrosis distal airway epithelia are dynamically and structurally dysfunctional. *Nat. Commun.* **2021**, *12*, 4566. [CrossRef] [PubMed]
104. Lange, A.W.; Sridharan, A.; Xu, Y.; Stripp, B.R.; Perl, A.-K.; Whitsett, J.A. Hippo/Yap signaling controls epithelial progenitor cell proliferation and differentiation in the embryonic and adult lung. *J. Mol. Cell Biol.* **2015**, *7*, 35–47. [CrossRef] [PubMed]
105. Choi, J.-Y.; Lee, H.; Kwon, E.-J.; Kong, H.-J.; Kwon, O.-S.; Cha, H.-J. TGFβ promotes YAP-dependent AXL induction in mesenchymal-type lung cancer cells. *Mol. Oncol.* **2021**, *15*, 679–696. [CrossRef] [PubMed]
106. Minutti, C.M.; Modak, R.V.; Macdonald, F.; Li, F.; Smyth, D.J.; Dorward, D.A.; Blair, N.; Husovsky, C.; Muir, A.; Giampazolias, E.; et al. A Macrophage-Pericyte Axis Directs Tissue Restoration via Amphiregulin-Induced Transforming Growth Factor Beta Activation. *Immunity* **2019**, *50*, 645–654.e6. [CrossRef] [PubMed]

107. Fukumoto, J.; Harada, C.; Kawaguchi, T.; Suetsugu, S.; Maeyama, T.; Inoshima, I.; Hamada, N.; Kuwano, K.; Nakanishi, Y. Amphiregulin attenuates bleomycin-induced pneumopathy in mice. *Am. J. Physiol.-Lung Cell. Mol. Physiol.* **2010**, *298*, L131–L138. [CrossRef] [PubMed]
108. Vermeer, P.D.; Einwalter, L.A.; Moninger, T.O.; Rokhlina, T.; Kern, J.A.; Zabner, J.; Welsh, M.J. Segregation of receptor and ligand regulates activation of epithelial growth factor receptor. *Nature* **2003**, *422*, 322–326. [CrossRef] [PubMed]
109. Nethery, D.E.; Moore, B.B.; Minowada, G.; Carroll, J.; Faress, J.A.; Kern, J.A. Expression of mutant human epidermal receptor 3 attenuates lung fibrosis and improves survival in mice. *J. Appl. Physiol.* **2005**, *99*, 298–307. [CrossRef]
110. Faress, J.A.; Nethery, D.E.; Kern, E.F.O.; Eisenberg, R.; Jacono, F.J.; Allen, C.L.; Kern, J.A. Bleomycin-induced pulmonary fibrosis is attenuated by a monoclonal antibody targeting HER2. *J. Appl. Physiol.* **2007**, *103*, 2077–2083. [CrossRef]
111. Plantier, L.; Crestani, B.; Wert, S.E.; Dehoux, M.; Zweytick, B.; Guenther, A.; Whitsett, J.A. Ectopic respiratory epithelial cell differentiation in bronchiolised distal airspaces in idiopathic pulmonary fibrosis. *Thorax* **2011**, *66*, 651–657. [CrossRef]
112. Rock, J.R.; Onaitis, M.W.; Rawlins, E.L.; Lu, Y.; Clark, C.P.; Xue, Y.; Randell, S.H.; Hogan, B.L.M. Basal cells as stem cells of the mouse trachea and human airway epithelium. *Proc. Natl. Acad. Sci. USA* **2009**, *106*, 12771–12775. [CrossRef] [PubMed]
113. Kettle, R.; Simmons, J.; Schindler, F.; Jones, P.; Dicker, T.; Dubois, G.; Giddings, J.; van Heeke, G.; Jones, C.E. Regulation of neuregulin 1beta1-induced MUC5AC and MUC5B expression in human airway epithelium. *Am. J. Respir. Cell Mol. Biol.* **2010**, *42*, 472–481. [CrossRef] [PubMed]

Article

FK506-Binding Protein 11 Is a Novel Plasma Cell-Specific Antibody Folding Catalyst with Increased Expression in Idiopathic Pulmonary Fibrosis

Stefan Preisendörfer [1], Yoshihiro Ishikawa [2,†], Elisabeth Hennen [1], Stephan Winklmeier [3], Jonas C. Schupp [4,5], Larissa Knüppel [1], Isis E. Fernandez [1,6], Leonhard Binzenhöfer [1], Andrew Flatley [7], Brenda M. Juan-Guardela [4], Clemens Ruppert [8], Andreas Guenther [8], Marion Frankenberger [1], Rudolf A. Hatz [9,10], Nikolaus Kneidinger [6], Jürgen Behr [6], Regina Feederle [7], Aloys Schepers [7,‡], Anne Hilgendorff [1], Naftali Kaminski [4], Edgar Meinl [3], Hans Peter Bächinger [2], Oliver Eickelberg [1,§] and Claudia A. Staab-Weijnitz [1,*]

[1] Institute of Lung Health and Immunity and Comprehensive Pneumology Center with the CPC-M bioArchive, Member of the German Center of Lung Research (DZL), Helmholtz-Zentrum München, 81377 Munich, Germany; preisendoerfer@dhm.mhn.de (S.P.); elisabeth.hennen@helmholtz-muenchen.de (E.H.); larissa.knueppel@secarna.com (L.K.); isis.fernandez@helmholtz-muenchen.de (I.E.F.); leonhard.binzenhoefer@med.uni-muenchen.de (L.B.); frankenberger@helmholtz-muenchen.de (M.F.); anne.hilgendorff@helmholtz-muenchen.de (A.H.); eickelbergo@upmc.edu (O.E.)

[2] Department of Biochemistry and Molecular Biology, Oregon Health & Science University, Portland, OR 97239, USA; yoshihiro.ishikawa@ucsf.edu (Y.I.); hanspeter.bachinger@gmail.com (H.P.B.)

[3] Institute of Clinical Neuroimmunology, Biomedical Center and LMU Klinikum, Ludwig-Maximilians-Universität München, 81377 Munich, Germany; stephan.winklmeier@med.uni-muenchen.de (S.W.); edgar.meinl@med.uni-muenchen.de (E.M.)

[4] Pulmonary, Critical Care and Sleep Medicine, Yale School of Medicine, New Haven, CT 06520, USA; jonas.schupp@yale.edu (J.C.S.); brendajuan@usf.edu (B.M.J.-G.); naftali.kaminski@yale.edu (N.K.)

[5] Department of Respiratory Medicine, Hannover Medical School, Biomedical Research in End-Stage and Obstructive Lung Disease Hannover, Member of the German Center for Lung Research (DZL), 30625 Hannover, Germany

[6] Department of Medicine V, LMU Klinikum, Ludwig-Maximilians-Universität München, Member of the German Center of Lung Research (DZL), 81377 Munich, Germany; nikolaus.kneidinger@med.uni-muenchen.de (N.K.); juergen.behr@med.uni-muenchen.de (J.B.)

[7] Monoclonal Antibody Core Facility, Institute for Diabetes and Obesity, Helmholtz-Zentrum München, 85764 Neuherberg, Germany; andrew.flatley@helmholtz-muenchen.de (A.F.); regina.feederle@helmholtz-muenchen.de (R.F.); schepers@helmholtz-munich.de (A.S.)

[8] Department of Internal Medicine, Medizinische Klinik II, Member of the German Center of Lung Research (DZL), 35392 Giessen, Germany; clemens.ruppert@innere.med.uni-giessen.de (C.R.); andreas.guenther@innere.med.uni-giessen.de (A.G.)

[9] Thoraxchirurgisches Zentrum, Klinik für Allgemeine-, Viszeral-, Transplantations-, Gefäß- und Thoraxchirurgie, LMU Klinikum, Ludwig-Maximilians-Universität München, 81377 Munich, Germany; rudolf.hatz@med.uni-muenchen.de

[10] Asklepios Fachkliniken München-Gauting, 82131 Gauting, Germany

* Correspondence: staab-weijnitz@helmholtz-muenchen.de

† Present address: Department of Ophthalmology, School of Medicine, University of California, San Francisco, CA 94117, USA.

‡ Present address: Institute of Epigenetics and Stem Cells, Helmholtz Zentrum München, 81377 Munich, Germany.

§ Present address: Pulmonary, Allergy and Critical Care Medicine, Department of Medicine, University of Pittsburgh Medical Center, Pittsburgh, PA 15213, USA.

Abstract: Antibodies are central effectors of the adaptive immune response, widespread used therapeutics, but also potentially disease-causing biomolecules. Antibody folding catalysts in the plasma cell are incompletely defined. Idiopathic pulmonary fibrosis (IPF) is a fatal chronic lung disease with increasingly recognized autoimmune features. We found elevated expression of FK506-binding protein 11 (*FKBP11*) in IPF lungs where FKBP11 specifically localized to antibody-producing plasma cells. Suggesting a general role in plasma cells, plasma cell-specific *FKBP11* expression was equally observed in lymphatic tissues, and in vitro B cell to plasma cell differentiation was accompanied by induction of *FKBP11* expression. Recombinant human FKBP11 was able to refold IgG antibody in vitro and inhibited by FK506, strongly supporting a function as antibody peptidyl-prolyl *cis-trans* isomerase. Induction of ER stress in cell lines demonstrated induction of *FKBP11* in the context of the unfolded protein response in an X-box-binding protein 1 (XBP1)-dependent manner. While deficiency of FKBP11 increased susceptibility to ER stress-mediated cell death in an alveolar epithelial cell line, FKBP11 knockdown in an antibody-producing hybridoma cell line neither induced cell death nor decreased expression or secretion of IgG antibody. Similarly, antibody secretion by the same hybridoma cell line was not affected by knockdown of the established antibody peptidyl-prolyl isomerase cyclophilin B. The results are consistent with FKBP11 as a novel XBP1-regulated antibody peptidyl-prolyl *cis-trans* isomerase and indicate significant redundancy in the ER-resident folding machinery of antibody-producing hybridoma cells.

Keywords: antibody folding; immunophilin; lung fibrosis; interstitial lung disease; ER stress; tacrolimus; FK506-binding protein; peptidyl-prolyl isomerase

1. Introduction

Plasma cell-secreted antibodies are ultimate effectors of the adaptive immune response and fundamentally important for the neutralization of pathogenic virus and bacteria [1]. Their activity relies on high-affinity binding to their cognate antigen, which requires correct folding into the functional three-dimensional structure in the endoplasmic reticulum (ER). This process is strictly dependent on an ER-resident protein folding machinery consisting of molecular chaperones, peptidyl-prolyl *cis-trans* isomerases (PPIases), disulfide isomerases, and glycosyl transferases [2,3]. During B-cell to plasma cell differentiation, components of this machinery are increased in the course of the so-called unfolded protein response (UPR) to accommodate the increasing burden of incoming nascent immunoglobulins and avoid accumulation of misfolded proteins in the ER [4,5]. X-box-binding protein 1 (XBP1) is a central transcription factor orchestrating the UPR by induction of chaperones and other protein folding catalysts during late-stage plasma cell differentiation [6–8].

Peptidyl-prolyl *cis-trans* isomerization often represents a rate-limiting step in protein folding. Prolines make up 5–10% of an antibody's primary sequence and facilitate the formation of turns connecting the β-strands in each immunoglobulin (Ig) fold. Two protein families collectively termed immunophilins exert PPIase activity in the ER, namely the FK506-binding proteins (FKBPs) and the cyclophilins [9]. Until now, limited evidence suggests that two PPIases may directly participate in antibody folding including peptidyl-prolyl *cis-trans* isomerase B (PPIB, also termed cyclophilin B, CypB) [10–13] and FKBP1A (also termed FKBP12) [14]. The latter, however, typically resides in the cytosol [15] and thus is unlikely to play a role in antibody folding in vivo.

FKBP11 (also termed FKBP19) was first described as predominantly expressed in secretory tissues including pancreas [16] and recent studies have suggested a role in beta cell survival under conditions of ER stress [17–19]. In addition, FKBP11 appears to play a role in osteoblasts and bone formation where it has been observed to associate with interferon-inducible transmembrane protein 5 (IFITM5) [20–22]. Other studies have proposed FKBP11 as a prognostic marker for hepatocellular carcinoma [23,24]. Many of the studies mentioned above point towards a role in the context of ER stress. Interestingly, gene expression profiling studies show upregulation of *FKBP11* during differentiation from B cells to antibody-secreting plasma cells and indicate that, in this context, *FKBP11* expression may be regulated by XBP1 [25,26]. Finally, overexpression of *FKBP11* in murine splenic B cells has been reported to increase initiation of plasma cell differentiation [27]. These observations suggest that FKBP11 may be involved in the plasma cell UPR and/or antibody folding but, to date, function and substrate of this protein have remained largely obscure.

Importantly, a profound understanding of mechanisms of plasma cell differentiation and antibody production may be beneficial for targeting autoimmune diseases where autoantibodies play a crucial pathogenetic role. Current treatment options include antibodies specifically targeting the B-cell lineage, the most prominent example being rituximab, a monoclonal antibody directed towards CD20, a pan B-cell surface protein [28], but B cell depletion shows a limited impact on the plasma cell population [29]. Other therapeutic options than complete B-cell depletion have proven successful in murine models of autoimmune disease, e.g., extracellular cleavage of autoantibodies [30]. Clearly, elucidation of the specific antibody folding machinery in plasma cells may contribute to the development of further therapeutic strategies. Notably, *FKBP11* is overexpressed in B-cells of patients suffering from Systemic Lupus Erythematosus, a chronic inflammatory autoimmune disease [27].

Idiopathic pulmonary fibrosis (IPF) is a fatal disease with median survival rates ranging from 3–5 years, increasing incidence worldwide, and limited treatment options [31,32]. Even if it is currently believed that IPF pathogenesis originates from micro-injuries to the airway and alveolar epithelium, the etiology of IPF is incompletely understood [33,34]. In contrast, it is well-known that many autoimmune diseases manifest in lung fibrosis [35] and studies in experimental mouse models have shown that autoantibodies can cause and promote lung fibrosis [36–39], while B-cell depletion is protective [40–42]. Notably, evidence is accumulating which also argues for significant autoimmune features in IPF: A recent proteomic study has revealed increased numbers of MZB1-positive plasma cells and higher IgG levels in tissue of patients suffering from various interstitial lung diseases (ILD) including IPF [43]. In blood of IPF patients, higher levels of circulating plasmablasts, several soluble factors that promote B cell growth and differentiation, and various autoantibodies towards lung antigens have been reported [44,45]. Finally, distinct (human leukocyte antigen (HLA) class II alleles are overrepresented in patients with IPF, thus equally supporting a role of autoimmunity in IPF aetiology [46,47].

Here, we report that FKBP11 is a novel antibody folding catalyst, levels of which are strongly increased in IPF, specifically produced by human plasma cells, and induced by the UPR in an XBP1-dependent manner.

Some of the results of these studies have been previously reported in the form of conference abstracts [48,49].

2. Materials and Methods

2.1. Patient Samples

Patient lung tissue and blood samples were obtained from the CPC-M bioArchive at the Comprehensive Pneumology Center (CPC) and from the UGMLC Giessen Biobank, member of the DZL platform biobanking. For samples from the CPC-M BioArchive and the biobank of the Institute of Clinical Neuroimmunology, the study was approved by the local Ethics Committee of Ludwig-Maximilians University of Munich, Germany (333-10, 382-10, and 163-16, respectively). Biomaterial collection by the UGMLC/DZL biobank was approved by votes from the Ethics Committee of the Justus-Liebig-University School of Medicine (111/08, and 58/15). Informed consent was obtained from each subject. The tissue microarray (Multi-normal human tissues, 96 samples, 35 organs/sites from three individuals) was from Abcam (ab178228) and contained only healthy specimens except for tonsils which were inflamed (tonsillitis).

2.2. Gene Expression Data

Gene expression data for *FKBP* genes in normal histology control ($n = 43$) and IPF lungs ($n = 99$) was extracted from microarray data generated by us on lung samples obtained from the National Lung, Heart, and Blood Institute-funded Tissue Resource Consortium (NLHBI LTRC), as described previously [50,51]. Gene expression microarray data (Agilent Technologies, Santa Clara, CA, USA) are available under accession number GSE47460 in the data set repository Gene Expression Omnibus (GEO). Significance was calculated using t statistics, and multiple testing was controlled by the false discovery rate method at 5% [52].

2.3. Cell Culture, Induction of ER Stress and Transfection

For details on culture, treatment, and transfection of A549 and Raji cells, see the online supplement. The mouse myeloma cell line P3X63-Ag8.653 (AG8) and mouse/rat hybridoma cell lines were maintained in the same manner as described for Raji cells (see online supplement).

Delivery of scrambled, anti-FKBP11, and anti-PPIB siRNA into the hybridoma cell line H3 was achieved by electroporation largely as described [53]. Briefly, hybridoma cells at a culture density between 3×10^5–5×10^5 cells/mL were spun down at $300 \times g$ and resuspended in fresh RPMI-1640 medium (Life Technologies, Carlsbad, CA, USA) without supplements at a concentration of 6×10^7 cells/mL. After addition of anti-FKBP11 siRNA (s82617, Life Technologies, targeting both rat and mouse FKBP11), anti-PPIB siRNA (s72031), or negative control siRNA No. 1 (Life Technologies) at a final concentration of 3 µM, 200 µL of the mixture were transferred to a 96-well electroporation plate (Bio-Rad, München, Germany). Electroporation was then carried out with a Gene Pulser (Bio-Rad, München) by application of a single exponential decay pulse at a capacity setting of 950 µF and a voltage of 300 V. Subsequently, cells were transferred to prewarmed full medium, incubated at 37 °C and cells and supernatant harvested after 48 h.

2.4. Plasma Cell Differentiation

PBMCs were isolated from blood of healthy volunteers using density gradient centrifugation (described in detail in the online supplement). PBMCs were transferred to prewarmed RPMI medium (Thermo Fisher Scientific, Schwerte, Germany) supplemented with 10% FBS, L-glutamine, sodium bicarbonate and non-essential amino acids and once washed. Afterwards, PBMCs were seeded in a cell culture dish at a concentration of 1×10^6 cells/mL and stimulated by 1000 U/mL of recombinant IL-2 (Roche) and 2.5 µg/mL TLR 7 + 8 ligand R848 (InvivoGen, San Diego, CA, USA), an established procedure for the induction of plasma cell transdifferentiation [54,55]. As a control, same volumes of diluents were added to PBMCs. After 7 days of incubation at 37 °C, supernatants were collected to determine IgG concentrations, cytospins were prepared, and RNA and protein was extracted from remaining cells.

For flow cytometric analysis of cell populations following stimulation, activated and differentiated cells were stained using anti-human CD3-Alexa Fluor 700 (OKT3; eBioscience, San Diego, CA, USA), CD19-APC/Fire 750 (HIB19; BioLegend, San Diego, CA, USA), CD27-Brilliant Violet 605 (O323; BioLegend), CD38-eFluor 450 (HB7; eBioscience), FcR blocking reagent (Miltenyi Biotec, Bergisch Gladbach, Germany) and TO-PRO-3 (Invitrogen, Eugene, OR, USA). Subsequently, cells were pre-gated on live and singlet cells and further gated on $CD3^-$ and $CD19^+$ B cells as described in Winklmeier et al. [56]. Plasmablasts ($CD19^+CD27^{high}CD38^{high}$) and non-plasmablast B cells ($CD19^+CD27^{low}CD38^{low}$) were bulk sorted using FACSAria Fusion (BD, Franklin Lakes, NJ, USA). In some experiments, $CD3^+$ T cells were removed before the FACS sorting using magnetic beads (EasySep™ Human CD3 Positive Selection Kit II, STEMCELL Technologies, Vancouver, Canada). Cells were lysed in RLT Plus buffer containing DTT according RNeasy Plus Mini Kit (QIAGEN, Hilden, Germany). Analysis of flow cytometry data was performed with FlowJo (V10.6.1, BD).

2.5. RNA Isolation and Real-Time Quantitative Reverse-Transcriptase PCR (qRT-PCR) Analysis

For details on isolation of RNA from cell cultures, reverse transcription and PCR analysis, see the online supplement.

2.6. Protein Isolation and Western Blot Analysis

For details on protein isolation and Western Blot analysis, see the online supplement.

2.7. Flow Cytometry Analysis

To assess the number of circulating plasma cells in blood of IPF patients in comparison with healthy donors, plasma cells from whole blood of IPF patients and healthy donors were sorted and identified as $CD20^-/CD3^-/CD27^+/CD38^+$ cells. First, venous blood from IPF patients or healthy individuals was collected in EDTA-coated vacutainer tubes (Sarstedt, Nümbrecht, Germany). For each staining, 100 µL of blood was incubated with antibodies (listed in Table S3) used to gate for plasma cells (see Figure S3 for gating strategy) for 20 min at 4 °C protected from light. In parallel, blood from the same specimen was stained with appropriate isotype controls. Next, lysis of erythrocytes was performed with a Coulter Q-Prep working station (Beckman Coulter, München, Germany) followed by data acquisition in a BD LSRII flow cytometer (Becton Dickinson, Heidelberg, Germany). FlowJo software (TreeStart Inc., Ashland, OR, USA) was used for data analysis. Data was presented as ratio $CD20^-/CD3^-/CD27^+/CD38^+$ cells of live cells. Negative thresholds for gating were set according to isotype-labelled controls.

2.8. Immunofluorescent Stainings

For details on immunofluorescent stainings of tissue sections and cytospins, please refer to the online supplement.

2.9. Unfolding and Refolding of Immunoglobulin G

Antibody refolding was performed essentially as described [14,57]. A monoclonal mouse anti-fibrillin-1 antibody [58] was denatured using 3 M guanidinium chloride pH 7.0, 0.1 M Tris, 0.005 M EDTA) for 24 h at an antibody concentration of 80 µg/mL at 4 °C. For initiation of refolding, the denatured antibody solution was diluted 10-fold under manual shaking in PBS containing a PPIase or a control protein (RNAse 45 µM, Sigma-Aldrich) at 10 °C, resulting in an antibody concentration of 8 µg/mL. Recombinant PPIases used were either PPIB (5 µM, positive control) or FKBP11 (45 µM) [59]. At given time points, aliquots of the refolding mixture were withdrawn and diluted 12-fold under vigorous stirring in a trypsin solution (300 U/mL trypsin, 5% milk, PBS) and kept on ice to stop further refolding. Final antibody concentrations were 0.66 µg/mL. After completion of the final time point, the amount of correctly refolded antibody was determined by ELISA (see below).

For experiments involving inhibition of PPIase activity, FKBP11 was preincubated for one hour with either FK506 (180 µM, Sigma-Aldrich, St. Louis, MO, USA) or DMSO (Sigma-Aldrich, St. Louis, MO, USA) as a negative control at +10 °C. Subsequently, antibody refolding was performed as described above.

2.10. ELISA

To assess the rate of correctly refolded IgG, a high binding ELISA plate was coated with recombinant fibrillin (fragment rf11) [58] overnight. After washing one time with TBS-Tween (0.025% Tween 20), the coated wells were blocked with 5% milk in PBS for one hour. Then, aliquots from the refolding experiment were incubated for one hour. The plate was washed once, followed by one hour of incubation with an HRP-linked anti-mouse antibody (Bio-Rad, Hercules). After rinsing the plate 5 times, 3,3′,5,5′-Tetramethylbenzidine (TMB) substrate (Sigma-Aldrich) was incubated for 20 min and the signal was read at 650 nm. In the graphs, values shown represent the optical density measured at 650 nm minus blank values (derived from incubation with trypsin solution without primary antibody).

For determination of yield and functionality of antibodies secreted from scr siRNA, FKBP11 siRNA or PPIB siRNA-transfected hybridoma H3 cells, ELISA plates were coated with a mixture of anti-κ LC (TIB172, ATCC) and anti-λ LC (mAb LA1B12 [60], both 5 µg/mL in 0.2 M carbonate buffer pH 9.5), the cognate antigen-GST fusion protein, or the untagged cognate antigen (each 10 µg/mL in 0.2 M carbonate buffer pH 9.5, in-house generated) overnight at 4 °C. After washing one time with PBS, the wells were blocked with PBS/2% fetal calf serum for 15 min. After blocking, a serial 2-fold dilution of supernatants (starting dilution 1:10) from siRNA-transfected hybridoma cells were added for 30 min. The plate was washed once, followed by 30 min of incubation with an HRP-linked mouse-anti-rat IgG2a, which is the IgG subclass of the antibody produced by this hybridoma cell line. After rinsing the plate 5 times with PBS, 3,3′,5,5′-Tetramethylbenzidine (TMB) substrate (Thermo Scientific/Pierce) was added, followed by incubation for 5 minutes and monitoring of absorbance at 650 nm.

3. Results

3.1. FKBP11 Expression Is Increased in IPF Lungs

As we had previously observed increased *FKBP10* expression in IPF [61], we set out to assess expression of other members of the *FKBP* family in IPF in microarray data of 99 IPF samples and 43 normal histology control samples [50,51]. With a false discovery rate of 5% [52], we found four more *FKBPs* to be significantly differentially expressed, namely *FKBP11*, *FKBP1A*, *FKBP5*, and *FKBP6*. *FKBP11* and *FKBP5*, but not *FKBP1A* and *FKBP6*, were expressed at comparably high abundance and altered more than two-fold, namely *FKBP11* with a Fold Change of +2.2 and *FKBP5* with a Fold Change of -3.4 (Figure 1A). Focusing on these two FKBPs, we found that, in contrast to transcript levels, FKBP5 protein levels were not decreased (Figure S1). However, immunoblot analysis demonstrated increased FKBP11 protein in IPF relative to healthy donor lung samples (Figure 1B,C).

Taking advantage of data available in the NLHBI LTRC data set [62], we correlated *FKBP11* expression with demographic and clinical parameters including age, sex, lung function, several readouts of quality of life and physical fitness as well as smoking history. We observed a significant ($p = 0.02$) but weak negative correlation with FVC (% of predicted) and a similar relationship with DLCO which, however, just failed significance ($p = 0.06$; Figure S2).

3.2. FKBP11 Localizes Mainly to CD27$^+$/CD38$^+$/CD138$^+$/CD20$^-$/CD45$^-$ Plasma Cells

We initially assessed whether *FKBP11*, like *FKBP10*, was expressed in primary human lung fibroblasts (phLF) and contributed to collagen synthesis and secretion [61]. Even if we detected FKBP11 in the microsomal fraction of phLF, in agreement with ER residence (Figure S3A), *FKBP11* was significantly less expressed in phLF than *FKBP10* (Figure S3B) and siRNA-mediated downregulation of FKBP11 did neither affect myofibroblast differentiation (as assessed by protein levels of α-smooth muscle actin, Figure S3C) nor collagen secretion from these cells (Figure S3D).

Immunofluorescent stainings of IPF lung tissue sections for different markers of the hematopoietic lineage revealed that FKBP11 specifically localizes to CD27$^+$/CD38$^+$/CD138$^+$/CD20$^-$/CD45$^-$ plasma cells in IPF lungs (Figure 2A,B). Our results further supported expression of *FKBP11* predominantly by IgG-producing plasma cells, but we also observed IgA/FKBP11 double-positive cells (Figure 2B). Elevated cell counts of FKBP11$^+$/CD38$^+$ plasma cells (Figure 2C) confirmed overexpression of *FBKP11* in IPF lungs and suggested that upregulation of *FKBP11* in IPF lung tissue is mostly due to increased prevalence of tissue-resident plasma cells. In agreement, *FKBP11* expression very strongly correlated with *MZB1*, an established marker of plasma cells [43], in IPF lung tissue, and not or only weakly with typical fibrotic markers such as *ACTA2*, *COL1A2*, and *COL3A1* (Figure S4). In contrast, proportions of CD38$^+$/CD27$^+$ cells in fresh whole blood samples analyzed by FACS analysis did not significantly differ between IPF and donor samples (Figure 2D, for gating strategy refer to Figure S5). We took advantage of a tissue microarray and observed that *FKBP11* was also expressed by CD38$^+$ plasma cells in primary and secondary lymphatic organs including thymus, spleen, tonsils and small intestine, suggesting that *FKBP11* expression is a common property of plasma cells (Figure 2E). We also found FKBP11$^+$/CD38$^-$ cells in pancreatic and gastric glands (Figure S6), in line with an important function of FKBP11 in secretory cells in other tissues. In contrast, on the same tissue microarray we did not detect neither FKBP11 nor CD38 in healthy human tissues such as muscle and lung (Figure S6).

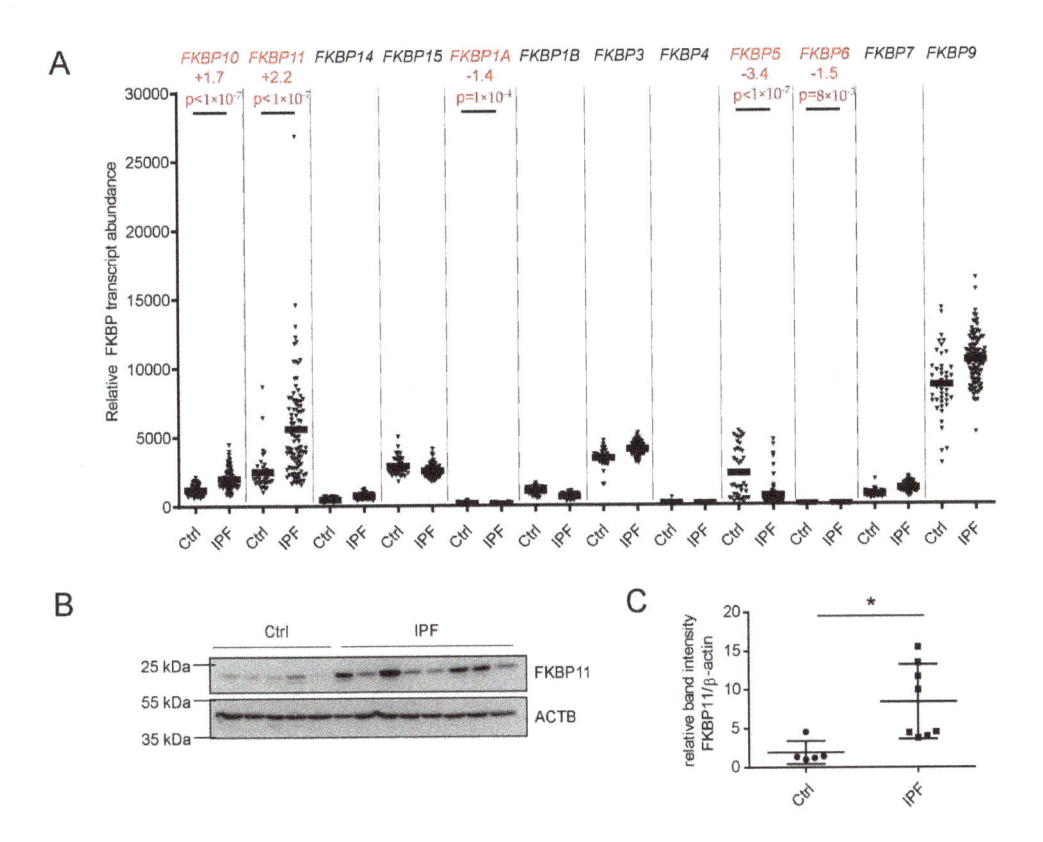

Figure 1. *FKBP11* is upregulated in idiopathic pulmonary fibrosis (IPF). (**A**) Scatter plot for *FKBP* gene expression data extracted from microarray data of normal histology control ($n = 43$) and samples from patients with IPF ($n = 99$) [50,51]. (**B**) Western blot analysis of total lung tissue homogenate showed upregulation of FKBP11 in patients with IPF ($n = 8$) relative to donor samples ($n = 5$). (**C**) Densitometric analysis of the Western blot from (**B**). For Western Blot analysis, data shown are mean ± SEM, and a two-tailed Mann-Whitney test was used for statistical analysis (* $p < 0.05$). ACTB = β-actin as loading control.

3.3. FKBP11 Is Upregulated during Plasma Cell Transdifferentiation

Isolation and subsequent 7-day treatment of peripheral blood mononuclear cells (PBMCs) from three independent healthy donors with a combination of IL2 and R848 led to transdifferentiation of memory B cells to IgG producing plasma cells (Figure 3A,B), as demonstrated before [43,54,55]. Upon treatment, immunofluorescent stainings of cytospins showed more IgG$^+$ cells than control (Figure 3A). In addition, transcript levels of PR domain zinc finger protein 1 (*PRDM1*, also termed BLIMP-1), a marker of B-cell activation [63], were significantly increased (Figure 3B). At the same time, B cell to plasma cell transdifferentiation was accompanied by an upregulation of FKBP11 on both transcript (Figure 3C) and protein level (Figure 3D). Upregulation of the ER chaperone HSPA5 (also termed BiP or GRP78) confirmed induction of the unfolded protein response (UPR) during differentiation to plasma cells (Figure 3D). In order to verify that upregulation of *FKBP11* indeed was due to B cell to plasmablast differentiation, we used flow cytometry to select the CD3$^-$CD19$^+$ B cell population from IL2/R848-activated cells, sorted those into plasmablasts (CD27^{high} CD38^{high}) and non-plasmablast B cells (CD27^{low} CD38^{low}), and directly compared *FKBP11* and *PRDM1* gene expression in these B cell populations (Figure 3E,F). Similar to *PRDM1*, *FKBP11* was highly enriched in the CD27^{high}CD38^{high} plasmablast population.

Finally, single cell-RNA-Seq analysis of healthy mouse lungs extracted from Angelidis et al [64] confirms plasma cells as the major source of *Fkbp11* in the lung (Figure S7), similar to *Mzb1*, which was previously reported by us as a plasma cell-specific protein upregulated in human lung fibrosis [43]. This data also showed marginal expression of *Fkbp11* in interstitial fibroblasts and alveolar epithelial cells, which is in agreement with our qRT-PCR and immunoblot results in phLF (Figure S3) and A549 (Figure 4). Notably, *PPIB*, typically stated to act as antibody peptidyl-prolyl isomerase [2], did not show similar specificity to plasma cells (Figure S7).

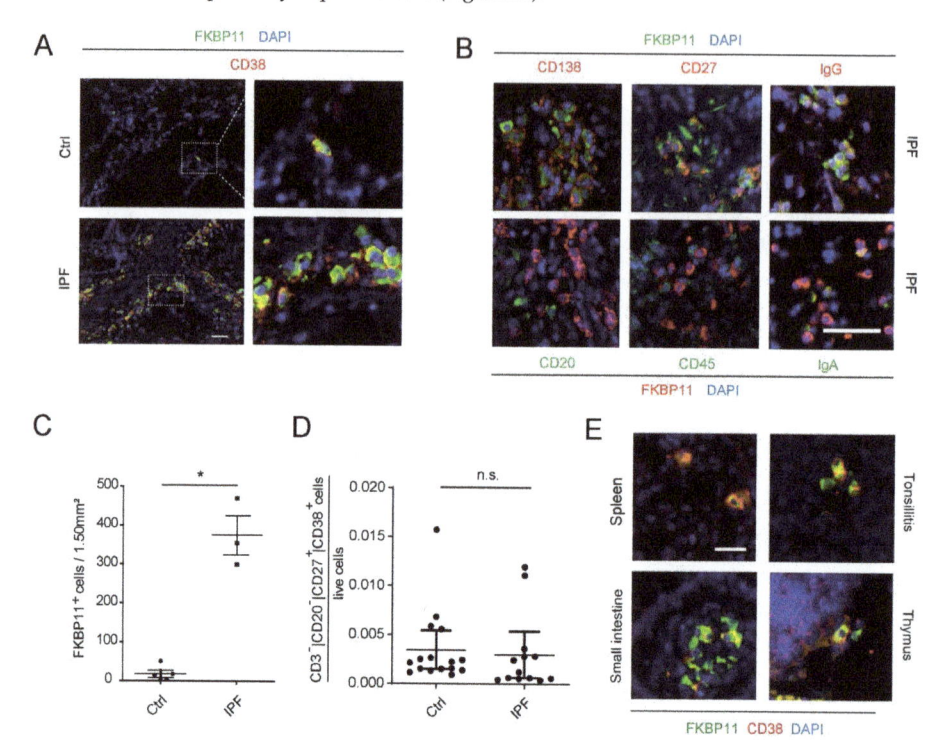

Figure 2. *FKBP11* is expressed by CD27$^+$/CD38$^+$/CD138$^+$/CD20$^-$/CD45$^-$ plasma cells. (**A**) Immunofluorescent stainings in control (Ctrl, upper panel) and IPF lung tissue sections (lower panel) demonstrate expression of FKBP11 in CD38$^+$ plasma cells. Stainings are representative for $n = 5$ (Ctrl) and $n = 3$ (IPF). Scale bar 40 µm. (**B**) Immunofluorescent stainings in IPF lung tissue sections further demonstrate that FKBP11$^+$ plasma cells are positive for CD138, CD27 (upper panel), but negative for CD20 and CD45 (lower panel) and produce mainly IgG (upper panel, far right), but also IgA (lower panel, far right). Note, that secondary antibody dyes for FKBP11 differ in upper and lower panel. Stainings of IPF lung sections are representative for $n = 2$ (CD138, CD27, CD20, CD45) and $n = 3$ (IgG, IgA). Scale bar, 40 µm. (**C**) Quantification of CD38/FKBP11 immunofluorescent stainings (**A**), based on lung sections from normal histology controls ($n = 5$) and IPF patients ($n = 3$, observer blinded to diagnosis), where FKBP11$^+$/CD38$^+$ cells from ten randomly selected images sized 1.5 mm^2 were counted and added up for all 10 images ($p = 0.0357$, two-tailed Mann-Whitney (**D**) Numbers of circulating CD20$^-$/CD27$^+$/CD38$^+$ plasma cells were not significantly changed ($p = 0.2680$, two-tailed Mann-Whitney test) between healthy subjects ($n = 20$) and IPF patients ($n = 13$). (**E**) Immunofluorescent stainings of a human tissue array demonstrated FKBP11$^+$/CD38$^+$ cells in other tissues than lung, namely spleen, tonsils, thymus, and small intestine. Scale bar 20 µm. * $p < 0.05$; n.s., not significant.

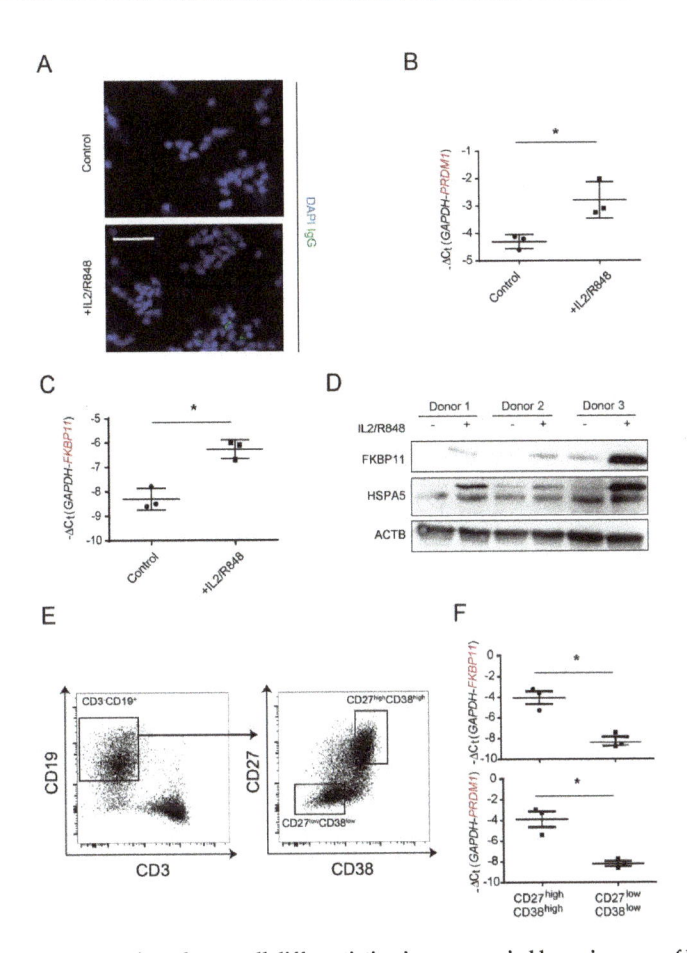

Figure 3. In vitro plasma cell differentiation is accompanied by an increase of FKBP11 expression. PBMCs from blood of three healthy volunteers were treated with interleukin-2 (IL2) and R848 to induce differentiation of memory B cells to antibody-producing plasma cells. (**A**) Increased IgG expression upon treatment was observed using immunofluorescence analysis of cytospins showing cells positive for intracellular IgG. Scale bar 50 μm. (**B**) IL2/R848 treatment led to increased levels of the B cell activation marker PR domain zinc finger protein 1 (PRDM1). (**C,D**) Expression of *FKBP11* at transcript (**C**) as well as protein (**D**) level was increased in the course of B cell to plasma cell differentiation. (**D**) Upregulation of the ER chaperone HSPA5 confirmed induction of the unfolded protein response (UPR) during B cell differentiation to plasma cells. (**E**) PBMCs of healthy donors were stimulated for 7 days with IL-2 and R848. Subsequently, the activated and differentiated cells were pre-gated on live and singlet cells and further gated on CD3$^-$ and CD19$^+$ B cells (left panel). Plasmablasts (CD19$^+$CD27^{high}CD38^{high}) and non-plasmablast B cells (CD19$^+$CD27^{low}CD38^{low}) were bulk sorted using FACSAria Fusion (right panel). Flow cytometry panels are displayed from one representative donor of three independent experiments. (**F**) Expression of *FKBP11* and *PRDM1* were analyzed by qPCR of the sorted cell fractions. ACTB = β-actin as loading control. For IgG concentrations and qPCR results, data shown are mean ± SEM, and a paired *t*-test was used for statistical analysis (* $p \leq 0.05$; exact *p*-values: B: $p = 0.0474$; C: $p = 0.0194$; F top panel (FKBP11): $p = 0.0180$; F bottom panel (PRDM1): $p = 0.0495$).

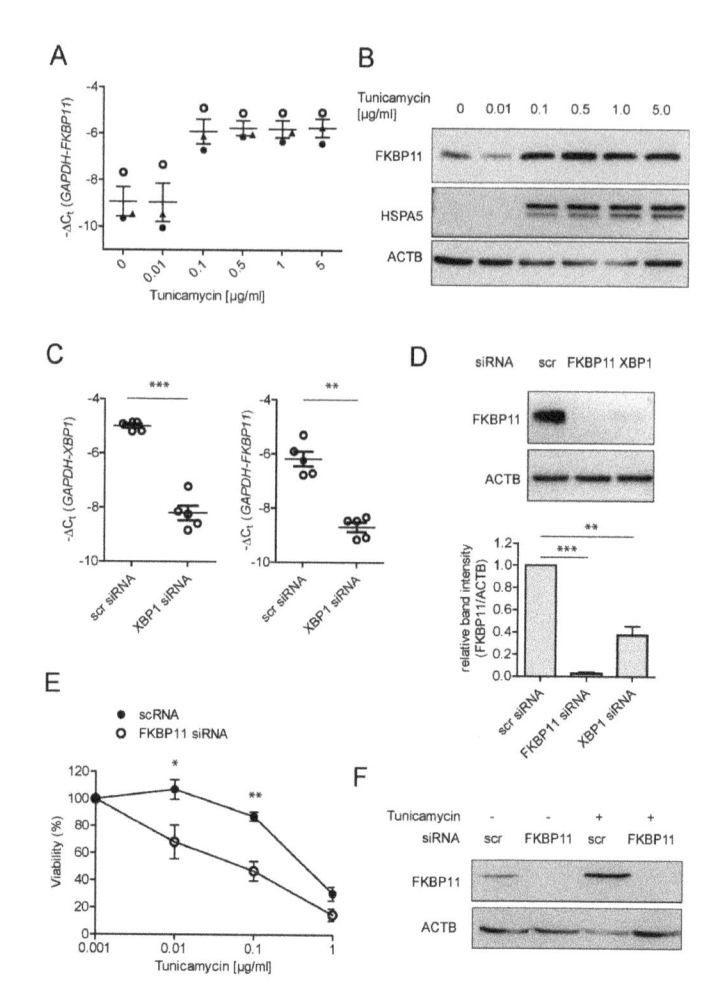

Figure 4. FKBP11 is induced by ER stress in an XBP1-dependent manner and protects from ER-stress induced cell death. (**A,B**) Treatment of A549 with the synthetic ER stress inducer tunicamycin led to a dose-dependent increase of *FKBP11* expression both on transcript (**A**) and on protein level (**B**). Upregulation of the ER chaperone HSPA5 confirmed induction of ER stress. ACTB = β-actin as loading control. (**C**) Knockdown of XBP1 in A549 cells treated with 0.1 μg/mL tunicamycin was efficient as assessed by qRT-PCR (left, $p = 0.0007$, paired *t*-test) and led to a drastic decrease of *FKBP11* transcript (right, $p = 0.0026$, paired *t*-test). (**D**) Knockdown of XBP1 equally led to loss of FKBP11 protein ($p = 0.0014$, paired *t*-test). This result is shown in comparison to FKBP11 knockdown under similar conditions ($p < 0.0001$, paired *t*-test); top panel, representative Western Blot; bottom panel corresponding densitometric analysis). (**E**) Combining FKBP11 knockdown with different concentrations of tunicamycin ranging from 1 ng/mL to 1 μg/mL and assessing cell viability by trypan blue exclusion showed that FKBP11 knockdown leads to higher susceptibility to ER stress-induced cell death (Exact *p*-values: 0.01 μg/mL: $p = 0.0414$; 0.1 μg/mL: $p = 0.0068$; paired *t*-test.) (**F**) Knockdown of FKBP11 in A549 cells was highly efficient in absence and presence of tunicamycin. For (**A,E**) data shown is based on three and four independent experiments, respectively, and given as mean ± SEM. (**B,F**) is representative for three independent experiments. For (**C,D**), data shown is based on five independent experiments and given as mean ± SEM. A paired *t*-test was used for statistical analysis (* $p < 0.05$; ** $p < 0.01$; *** $p < 0.001$).

3.4. Expression of FKBP11 Is Induced by the Transcription Factor X-Box Binding Protein 1 (XBP1) and Protects an Alveolar Cell Line from ER-Stress Induced Cell Death

Plasma cell differentiation requires the activation of the unfolded protein response (UPR) [65], an ER stress-induced signaling pathway, and FKBP11 has been described as an ER-resident peptidyl prolyl isomerase [59]. We therefore assessed, using treatment with the ER stress inducer tunicamycin and subcellular fractionation, whether FKBP11 localized to the ER and was upregulated by ER stress in the B lymphocyte cell line Raji (derived from Burkitt's lymphoma) and in A549 cells (derived from lung adenocarcinoma). In both cell types, the subcellular fractionation pattern of FKBP11 protein was consistent with ER residence, as judged by predominance in the microsomal fraction and colocalization with PDIA3 (Figure S8A, see also Figure S3A in phLF). The ER stress inducer tunicamycin upregulated *FKBP11* expression in a dose-dependent manner, in parallel to the well-established UPR target protein HSPA5 (A549, Figure 4A,B; Raji, Figure S8B,C). In A549, a tunicamycin concentration of 0.1 µg/mL was sufficient to reproducibly induce the UPR (Figure 4A,B). Therefore, subsequent experiments for regulation of *FKBP11* expression in A549 were conducted in presence of 0.1 µg/mL tunicamycin to induce ER stress. The transcription factor X-box binding protein 1 (XBP1), a critical regulator of the UPR which governs late events of plasma cell differentiation [7,8,66], has been described to regulate expression of a subset of protein folding catalysts in this context [67]. Hence, we assessed whether also *FKBP11* is regulated in an XBP1-dependent manner. Indeed, siRNA-mediated knockdown of XBP1 in A549 cells after induction of ER stress by tunicamycin treatment, resulted in significant downregulation of *FKBP11* expression on transcript and protein level (Figure 4C,D). In agreement with a protective role under conditions of ER stress, knockdown of FKBP11 in A549 resulted in a higher susceptibility to tunicamycin-induced cell death (Figure 4E,F).

3.5. Recombinant FKBP11 Folds IgG Antibody In Vitro

Given ER residence and expression of *FKBP11* in antibody-producing plasma cells, we hypothesized that FKBP11 functions as an antibody foldase. To address this hypothesis, we took advantage of an in vitro antibody refolding assay, where, after full denaturation of IgG with guanidinium chloride, refolding kinetics in absence and presence of the purified recombinant FKBP domain of human FKBP11 was monitored by an IgG ELISA. As antigen-antibody binding strictly relies on the native three-dimensional structure, ELISA readouts are a measure of correctly folded IgG [14,57]. Recombinant PPIB, commonly accepted as antibody peptidyl-prolyl isomerase (PPIase) [2], was used as positive control. Addition of the recombinant FKBP domain of FKBP11 (amino acids Gly28 - Ala146 as described in Ishikawa et al. [59], for FKBP11 domain structure see Figure 5A) to denatured IgG resulted in an increase of both rate of refolding and total yield of refolded IgG as compared to negative controls (RNase and PBS, Figure 5B). This effect was inhibited by tacrolimus (FK506), a known inhibitor of many FKBPs, which binds to the PPIase activity-bearing FKBP domain [68] (Figure 5C). In comparison to the established antibody PPIase PPIB, considerably higher concentrations of FKBP11 (45 µM FKBP11 in comparison to 5 µM PPIB, see Figure 5B) were needed to demonstrate similar refolding activity.

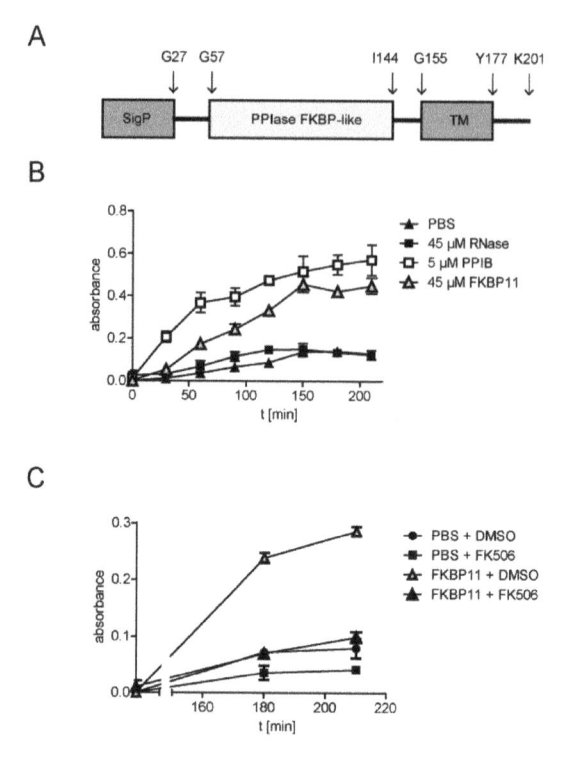

Figure 5. Recombinant FKBP11 folds IgG antibody in vitro. (**A**) Schematic representation of FKBP11 domain structure. For these experiments, the purified FKBP domain of FKBP11 (amino acids G28 - A146) without the N-terminal signal peptide (SigP) and the C-terminal transmembrane region (TM) was used. (**B**) In vitro antibody refolding kinetics in absence and presence of FKBP11 and recombinant PPIB as positive control. (**C**) Antibody refolding by FKBP11 was inhibited by tacrolimus (FK506). Data shown is based on three independent experiments and given as mean ± SEM; error bars are missing when they were smaller than the size of the data symbols.

3.6. Neither Knockdown of FKBP11 Nor Knockdown of Cyclophilin B Affects IgG Yield of an Antibody-Producing Hybridoma Cell Line

The fusion of splenocytes from immunized mice or rats with a mouse myeloma cell line, the hybridoma technology, is a well-established method to generate cell lines for reproducible production of specific monoclonal antibodies, also at large-scale. In efforts to screen for a suitable hybridoma cell line for loss-of-function experiments, we first determined levels of FKBP11 and rat IgG in three hybridoma cell lines created by fusion of the mouse myeloma cell line P3X63-Ag8.653 (AG8) with splenocytes of differently immunized rats (H1-H3, Figure 6A). We verified expression of *Fkbp11* in all of these cell lines, but observed the highest protein levels of FKBP11 and rat IgG in the hybridoma cell line H3. We therefore chose H3 for loss-of-function experiments. ER residence of FKBP11 in H3 was confirmed by colocalization with concanavalin A using confocal microscopy (Figure 6B) and by subcellular fractionation, where FKBP11 showed the same enrichment pattern as the ER marker calreticulin (CALR, Figure 6C). While the subcellular fractionation results also indicated a nuclear localization of FKBP11, this could not be confirmed by confocal microscopy (no colocalization with DAPI in Figure 6B). Therefore, enrichment of FKBP11 and CALR in the nuclear fraction probably represent some contamination of the nuclear fraction by ER-resident proteins.

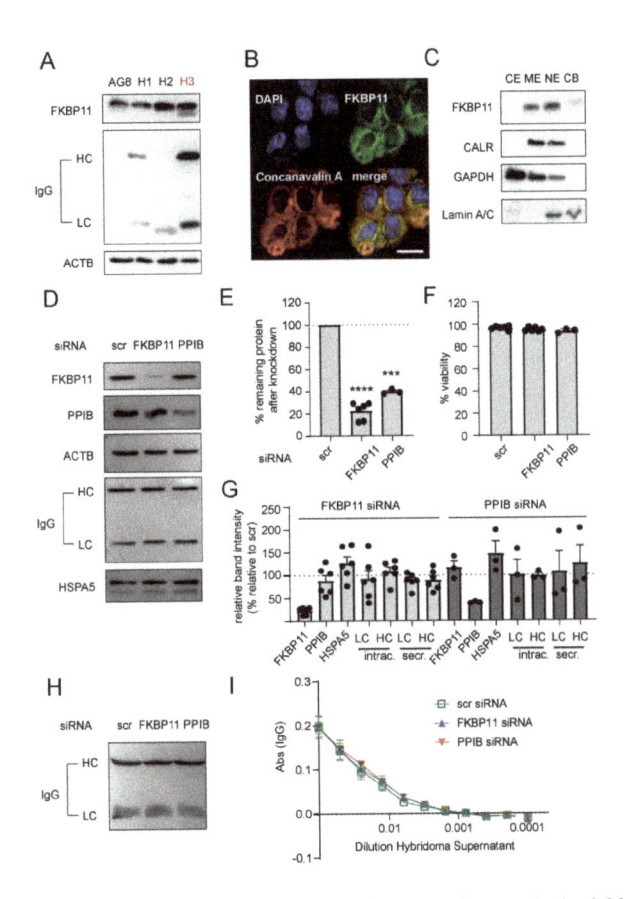

Figure 6. **Knockdown of FKBP11 or PPIB does not reduce antibody yield of a hybridoma cell line.** (**A**) Protein levels of FKBP11 and rat IgG in three different rat/mouse hybridoma cell lines (H1–H3) and the mouse myeloma cell line P3X63-Ag8.653 (AG8) used for fusion. H3 was chosen for subsequent experiments. (**B**) Confocal microscopy demonstrated colocalization of FKBP11 with the ER marker concanavalin A. Scale bar 20 μm. (**C**) Subcellular fractionation showed a similar enrichment pattern for FKBP11 as for the ER-resident protein calreticulin (CALR), with main localization in the microsomal (ME) and the nuclear extract (NE), but little to no detection in the cytosolic extract (CE) and the chromatin-bound fraction (CB). (**D**) Representative Western Blot analysis showing levels of FKBP11, the known antibody folding catalyst PPIB, loading control β-actin (ACTB), intracellular IgG antibody heavy (HC) and light chain (LC), and ER chaperone HSPA5, following siRNA-mediated knockdown of FKBP11 or PPIB in hybridoma cell line H3. (**E**) Mean FKBP11 knockdown efficiency in the rat hybridoma cell line H3 was 78 ± 3% ($n = 6$; paired t-test; **** $p < 0.0001$), mean PPIB knockdown efficiency in the same cell line was 60 ± 1% ($n = 3$; paired t-test; *** $p < 0.001$). (**F**) Knockdown of FKBP11 ($n = 6$) or PPIB ($n = 3$) did not affect cell viability relative to scr siRNA control. (**G**) Quantification of immunoblot band intensities (see representative immunoblots for intracellular protein in panel **D**, for secreted IgG in panel **H**) following FKBP11 or PPIB knockdown revealed no significant changes except for the siRNA targets FKBP11 and PPIB; data for the latter two is identical to panel E; intrac., intracellular; secr., secreted. (**H**) Representative Western Blot analysis showing levels of secreted IgG antibody heavy (HC) and light chain (LC), following siRNA-mediated knockdown of FKBP11 or PPIB in hybridoma cell line H3. Quantification is given in panel G (secr. IgG, LC, HC). (**I**) ELISA-based IgG quantification showed no significant effect on antibody secretion from FKBP11-, PPIB- or scr siRNA-transfected H3 cells ($n = 3$).

Delivery of *Fkbp11*- and *Ppib*-specific siRNA into H3 by electroporation resulted in acceptable knockdown efficiencies (Figure 6E), without affecting cell viability in comparison to non-targeting scrambled siRNA (scr, Figure 6F). Neither *Fkbp11*- nor *Ppib*-specific siRNA affected levels of intracellular IgG heavy (HC) or light chain (LC, Figure 6D, quantified in Figure 6G). Also levels of the ER stress marker HSPA5 were not altered by reductions in *Fkbp11* or *Ppib* expression (Figure 6D, quantified in Figure 6G). While we observed a small non-significant trend for decreased transcript for IgG HC in response to PPIB knockdown, the same remained unchanged in response to FKBP11 knockdown (Figure S9A). Furthermore, knockdown of FKBP11 did not alter the subcellular fractionation pattern of IgG chains, which could have indicated accumulation of misfolded protein in the ER (Figure S9B). Western Blot analysis of the hybridoma supernatants suggested a weak reduction of secreted IgG antibody chains for FKBP11 knockdown which, however, failed to reach significance (LC, $p = 0.1203$; HC, $p = 0.2650$; paired *t*-test; Figure 6H, quantified in Figure 6G, secreted LC/HC). For a more rigorous quantification of IgG in the hybridoma supernatants, we compared IgG levels after transfection of hybridoma cells with control, FKBP11 and PPIB siRNA by ELISA using serial dilutions of the hybridoma supernatants. Here, we observed no differences of IgG concentrations relative to control siRNA (Figure 6I). Finally, using a similar ELISA approach, we also assessed whether knockdown of FKBP11 or PPIB affected binding of secreted IgG to the cognate antigen and again found that there was no difference relative to control siRNA (Figure S9D,E).

4. Discussion

A profound understanding of mechanisms of plasma cell differentiation and antibody folding is beneficial not only for the development and production of antibody-based therapeutics but also for targeting autoimmune diseases. In the current study, we identified the immunophilin FKBP11 as a novel plasma cell-specific antibody folding catalyst. Expression of *FKBP11* was increased in lungs with IPF, a fatal fibrotic disease with autoimmune features [43–45], and localized specifically to tissue-resident plasma cells in IPF lung as well as primary and secondary lymphatic organs. *FKBP11* was upregulated upon differentiation of B cells into antibody-secreting plasma cells and upon induction of ER stress in an XBP1-dependent manner in vitro. The purified FKBP domain of human FKBP11, which carries the PPIase activity, catalysed antibody refolding. While FKBP11 knockdown resulted in higher susceptibility to ER stress-induced cell death in A549 cells, viability and antibody yield of a hybridoma cell line was not affected relative to control siRNA.

Antibody function is strictly dependent on correct folding of the three-dimensional structure and peptidyl-prolyl isomerization is the rate-limiting step in the process of IgG folding [2]. However, the knowledge on PPIases catalysing this step is much based on circumstantial evidence and PPIases in the human plasma cell have not been well-described. In our study, we provide strong in vivo and in vitro evidence that human FKBP11 is a novel plasma cell-specific antibody PPIase. To date, two other PPIases have been proposed in the context of antibody folding, namely FKBP1A (FKBP12) and PPIB. Lilie et al. [14] provided the first conceptual evidence that immunophilins of the FKBP family may contribute to antibody folding, showing that purified FKBP1A acts as antibody PPIase in vitro. The authors used the recombinant protein and an IgG Fab fragment refolding assay [14], very similar to the one that we used (Figure 5B,C). However, FKBP1A is a cytosolic protein [15] and therefore unlikely to contribute to antibody folding in the ER in vivo.

PPIB is commonly accepted as antibody PPIase [2], a concept which, however, is still based on relatively few key indications: First, purified PPIB has been shown by Feige et al. [11] to catalyse immunoglobulin folding in vitro, a finding which we confirm in our study (Figure 5B). Second, using a chemical crosslinking approach in mouse lymphoma cell lines followed by mass spectrometry-based identification, PPIB was found to reside in a complex associated with unassembled, incompletely folded immunoglobulin heavy chains [10]. More recently, using a combination of ER-specific pull-down and a yeast-two hybrid system, Jansen et al. were able to map multiple interactions between ER foldases, and identified a novel complex between PPIB and the oxidoreductase ERp72 (encoded by *PDIA4*) [13]. In a folding assay which monitored disulphide bond formation between the constant parts of the IgG heavy and light chain, a C_H1-C_L assembly assay [11], the authors could show that PPIB potentiates disulphide isomerase activity of Erp72 [13]. However, PPIB is a general ER-resident folding catalyst, for instance with an established role in collagen triple helix formation [69]; indeed sc-RNA-Seq data from mouse lungs (Supplementary Figure S7) confirms that PPIB is abundantly expressed in almost all cell types. In the present study, by contrast, we not only show that FKBP11 directly catalyses antibody folding, but provide multiple evidence for plasma cell-specific upregulation in patient material and human test systems and demonstrate that *FKBP11* expression is induced by the UPR in an XBP1-dependent manner, a pathway crucial for late events in the course of B cell differentiation to antibody-producing plasma cells. Notably, our findings are backed up by previous transcriptomic studies on UPR-induced gene expression in the lymphoma cell line Raji and in fibroblasts, which also show upregulation of FKBP11 transcript [70,71]. In addition, we confirm ER residence of FKBP11 [72] and show that FKBP11 colocalizes in plasma cells with at least two major immunoglobulin classes, namely IgG and IgA. Our observations thus support a critical and specific function of FKBP11 in general plasma cell biology. In agreement, in work using a lentiviral transgenic mouse model, Ruer-Laventie et al. have provided evidence that *FKBP11* overexpression initiates plasma cell differentiation and results in higher serum levels of basal IgG3 [27]. Also, *FKBP11* expression in peripheral B cells from Systemic Lupus Erythematosus (SLE) patients, a severe and prototypic autoimmune disease, has been found to correlate with increased numbers of peripheral plasmablasts [27].

While our results of the IgG refolding assay establish FKBP11 as a novel plasma cell antibody foldase, knocking down FKBP11 in a hybridoma cell line was not sufficient to affect antibody yield or functionality. Notably, in our hands, the same was true for the established antibody foldase PPIB. We believe that this observation does not contradict a function as antibody foldase for FKBP11, but may rather reflect considerable redundancy in the antibody folding capacity in hybridoma cell lines. Overall, this underlines the general importance of the UPR, inducing a plethora of chaperones and folding catalysts, which collectively protect unfolded proteins from aggregation. Furthermore, it is important to acknowledge that, while PPIases typically accelerate folding kinetics, their absence does not much affect overall yield of correctly folded antibody fragments after denaturation and refolding in vitro [11,73], indicating considerable, albeit slow, auto-catalysis. Hence, therapeutic application of our findings for treatment of autoimmune disease may require additional targets for the depletion of plasma cells, but, given the comparably high level of plasma cell specificity, FKBP11-directed drugs could be used to specifically target the ER-resident folding machinery in plasma cells.

Our finding that PPIB knockdown was not sufficient to decrease antibody yield is in part contradictory to a previous study, which reported that knockdown of PPIB, with similar knockdown efficiency as shown here, in murine hybridoma and primary B cells impaired IgG synthesis [12]. Unfortunately, the authors did not assess secreted IgG in that assay and the robustness of the latter findings remains unclear as only representative results without statistical analysis are given.

FKBP2 (also termed FKBP13) is another immunophilin that recently has received attention in the context of plasma cell biology and IPF. While a direct antibody folding activity has to date not been reported, findings reported by Jeong et al. suggest that FKBP2 is also regulated by XBP1, directly interacts with immunoglobulins in the ER, but targets them for proteasome-mediated degradation and thereby reduces the overall level of ER stress [74]. Similar to *PPIB*, however, expression of *FKBP2* is not restricted to plasma cells, at least not in the lung (Figure S5) [64,75]. FKBP2 was enriched in fibrotic regions in IPF lungs, while, in the bleomycin-induced mouse model of lung fibrosis, deficiency of FKBP2 aggravated fibrogenesis and impaired resolution of fibrosis [75]. Overall, these findings rather point towards a protective role of FKBP2 in the context of fibrosis.

As FKBP11 was exclusively expressed by $CD3^-/CD20^-/CD38^+/CD27^+$ plasma cells in IPF lung tissue, we quantified this cell population in plasma of IPF patients. Here, in contrast to other studies [27,44], we did not gate for $CD19^+$ cells and normalize to the total B cell population, as it has been reported that a significant proportion of plasma cells lose CD19 expression [76,77]. Therefore a direct comparison of our results with the published ones [27,44] is not possible. With an average of around 0.3% of all live cells, the resulting population was very small and we did not observe an increase as compared to healthy control blood samples (Figure 2C). This suggested that the majority of plasma cells in IPF lungs did not derive from peripheral organs but differentiated from local B cells within the fibrotic lung tissue.

Several studies have indicated the presence of circulating autoantibodies and increased levels of B-lymphocyte stimulator factor (BLyS) in plasma of IPF patients [44,78]. In a recent proteomic study, we could show that upregulation of the plasma cell-specific protein MZB1 is a common feature of fibrotic lung diseases including IPF and, notably, also FKBP11 was among the significantly upregulated proteins in this study [43]. Even if our study provides circumstantial support for the autoimmune hypothesis in IPF, it still remains unclear at present whether these observations represent epiphenomena or actually reflect disease-causing autoimmune mechanisms. Our correlations of *FKBP11* transcript abundance with lung function and transcript abundance of typical fibrotic markers in IPF lungs suggest that there is no strong direct relationship between the level of scarring and the presence of $FKBP11^+$ plasma cells (Figure S4), but a time- and space-resolved analysis of interstitial scarring and lung-resident plasma cell differentiation would be necessary to draw robust conclusions in terms of cause or consequence. Auto-antibody-targeted treatments, including therapeutic plasma exchange, have been beneficial in acute exacerbations of IPF [79] and a clinical phase II study is currently ongoing to evaluate the potential therapeutic efficacy of rituximab, a CD20 antibody which specifically targets B lymphocytes (ClinicalTrials.gov Identifier NCT01969409), in IPF patients. Our study suggests that it may be beneficial to evaluate the potential of more plasma cell-specific treatments, e.g., by use of CD38-specific antibodies some of which are currently in clinical trials for treatment of multiple myeloma [80].

Our study has several limitations. First, we used a mouse/rat hybridoma cell line as model for antibody secretion and not human plasma cells or an antibody-secreting plasmacytoma cell line. This was primarily due to the well-known technical challenges of electroporation/nucleofection of B-, plasma and myeloma cells [81]. While we, after multiple rounds of optimization, succeeded to achieve an acceptable and consistent knockdown efficiency for both FKBP11 and PPIB in the hybridoma cell line, we failed doing so for the plasma cell myeloma cell line JK-6L. Unfortunately, while the yield of our plasma cell differentiation assay (Figure 3) was sufficient for subsequent FACS sorting and qRT-PCR analysis of the resulting subpopulations, it did not allow for testing downstream genetic manipulation assays and effects on antibody yield. We considered using a Crispr-Cas9 approach in the hybridoma cell line for a clean knockout of FKBP11, which ultimately may have led to more conclusive results on the role of FKBP11 in antibody synthesis and secretion. But as CrisprCas9 approaches are a challenging task in polyploid cells, we ultimately decided against that, given the polyploid nature of the hybridoma cell line [82]. As to in vivo models, the FKBP11 knockout mouse is, to the best of our knowledge, not yet commercially available. Future studies using more efficient genetic manipulation approaches, human cells, and animal models are needed to further elucidate the role of FKBP11 in plasma cells.

Second, our study does not establish whether FKBP11 is protective from fibrosis or contributes to disease development. Our observation that knockdown of FKBP11 increases susceptibility to cell death in the alveolar epithelial cell line A549, raises an important concern when considering FKBP11 inhibition as a therapeutic target in IPF. ER stress-induced apoptosis of alveolar epithelial cells is believed to be a triggering profibrotic event in IPF [83–85] and scRNA-Seq data demonstrate—comparatively weak, but detectable-expression of *FKBP11* in type I and II alveolar epithelial cells (type I and II pneumocytes). Targeting FKBP11 may therefore increase susceptibility to ER stress in remaining alveolar type II cells, perpetuating disease progression rather than halting it.

Of note, there is increasing evidence of involvement of multiple FKBPs in human disease. While FKBP10 [61], FKBP11 (this study), and FKBP2 [75] have been reported in the context of IPF, others have demonstrated a role of FKBP11 in autoimmune disease [27]. Additional FKBPs have been put forward as potential drug targets in steroid hormone-associated cancer and psychotic disorders (FKBP4, 5, 8), and Alzheimer's disease (FKBP1A, 4, 5) [15,72,86]. Overall, it is becoming increasingly clear, that a systematic and detailed analysis of FK506 and FK506 analogues and their relative contribution to FKBP inhibition is warranted for the development of multiple novel therapeutic agents including the development of agents that lack FKBP1A-binding and calcineurin-inhibiting T cell suppressive activity.

5. Conclusions

Using a combination of patient material, human cell culture systems, and an in vitro refolding assay, the present study has identified *FKBP11* as an XBP1-driven UPR gene, which is highly expressed by plasma cells and encodes a peptidyl prolyl isomerase, which folds antibodies in vitro. Neither knockdown of FKBP11 nor PPIB in an antibody-producing hybridoma cell line affected antibody yield and functionality, indicating considerable redundancy in antibody folding mechanisms. Finally, the results also strengthen the underappreciated concept of autoimmune features in IPF.

Supplementary Materials: The following supporting information can be downloaded at: https://www.mdpi.com/article/10.3390/cells11081341/s1, Supplementary Methods; Table S1: Primer table for qRT-PCR. Table S2: Primary antibodies; Table S3: Antibodies used for Flow Cytometry; Figure S1: Protein levels of FKBP5 are not altered in IPF; Figure S2: Correlation of *FKBP11* expression with demographic and clinical parameters.; Figure S3: FKBP11 localizes to the ER in primary human lung fibroblasts, but *FKBP11* shows much lower expression than FKBP10, and FKBP11 deficiency does not affect myofibroblast differentiation and collagen secretion.; Figure S4: Correlation of *FKBP11* expression with *MZB1*, *ACTA2*, *COL1A2*, and *COL3A1* expression.; Figure S5: Gating strategy for quantification of plasma cells in peripheral blood of IPF patients in comparison to healthy control.; Figure S6: FKBP11 is also detected in non-plasma (CD38$^-$) cells in pancreas and stomach, but not in other healthy human tissue like muscle and lung.; Figure S7: Single cell-RNA-Seq analysis of mouse lungs confirms high plasma cell specificity for *Fkbp11*.; Figure S8: FKBP11 localizes to the ER in A549 and Raji cells and is induced by the UPR also in Raji cells.; Figure S9: FKBP11 knockdown affects neither IgG HC transcription, nor IgG levels in the ER, nor antibody binding affinity in the assessed hybridoma cell line H3.; Supplementary references.

Author Contributions: Conceptualization: C.A.S.-W., O.E., H.P.B.; Investigation: S.P., Y.I., E.H., S.W., L.K., I.E.F., L.B., A.F.; Data curation: J.C.S., B.M.J.-G.; Formal Analysis: S.P., Y.I., E.H., S.W., J.C.S., L.K., I.E.F., L.B., B.M.J.-G., R.F., A.S., E.M., H.P.B., C.A.S.-W.; Visualization: S.P., Y.I., E.H., S.W., J.C.S., C.A.S.-W.; Resources: C.R., A.G., M.F., R.A.H., N.K. (Nikolaus Kneidinger), J.B., R.F., A.S., A.H., E.M., H.P.B., O.E.; Project Administration: C.R., A.G., M.F., R.A.H., N.K. (Nikolaus Kneidinger), J.B., A.H., N.K. (Naftali Kaminski), E.M., H.P.B., C.A.S.-W.; Supervision: N.K. (Nikolaus Kneidinger), J.B., A.H., N.K. (Naftali Kaminski), E.M., H.P.B., O.E., C.A.S.-W.; Methodology: N.K. (Naftali Kaminski), E.M., H.P.B.; Funding Acquisiton: N.K. (Naftali Kaminski), E.M., H.P.B., O.E., C.A.S.-W.; Writing-original draft: S.P., C.A.S.-W.; Writing-review & editing: all. All authors have read and agreed to the published version of the manuscript.

Funding: This work was supported by the Friedrich-Baur-Stiftung (grant to C.A.S.-W., 51/16), the Helmholtz Association, the German Center for Lung Research (DZL), the Deutsche Forschungsgemeinschaft (DFG) within the Research Training Group GRK2338 (C.A.S.-W.), National Institutes of Health grants RO1HL108642 and RC2HL101715 (grants to Na.K.), and a grant from Shriners Hospital for Children (to H.P.B.). The CPC Research School funded S.P.'s stay in the H.P.B. lab and E.M. is supported by the DFG (SFB-TR128). J.C.S. is supported by the Else Kröner-Fresenius Foundation (2021_EKEA.16) and O.E. by the NIH (U54 AG075931 and R01 HL146519).

Institutional Review Board Statement: The study was conducted in accordance with the Declaration of Helsinki, and approved by the local Ethics Committee of the Ludwig-Maximilians University of Munich, Germany (333-10, 382-10, and 163-16), and the Ethics Committee of the Justus-Liebig-University School of Medicine (111/08, and 58/15).

Informed Consent Statement: Informed consent was obtained from all subjects involved in the study.

Data Availability Statement: Gene expression microarray data (Agilent Technologies, Santa Clara, CA) have been deposited under accession number GSE47460 in the data repository Gene Expression Omnibus (GEO, NCBI).

Acknowledgments: We gratefully acknowledge the provision of human biomaterial from the CPC-M bioArchive and its partners at the Asklepios Biobank Gauting, the Klinikum der Universität München, and the Ludwig-Maximilians-Universität München. We are equally grateful to the UGMLC biobank for the provision of material for validation in an independent cohort. The authors thank Daniela Dietel for excellent technical assistance, Flavia Greiffo for help with FACS analysis, and Herbert Schiller for providing single cell analysis data. We further acknowledge the Core Facility Flow Cytometry at the Biomedical Center, Ludwig-Maxmilians-Universität München, for providing us with the FACSAria Fusion.

Conflicts of Interest: N.K. (Naftali Kaminski) served as a consultant to Boehringer Ingelheim, Third Rock, Pliant, Samumed, NuMedii, Theravance, LifeMax, Three Lake Partners, Optikira, Astra Zeneca, RohBar, Veracyte, Augmanity, CSL Behring, Galapagos, Gilead and Thyron over the last 3 years, reports Equity in Pliant and Thyron, and a grant from Veracyte, Boehringer Ingelheim, BMS and non-financial support from MiRagen and Astra Zeneca. N.K. (Naftali Kaminski) has IP on novel biomarkers and therapeutics in IPF licensed to Biotech. E.M. received honorarium from Roche, Novartis, Merck, Sanofi, Biogen, and Bioeq and grant support from Novartis, Sanofi, Roche and Merck. O.E. is supported by Bristol Myers Squibb (FP00018992) and serves in advisory capacity to Pieris Pharmaceuticals, Blade Therapeutics, Delta 4 and YAP Therapeutics. L.K. is employee of Secarna Pharmaceuticals, but was still Ph.D. candidate in Staab-Weijnitz Lab when she contributed to the study. The funders had no role in the design of the study; in the collection, analyses, or interpretation of data; in the writing of the manuscript, or in the decision to publish the results. All other authors declare no conflict of interest.

References

1. Flajnik, M.F.; Kasahara, M. Origin and evolution of the adaptive immune system: Genetic events and selective pressures. *Nat. Rev. Genet.* **2010**, *11*, 47–59. [CrossRef] [PubMed]
2. Feige, M.J.; Hendershot, L.M.; Buchner, J. How antibodies fold. *Trends Biochem. Sci.* **2010**, *35*, 189–198. [CrossRef] [PubMed]
3. Feige, M.J.; Buchner, J. Principles and engineering of antibody folding and assembly. *Biochim. Biophys. Acta* **2014**, *1844*, 2024–2031. [CrossRef] [PubMed]
4. Moore, K.A.; Hollien, J. The unfolded protein response in secretory cell function. *Annu. Rev. Genet.* **2012**, *46*, 165–183. [CrossRef]
5. Todd, D.J.; Lee, A.H.; Glimcher, L.H. The endoplasmic reticulum stress response in immunity and autoimmunity. *Nat. Rev. Immunol.* **2008**, *8*, 663–674. [CrossRef]
6. Janssens, S.; Pulendran, B.; Lambrecht, B.N. Emerging functions of the unfolded protein response in immunity. *Nat. Immunol.* **2014**, *15*, 910–919. [CrossRef]
7. Taubenheim, N.; Tarlinton, D.M.; Crawford, S.; Corcoran, L.M.; Hodgkin, P.D.; Nutt, S.L. High rate of antibody secretion is not integral to plasma cell differentiation as revealed by XBP-1 deficiency. *J. Immunol.* **2012**, *189*, 3328–3338. [CrossRef]
8. Todd, D.J.; McHeyzer-Williams, L.J.; Kowal, C.; Lee, A.H.; Volpe, B.T.; Diamond, B.; McHeyzer-Williams, M.G.; Glimcher, L.H. XBP1 governs late events in plasma cell differentiation and is not required for antigen-specific memory B cell development. *J. Exp. Med.* **2009**, *206*, 2151–2159. [CrossRef]
9. Harikishore, A.; Yoon, H.S. Immunophilins: Structures, Mechanisms and Ligands. *Curr. Mol. Pharmacol.* **2015**, *9*, 37–47. [CrossRef]
10. Meunier, L.; Usherwood, Y.K.; Chung, K.T.; Hendershot, L.M. A subset of chaperones and folding enzymes form multiprotein complexes in endoplasmic reticulum to bind nascent proteins. *Mol. Biol. Cell* **2002**, *13*, 4456–4469. [CrossRef]
11. Feige, M.J.; Groscurth, S.; Marcinowski, M.; Shimizu, Y.; Kessler, H.; Hendershot, L.M.; Buchner, J. An unfolded CH1 domain controls the assembly and secretion of IgG antibodies. *Mol. Cell* **2009**, *34*, 569–579. [CrossRef] [PubMed]
12. Lee, J.; Choi, T.G.; Ha, J.; Kim, S.S. Cyclosporine A suppresses immunoglobulin G biosynthesis via inhibition of cyclophilin B in murine hybridomas and B cells. *Int. Immunopharmacol.* **2012**, *12*, 42–49. [CrossRef] [PubMed]
13. Jansen, G.; Maattanen, P.; Denisov, A.Y.; Scarffe, L.; Schade, B.; Balghi, H.; Dejgaard, K.; Chen, L.Y.; Muller, W.J.; Gehring, K.; et al. An interaction map of endoplasmic reticulum chaperones and foldases. *Mol. Cell. Proteom.* **2012**, *11*, 710–723. [CrossRef] [PubMed]

14. Lilie, H.; Lang, K.; Rudolph, R.; Buchner, J. Prolyl isomerases catalyze antibody folding in vitro. *Protein Sci.* **1993**, *2*, 1490–1496. [CrossRef] [PubMed]
15. Tong, M.; Jiang, Y. FK506-Binding Proteins and Their Diverse Functions. *Curr. Mol. Pharmacol.* **2015**, *9*, 48–65. [CrossRef] [PubMed]
16. Rulten, S.L.; Kinloch, R.A.; Tateossian, H.; Robinson, C.; Gettins, L.; Kay, J.E. The human FK506-binding proteins: Characterization of human FKBP19. *Mamm. Genome* **2006**, *17*, 322–331. [CrossRef] [PubMed]
17. Bensellam, M.; Chan, J.Y.; Lee, K.; Joglekar, M.V.; Hardikar, A.A.; Loudovaris, T.; Thomas, H.E.; Jonas, J.C.; Laybutt, D.R. Phlda3 regulates beta cell survival during stress. *Sci. Rep.* **2019**, *9*, 12827. [CrossRef]
18. Chan, J.Y.; Lee, K.; Maxwell, E.L.; Liang, C.; Laybutt, D.R. Macrophage alterations in islets of obese mice linked to beta cell disruption in diabetes. *Diabetologia* **2019**, *62*, 993–999. [CrossRef]
19. Bensellam, M.; Maxwell, E.L.; Chan, J.Y.; Luzuriaga, J.; West, P.K.; Jonas, J.C.; Gunton, J.E.; Laybutt, D.R. Hypoxia reduces ER-to-Golgi protein trafficking and increases cell death by inhibiting the adaptive unfolded protein response in mouse beta cells. *Diabetologia* **2016**, *59*, 1492–1502. [CrossRef]
20. Hanagata, N.; Li, X. Osteoblast-enriched membrane protein IFITM5 regulates the association of CD9 with an FKBP11-CD81-FPRP complex and stimulates expression of interferon-induced genes. *Biochem. Biophys. Res. Commun.* **2011**, *409*, 378–384. [CrossRef]
21. Hanagata, N.; Li, X.; Morita, H.; Takemura, T.; Li, J.; Minowa, T. Characterization of the osteoblast-specific transmembrane protein IFITM5 and analysis of IFITM5-deficient mice. *J. Bone Mineral. Metab.* **2011**, *29*, 279–290. [CrossRef] [PubMed]
22. Tsukamoto, T.; Li, X.; Morita, H.; Minowa, T.; Aizawa, T.; Hanagata, N.; Demura, M. Role of S-palmitoylation on IFITM5 for the interaction with FKBP11 in osteoblast cells. *PLoS ONE* **2013**, *8*, e75831. [CrossRef] [PubMed]
23. Wang, W.; Li, Q.; Huang, G.; Lin, B.Y.; Lin, D.; Ma, Y.; Zhang, Z.; Chen, T.; Zhou, J. Tandem Mass Tag-Based Proteomic Analysis of Potential Biomarkers for Hepatocellular Carcinoma Differentiation. *Onco Targets Ther.* **2021**, *14*, 1007–1020. [CrossRef] [PubMed]
24. Lin, I.Y.; Yen, C.H.; Liao, Y.J.; Lin, S.E.; Ma, H.P.; Chan, Y.J.; Chen, Y.M. Identification of FKBP11 as a biomarker for hepatocellular carcinoma. *Anticancer Res.* **2013**, *33*, 2763–2769. [PubMed]
25. Shi, W.; Liao, Y.; Willis, S.N.; Taubenheim, N.; Inouye, M.; Tarlinton, D.M.; Smyth, G.K.; Hodgkin, P.D.; Nutt, S.L.; Corcoran, L.M. Transcriptional profiling of mouse B cell terminal differentiation defines a signature for antibody-secreting plasma cells. *Nat. Immunol.* **2015**, *16*, 663–673. [CrossRef]
26. Tellier, J.; Shi, W.; Minnich, M.; Liao, Y.; Crawford, S.; Smyth, G.K.; Kallies, A.; Busslinger, M.; Nutt, S.L. Blimp-1 controls plasma cell function through the regulation of immunoglobulin secretion and the unfolded protein response. *Nat. Immunol.* **2016**, *17*, 323–330. [CrossRef]
27. Ruer-Laventie, J.; Simoni, L.; Schickel, J.N.; Soley, A.; Duval, M.; Knapp, A.M.; Marcellin, L.; Lamon, D.; Korganow, A.S.; Martin, T.; et al. Overexpression of Fkbp11, a feature of lupus B cells, leads to B cell tolerance breakdown and initiates plasma cell differentiation. *Immun. Inflamm. Dis.* **2015**, *3*, 265–279. [CrossRef]
28. Hofmann, K.; Clauder, A.K.; Manz, R.A. Targeting B Cells and Plasma Cells in Autoimmune Diseases. *Front. Immunol.* **2018**, *9*, 835. [CrossRef]
29. Lee, D.S.W.; Rojas, O.L.; Gommerman, J.L. B cell depletion therapies in autoimmune disease: Advances and mechanistic insights. *Nat. Rev. Drug Discov.* **2021**, *20*, 179–199. [CrossRef]
30. Kao, D.; Lux, A.; Schwab, I.; Nimmerjahn, F. Targeting B cells and autoantibodies in the therapy of autoimmune diseases. *Semin. Immunopathol.* **2014**, *36*, 289–299. [CrossRef]
31. Hutchinson, J.; Fogarty, A.; Hubbard, R.; McKeever, T. Global incidence and mortality of idiopathic pulmonary fibrosis: A systematic review. *Eur. Respir. J.* **2015**, *46*, 795–806. [CrossRef] [PubMed]
32. King, T.E., Jr.; Pardo, A.; Selman, M. Idiopathic pulmonary fibrosis. *Lancet* **2011**, *378*, 1949–1961. [CrossRef]
33. Fernandez, I.E.; Eickelberg, O. New cellular and molecular mechanisms of lung injury and fibrosis in idiopathic pulmonary fibrosis. *Lancet* **2012**, *380*, 680–688. [CrossRef]
34. Chakraborty, A.; Mastalerz, M.; Ansari, M.; Schiller, H.B.; Staab-Weijnitz, C.A. Emerging Roles of Airway Epithelial Cells in Idiopathic Pulmonary Fibrosis. *Cells* **2022**, *11*, 1050. [CrossRef]
35. Wells, A.U.; Denton, C.P. Interstitial lung disease in connective tissue disease—mechanisms and management. *Nat. Rev. Rheumatol.* **2014**, *10*, 728–739. [CrossRef]
36. Komura, K.; Yanaba, K.; Horikawa, M.; Ogawa, F.; Fujimoto, M.; Tedder, T.F.; Sato, S. CD19 regulates the development of bleomycin-induced pulmonary fibrosis in a mouse model. *Arthritis Rheum.* **2008**, *58*, 3574–3584. [CrossRef]
37. Vittal, R.; Mickler, E.A.; Fisher, A.J.; Zhang, C.; Rothhaar, K.; Gu, H.; Brown, K.M.; Emtiazdjoo, A.; Lott, J.M.; Frye, S.B.; et al. Type V collagen induced tolerance suppresses collagen deposition, TGF-beta and associated transcripts in pulmonary fibrosis. *PLoS ONE* **2013**, *8*, e76451. [CrossRef]
38. Shum, A.K.; Alimohammadi, M.; Tan, C.L.; Cheng, M.H.; Metzger, T.C.; Law, C.S.; Lwin, W.; Perheentupa, J.; Bour-Jordan, H.; Carel, J.C.; et al. BPIFB1 is a lung-specific autoantigen associated with interstitial lung disease. *Sci. Transl. Med.* **2013**, *5*, 206ra139. [CrossRef]
39. Mehta, H.; Goulet, P.O.; Nguyen, V.; Perez, G.; Koenig, M.; Senecal, J.L.; Sarfati, M. Topoisomerase I peptide-loaded dendritic cells induce autoantibody response as well as skin and lung fibrosis. *Autoimmunity* **2016**, *49*, 503–513. [CrossRef]

40. Yoshizaki, A.; Iwata, Y.; Komura, K.; Ogawa, F.; Hara, T.; Muroi, E.; Takenaka, M.; Shimizu, K.; Hasegawa, M.; Fujimoto, M.; et al. CD19 regulates skin and lung fibrosis via Toll-like receptor signaling in a model of bleomycin-induced scleroderma. *Am. J. Pathol.* **2008**, *172*, 1650–1663. [CrossRef]
41. Francois, A.; Gombault, A.; Villeret, B.; Alsaleh, G.; Fanny, M.; Gasse, P.; Adam, S.M.; Crestani, B.; Sibilia, J.; Schneider, P.; et al. B cell activating factor is central to bleomycin- and IL-17-mediated experimental pulmonary fibrosis. *J. Autoimmun.* **2015**, *56*, 1–11. [CrossRef] [PubMed]
42. Matsushita, T.; Kobayashi, T.; Mizumaki, K.; Kano, M.; Sawada, T.; Tennichi, M.; Okamura, A.; Hamaguchi, Y.; Iwakura, Y.; Hasegawa, M.; et al. BAFF inhibition attenuates fibrosis in scleroderma by modulating the regulatory and effector B cell balance. *Sci. Adv.* **2018**, *4*, eaas9944. [CrossRef] [PubMed]
43. Schiller, H.B.; Mayr, C.H.; Leuschner, G.; Strunz, M.; Staab-Weijnitz, C.; Preisendorfer, S.; Eckes, B.; Moinzadeh, P.; Krieg, T.; Schwartz, D.A.; et al. Deep Proteome Profiling Reveals Common Prevalence of MZB1-Positive Plasma B Cells in Human Lung and Skin Fibrosis. *Am. J. Respir. Crit. Care Med.* **2017**, *196*, 1298–1310. [CrossRef] [PubMed]
44. Xue, J.; Kass, D.J.; Bon, J.; Vuga, L.; Tan, J.; Csizmadia, E.; Otterbein, L.; Soejima, M.; Levesque, M.C.; Gibson, K.F.; et al. Plasma B lymphocyte stimulator and B cell differentiation in idiopathic pulmonary fibrosis patients. *J. Immunol.* **2013**, *191*, 2089–2095. [CrossRef]
45. Hoyne, G.F.; Elliott, H.; Mutsaers, S.E.; Prele, C.M. Idiopathic pulmonary fibrosis and a role for autoimmunity. *Immunol. Cell Biol.* **2017**, *95*, 577–583. [CrossRef]
46. Xue, J.; Gochuico, B.R.; Alawad, A.S.; Feghali-Bostwick, C.A.; Noth, I.; Nathan, S.D.; Rosen, G.D.; Rosas, I.O.; Dacic, S.; Ocak, I.; et al. The HLA class II Allele DRB1*1501 is over-represented in patients with idiopathic pulmonary fibrosis. *PLoS ONE* **2011**, *6*, e14715. [CrossRef]
47. Fingerlin, T.E.; Zhang, W.; Yang, I.V.; Ainsworth, H.C.; Russell, P.H.; Blumhagen, R.Z.; Schwarz, M.I.; Brown, K.K.; Steele, M.P.; Loyd, J.E.; et al. Genome-wide imputation study identifies novel HLA locus for pulmonary fibrosis and potential role for auto-immunity in fibrotic idiopathic interstitial pneumonia. *BMC Genet.* **2016**, *17*, 74. [CrossRef]
48. Preisendörfer, S.; Ishikawa, Y.; Knüppel, L.; Fernandez, I.; Binzenhofer, L.; Juan-Guardela, B.; Hennen, E.; Ruppert, C.; Guenther, A.; Kneidinger, N.; et al. FK506-binding protein 11, a novel plasma cell specific antibody folding catalyst, is increased in idiopathic pulmonary fibrosis. *Eur. Respir. J.* **2020**, *56*, 2293. [CrossRef]
49. Preisendörfer, S.; Knüppel, L.; Ishikawa, Y.; Binzenhofer, L.; Fernandez, I.E.; Juan-Guardela, B.M.; Ruppert, C.; Guenther, A.; Hatz, R.; Behr, J.; et al. FK506 Binding Protein 11, a Plasma Cell-Specific Antibody Folding Catalyst, Is Increased in Pulmonary Fibrosis. *Am. J. Respir. Crit. Care Med.* **2018**, *197*, A2204.
50. Bauer, Y.; Tedrow, J.; de Bernard, S.; Birker-Robaczewska, M.; Gibson, K.F.; Guardela, B.J.; Hess, P.; Klenk, A.; Lindell, K.O.; Poirey, S.; et al. A novel genomic signature with translational significance for human idiopathic pulmonary fibrosis. *Am. J. Respir. Cell Mol. Biol.* **2015**, *52*, 217–231. [CrossRef]
51. Yang, I.V.; Pedersen, B.S.; Rabinovich, E.; Hennessy, C.E.; Davidson, E.J.; Murphy, E.; Guardela, B.J.; Tedrow, J.R.; Zhang, Y.; Singh, M.K.; et al. Relationship of DNA methylation and gene expression in idiopathic pulmonary fibrosis. *Am. J. Respir. Crit. Care Med.* **2014**, *190*, 1263–1272. [CrossRef] [PubMed]
52. Herazo-Maya, J.D.; Noth, I.; Duncan, S.R.; Kim, S.; Ma, S.F.; Tseng, G.C.; Feingold, E.; Juan-Guardela, B.M.; Richards, T.J.; Lussier, Y.; et al. Peripheral blood mononuclear cell gene expression profiles predict poor outcome in idiopathic pulmonary fibrosis. *Sci. Transl. Med.* **2013**, *5*, 205ra136. [CrossRef] [PubMed]
53. Steinbrunn, T.; Chatterjee, M.; Bargou, R.C.; Stuhmer, T. Efficient transient transfection of human multiple myeloma cells by electroporation–an appraisal. *PLoS ONE* **2014**, *9*, e97443. [CrossRef] [PubMed]
54. Pinna, D.; Corti, D.; Jarrossay, D.; Sallusto, F.; Lanzavecchia, A. A Clonal dissection of the human memory B-cell repertoire following infection and vaccination. *Eur. J. Immunol.* **2009**, *39*, 1260–1270. [CrossRef]
55. Laurent, S.A.; Hoffmann, F.S.; Kuhn, P.H.; Cheng, Q.; Chu, Y.; Schmidt-Supprian, M.; Hauck, S.M.; Schuh, E.; Krumbholz, M.; Rubsamen, H.; et al. gamma-Secretase directly sheds the survival receptor BCMA from plasma cells. *Nat. Commun.* **2015**, *6*, 7333. [CrossRef]
56. Winklmeier, S.; Schluter, M.; Spadaro, M.; Thaler, F.S.; Vural, A.; Gerhards, R.; Macrini, C.; Mader, S.; Kurne, A.; Inan, B.; et al. Identification of circulating MOG-specific B cells in patients with MOG antibodies. *Neurol. Neuroimmunol. Neuroinflamm.* **2019**, *6*, 625. [CrossRef]
57. Lilie, H. Folding of the Fab fragment within the intact antibody. *FEBS Lett.* **1997**, *417*, 239–242. [CrossRef]
58. Reinhardt, D.P.; Keene, D.R.; Corson, G.M.; Poschl, E.; Bachinger, H.P.; Gambee, J.E.; Sakai, L.Y. Fibrillin-1: Organization in microfibrils and structural properties. *J. Mol. Biol.* **1996**, *258*, 104–116. [CrossRef]
59. Ishikawa, Y.; Mizuno, K.; Bächinger, H.P. Ziploc-ing the structure 2.0: Endoplasmic reticulum-resident peptidyl prolyl isomerases show different activities toward hydroxyproline. *J. Biol. Chem.* **2017**, *292*, 9273–9282. [CrossRef]
60. Krämer, P.M.; Weber, C.M.; Forster, S.; Rauch, P.; Kremmer, E. Analysis of DDT isomers with enzyme-linked immunosorbent assay and optical immunosensor based on rat monoclonal antibodies as biological recognition elements. *J. AOAC Int.* **2010**, *93*, 44–58. [CrossRef]
61. Staab-Weijnitz, C.A.; Fernandez, I.E.; Knüppel, L.; Maul, J.; Heinzelmann, K.; Juan-Guardela, B.M.; Hennen, E.; Preissler, G.; Winter, H.; Neurohr, C.; et al. FK506-Binding Protein 10, a Potential Novel Drug Target for Idiopathic Pulmonary Fibrosis. *Am. J. Respir. Crit. Care Med.* **2015**, *192*, 455–467. [CrossRef] [PubMed]

62. Kim, S.; Herazo-Maya, J.D.; Kang, D.D.; Juan-Guardela, B.M.; Tedrow, J.; Martinez, F.J.; Sciurba, F.C.; Tseng, G.C.; Kaminski, N. Integrative phenotyping framework (iPF): Integrative clustering of multiple omics data identifies novel lung disease subphenotypes. *BMC Genom.* **2015**, *16*, 924. [CrossRef] [PubMed]
63. Angelin-Duclos, C.; Cattoretti, G.; Lin, K.I.; Calame, K. Commitment of B lymphocytes to a plasma cell fate is associated with Blimp-1 expression in vivo. *J. Immunol.* **2000**, *165*, 5462–5471. [CrossRef]
64. Angelidis, I.; Simon, L.M.; Fernandez, I.E.; Strunz, M.; Mayr, C.H.; Greiffo, F.R.; Tsitsiridis, G.; Ansari, M.; Graf, E.; Strom, T.M.; et al. An atlas of the aging lung mapped by single cell transcriptomics and deep tissue proteomics. *Nat. Commun.* **2019**, *10*, 963. [CrossRef] [PubMed]
65. Gass, J.N.; Gunn, K.E.; Sriburi, R.; Brewer, J.W. Stressed-out B cells? Plasma-cell differentiation and the unfolded protein response. *Trends Immunol.* **2004**, *25*, 17–24. [CrossRef] [PubMed]
66. Iwakoshi, N.N.; Lee, A.H.; Glimcher, L.H. The X-box binding protein-1 transcription factor is required for plasma cell differentiation and the unfolded protein response. *Immunol. Rev.* **2003**, *194*, 29–38. [CrossRef]
67. Lee, A.H.; Iwakoshi, N.N.; Glimcher, L.H. XBP-1 regulates a subset of endoplasmic reticulum resident chaperone genes in the unfolded protein response. *Mol. Cell. Biol.* **2003**, *23*, 7448–7459. [CrossRef]
68. Kay, J.E. Structure-function relationships in the FK506-binding protein (FKBP) family of peptidylprolyl cis-trans isomerases. *Biochem. J.* **1996**, *314 Pt 2*, 361–385. [CrossRef]
69. Ishikawa, Y.; Bachinger, H.P. A molecular ensemble in the rER for procollagen maturation. *Biochim. Biophys. Acta* **2013**, *1833*, 2479–2491. [CrossRef]
70. Lecca, M.R.; Wagner, U.; Patrignani, A.; Berger, E.G.; Hennet, T. Genome-wide analysis of the unfolded protein response in fibroblasts from congenital disorders of glycosylation type-I patients. *FASEB J.* **2005**, *19*, 240–242. [CrossRef]
71. Shaffer, A.L.; Shapiro-Shelef, M.; Iwakoshi, N.N.; Lee, A.H.; Qian, S.B.; Zhao, H.; Yu, X.; Yang, L.; Tan, B.K.; Rosenwald, A.; et al. XBP1, downstream of Blimp-1, expands the secretory apparatus and other organelles, and increases protein synthesis in plasma cell differentiation. *Immunity* **2004**, *21*, 81–93. [CrossRef] [PubMed]
72. Bonner, J.M.; Boulianne, G.L. Diverse structures, functions and uses of FK506 binding proteins. *Cell. Signal.* **2017**, *38*, 97–105. [CrossRef] [PubMed]
73. Lilie, H.; Rudolph, R.; Buchner, J. Association of antibody chains at different stages of folding: Prolyl isomerization occurs after formation of quaternary structure. *J. Mol. Biol.* **1995**, *248*, 190–201. [CrossRef] [PubMed]
74. Jeong, M.; Jang, E.; Choi, S.S.; Ji, C.; Lee, K.; Youn, J. The Function of FK506-Binding Protein 13 in Protein Quality Control Protects Plasma Cells from Endoplasmic Reticulum Stress-Associated Apoptosis. *Front. Immunol.* **2017**, *8*, 222. [CrossRef]
75. Tat, V.; Ayaub, E.A.; Ayoub, A.; Vierhout, M.; Naiel, S.; Padwal, M.K.; Abed, S.; Mekhael, O.; Tandon, K.; Revill, S.D.; et al. FK506-Binding Protein 13 Expression Is Upregulated in Interstitial Lung Disease and Correlated with Clinical Severity. A Potentially Protective Role. *Am. J. Respir. Cell Mol. Biol.* **2021**, *64*, 235–246. [CrossRef]
76. Calame, K.L. Plasma cells: Finding new light at the end of B cell development. *Nat. Immunol.* **2001**, *2*, 1103–1108. [CrossRef]
77. Caraux, A.; Klein, B.; Paiva, B.; Bret, C.; Schmitz, A.; Fuhler, G.M.; Bos, N.A.; Johnsen, H.E.; Orfao, A.; Perez-Andres, M.; et al. Circulating human B and plasma cells. Age-associated changes in counts and detailed characterization of circulating normal CD138- and CD138+ plasma cells. *Haematologica* **2010**, *95*, 1016–1020. [CrossRef]
78. Feghali-Bostwick, C.A.; Wilkes, D.S. Autoimmunity in idiopathic pulmonary fibrosis: Are circulating autoantibodies pathogenic or epiphenomena? *Am. J. Respir. Crit. Care Med.* **2011**, *183*, 692–693. [CrossRef]
79. Donahoe, M.; Valentine, V.G.; Chien, N.; Gibson, K.F.; Raval, J.S.; Saul, M.; Xue, J.; Zhang, Y.; Duncan, S.R. Autoantibody-Targeted Treatments for Acute Exacerbations of Idiopathic Pulmonary Fibrosis. *PLoS ONE* **2015**, *10*, e0127771. [CrossRef]
80. van de Donk, N.W.; Janmaat, M.L.; Mutis, T.; Lammerts van Bueren, J.J.; Ahmadi, T.; Sasser, A.K.; Lokhorst, H.M.; Parren, P.W. Monoclonal antibodies targeting CD38 in hematological malignancies and beyond. *Immunol. Rev.* **2016**, *270*, 95–112. [CrossRef]
81. Shih, T.; De, S.; Barnes, B.J. RNAi Transfection Optimized in Primary Naive B Cells for the Targeted Analysis of Human Plasma Cell Differentiation. *Front. Immunol.* **2019**, *10*, 1652. [CrossRef] [PubMed]
82. Xia, B.; Amador, G.; Viswanatha, R.; Zirin, J.; Mohr, S.E.; Perrimon, N. CRISPR-based engineering of gene knockout cells by homology-directed insertion in polyploid Drosophila S2R+ cells. *Nat. Protoc.* **2020**, *15*, 3478–3498. [CrossRef]
83. Korfei, M.; Ruppert, C.; Mahavadi, P.; Henneke, I.; Markart, P.; Koch, M.; Lang, G.; Fink, L.; Bohle, R.M.; Seeger, W.; et al. Epithelial endoplasmic reticulum stress and apoptosis in sporadic idiopathic pulmonary fibrosis. *Am. J. Respir. Crit. Care Med.* **2008**, *178*, 838–846. [CrossRef] [PubMed]
84. Lawson, W.E.; Crossno, P.F.; Polosukhin, V.V.; Roldan, J.; Cheng, D.S.; Lane, K.B.; Blackwell, T.R.; Xu, C.; Markin, C.; Ware, L.B.; et al. Endoplasmic reticulum stress in alveolar epithelial cells is prominent in IPF: Association with altered surfactant protein processing and herpesvirus infection. *Am. J. Physiol. Lung Cell Mol. Physiol.* **2008**, *294*, L1119–L1126. [CrossRef] [PubMed]
85. Tanjore, H.; Lawson, W.E.; Blackwell, T.S. Endoplasmic reticulum stress as a pro-fibrotic stimulus. *Biochim. Biophys. Acta* **2013**, *1832*, 940–947. [CrossRef] [PubMed]
86. Ghartey-Kwansah, G.; Li, Z.; Feng, R.; Wang, L.; Zhou, X.; Chen, F.Z.; Xu, M.M.; Jones, O.; Mu, Y.; Chen, S.; et al. Comparative analysis of FKBP family protein: Evaluation, structure, and function in mammals and Drosophila melanogaster. *BMC Dev. Biol.* **2018**, *18*, 7. [CrossRef]

cells

Article

Transcriptional Profiling of Insulin-like Growth Factor Signaling Components in Embryonic Lung Development and Idiopathic Pulmonary Fibrosis

Vahid Kheirollahi [1,2,3,4,†], Ali Khadim [1,2,3,4,†], Georgios Kiliaris [1,2,3,4], Martina Korfei [1,3,4], Margarida Maria Barroso [1,2,3,4], Ioannis Alexopoulos [1,2,3,4], Ana Ivonne Vazquez-Armendariz [1,2,3,4], Malgorzata Wygrecka [1,2,3], Clemens Ruppert [1,3], Andreas Guenther [1,3,4], Werner Seeger [1,2,3,4], Susanne Herold [1,2,3,4] and Elie El Agha [1,2,3,4,*]

[1] Department of Medicine II, Internal Medicine, Pulmonary and Critical Care, Universities of Giessen and Marburg Lung Center (UGMLC), Member of the German Center for Lung Research (DZL), Justus-Liebig University Giessen, 35392 Giessen, Germany; vkheirollahi@gmail.com (V.K.); ali.khadim@innere.med.uni-giessen.de (A.K.); georgios.kiliaris@innere.med.uni-giessen.de (G.K.); martina.korfei@innere.med.uni-giessen.de (M.K.); margarida.barroso@innere.med.uni-giessen.de (M.M.B.); ioannis.alexopoulos@innere.med.uni-giessen.de (I.A.); ana.i.vazquez-armendariz@innere.med.uni-giessen.de (A.I.V.-A.); malgorzata.wygrecka@innere.med.uni-giessen.de (M.W.); clemens.ruppert@innere.med.uni-giessen.de (C.R.); andreas.guenther@innere.med.uni-giessen.de (A.G.); werner.seeger@innere.med.uni-giessen.de (W.S.); susanne.herold@innere.med.uni-giessen.de (S.H.)
[2] Department of Medicine V, Internal Medicine, Infectious Diseases and Infection Control, Universities of Giessen and Marburg Lung Center (UGMLC), Member of the German Center for Lung Research (DZL), Justus-Liebig University Giessen, 35392 Giessen, Germany
[3] Cardio-Pulmonary Institute (CPI), Justus-Liebig University Giessen, 35392 Giessen, Germany
[4] Institute for Lung Health (ILH), Justus-Liebig University Giessen, 35392 Giessen, Germany
* Correspondence: elie.el-agha@innere.med.uni-giessen.de
† These authors contributed equally to this work.

Abstract: Insulin-like growth factor (IGF) signaling controls the development and growth of many organs, including the lung. Loss of function of *Igf1* or its receptor *Igf1r* impairs lung development and leads to neonatal respiratory distress in mice. Although many components of the IGF signaling pathway have shown to be dysregulated in idiopathic pulmonary fibrosis (IPF), the expression pattern of such components in different cellular compartments of the developing and/or fibrotic lung has been elusive. In this study, we provide a comprehensive transcriptional profile for such signaling components during embryonic lung development in mice, bleomycin-induced pulmonary fibrosis in mice and in human IPF lung explants. During late gestation, we found that *Igf1* is upregulated in parallel to *Igf1r* downregulation in the lung mesenchyme. Lung tissues derived from bleomycin-treated mice and explanted IPF lungs revealed upregulation of IGF1 in parallel to downregulation of IGF1R, in addition to upregulation of several IGF binding proteins (IGFBPs) in lung fibrosis. Finally, treatment of IPF lung fibroblasts with recombinant IGF1 led to myogenic differentiation. Our data serve as a resource for the transcriptional profile of IGF signaling components and warrant further research on the involvement of this pathway in both lung development and pulmonary disease.

Keywords: IGF1; IGF1R; lung development; bleomycin-induced pulmonary fibrosis; idiopathic pulmonary fibrosis

1. Introduction

The insulin-like growth factor (IGF) family consists of two ligands (IGF1 and IGF2), two receptors (IGF1R and IGF2R), six IGF-binding proteins (IGFBP1-6) and one IGFBP-related protein (IGFBP-rP1 or IGFBP7). IGFBPs regulate the bioavailability of IGF ligands in the blood stream. As the name suggests, IGF shares structural homology with insulin and can therefore bind to and activate the insulin receptor, albeit with lower affinity than insulin. Although it is expressed in most tissues, IGF1 is mainly produced by the liver upon growth hormone (GH) stimulation. In fact, IGF1 functions as a growth hormone and *IGF1* deficiency is linked to dwarfism in mice and humans [1–4]. IGF1 is regarded as the natural ligand for IGF1R, and therefore transduces mitogenic and survival signals by activating MAPK, PI3K/AKT and mTOR signaling pathways [5]. On the other hand, IGF2 binds to IGF1R and IGF2R, with the latter functioning as a clearance receptor for IGF2 [6].

IGF signaling has been shown to be involved in murine lung organogenesis. *Igf1*-knockout newborn pups suffer from disproportional lung hypoplasia and die due to respiratory distress [1,7]. These mutants display thickened mesenchyme, alterations in extracellular matrix (ECM) protein deposition, thin smooth muscle and dilated blood vessels, indicating delayed lung development [1,7]. Using a hypomorphic *Igf1r^{neo}* allele that yields an 80% reduction in *Igf1r* expression, it was shown that reduced expression of *Igf1r* does not lead to an obvious phenotype [8]. On the other hand, *Igf1r*-knockout mouse embryos suffer from general organ hypoplasia including severe lung hypoplasia and underdeveloped diaphragms. These mutants die shortly after birth due to respiratory distress [1,8]. Histological analysis during late gestation showed that *Igf1r*-knockout mouse lungs display thickened intersaccular mesenchyme and delayed development [8]. *Igf2*-kockout pups also display delayed lung development at the end of gestation [9]. These pups display lower plasma corticosterone levels, and supplementing pregnant mice carrying *Igf2*-knockout pups with corticosterone rescues delayed lung development [9].

IGF1/IGF1R signaling has also been studied in the context of mouse models of lung injury and repair. For instance, *Igf1r* deficiency improves survival and ameliorates lung injury in response to hyperoxia [10]. IGF1R signaling controls the kinetics of cell proliferation and differentiation during airway epithelial regeneration [11]. Moreover, smooth muscle-derived IGF1 has been implicated in pulmonary hypertension development in response to hypoxia [12]. Last but not least, intervention with monoclonal antibodies against IGF1R attenuates bleomycin-induced pulmonary fibrosis [13].

Lipofibroblasts are adipocyte-like cells that not only transfer triglycerides to adjacent type 2 alveolar epithelial cells (AT2) to assist them in the process of surfactant production, but are also regarded as a niche that maintains AT2 stemness [14–16]. We have previously shown that lipofibroblasts are a source of myofibroblasts in lung fibrosis and that myofibroblast-to-lipofibroblast transdifferentiation represents a route for fibrosis resolution [17–19]. Since insulin signaling is integral to the differentiation of preadipocytes to adipocytes [20], and given that decreased IGF signaling is linked to impaired alveolar maturation, the question arose whether IGF signaling is involved in lipofibroblast formation. In this study, we provide a transcriptional profile for IGF family components at various stages of embryonic murine lung development, murine lung fibrosis and lung samples derived from idiopathic pulmonary fibrosis (IPF) patients. We also provide in vitro data on the effect of recombinant IGF1 on primary cultures of human IPF lung fibroblasts.

2. Materials and Methods

2.1. Animal Experiments

All animal experiments were approved by the local authorities. Mice were housed in a specific-pathogen-free (SPF) environment with free access to food and water. RjOrl:SWISS mice were obtained from Janvier Labs and timed pregnant females were used to collect embryonic tissues at the indicated timepoints (Approval number: 437_M). In bleomycin experiments, C57BL6/J female mice were subjected to a single intratracheal injection of saline (SAL; $n = 6$) or bleomycin (BLM; 2.5 U/Kg), and mice were euthanized after 7 (BLM d7; $n = 5$) or 14 days (BLM d14; $n = 5$) (Approval number: Gi20/10, No.: 109/2011, JLU-number: 594_GP). Protein lysates were used for western blotting and lung sections were used for histological analysis. Lung tissues were also used for RNA extraction and gene expression analysis.

2.2. Human-Derived Lung Material

Lung tissues and interstitial fibroblasts were isolated from explanted IPF and control lungs, collected in frame of the European IPF registry (eurIPFreg) and provided by the UGMLC Giessen Biobank, member of the DZL Platform Biobanking. The Ethics Committee of the Justus-Liebig University has approved the biospecimen collection of the UGMLC/DZL biobank under the ethics vote number 58/15. The patients have been informed and given their written consent for the use of biospecimen for research purposes. All studies and procedures to obtain human specimen were conducted according to the Declaration of Helsinki.

2.3. Primary Culture of Murine Lung Fibroblasts

Primary murine lung fibroblasts were cultured by differential adhesion as previously described [21]. Embryonic lungs were harvested and minced into fine pieces using blades, followed by digestion in 0.5% (w/v) collagenase IV (Thermo Fisher Scientific, Schwerte, Germany) for 45 min with slight agitation. Digested suspensions were then aspirated through 18G, 20G and 24G needles before being passed through 70 μm and 40 μm cell strainers (Sarstedt, Nümbrecht, Germany). Single-cell suspensions were allowed to adhere onto six-well plates for 17 min before washing with PBS. Cells were allowed to grow in DMEM (low glucose, GlutaMAX^{TM} Supplement, pyruvate) (Thermo Fisher Scientific) supplemented with 10% bovine calf serum (BCS) (Thermo Fisher Scientific) for the next 24 h before fresh culture medium was added.

2.4. Primary Culture of Human Lung Fibroblasts

Primary human lung fibroblasts derived from IPF patients were maintained in DMEM (Thermo Fisher Scientific) supplemented with 10% BCS (Thermo Fisher Scientific). Cells between passages three and five were used for experiments. Three hundred thousand cells were plated per well in six-well plates. After 24 h, cells were starved by replacing culture media by serum-free media for 24 h. Cells were then treated with recombinant human IGF1 (rhIGF1, 250 ng/mL) (R&D systems, Wiesbaden, Germany) or vehicle (phosphate-buffered saline, PBS) for 72 h. Cells derived from the same patients were used as controls. In the designated experiments, cells were cultured on CytoSoft plates with elastic modulus of 16 kPa (Sigma-Aldrich, St. Louis, MO, USA).

2.5. RNA Extraction, cDNA Synthesis and qPCR

RNeasy mini kit (Qiagen, Hilden, Germany) was used for RNA extraction followed by cDNA synthesis using Quantitect reverse transcription kit (Qiagen) according to the manufacturer's protocol. Quantitative real-time PCR (qPCR) was carried out using PowerUp SYBR green master mix (Thermo Fisher Scientific) and LightCycler 480 II machine (Roche Applied Science, Mannheim, Germany). Primer sequences are listed in Table 1.

Table 1. Primers used for qPCR.

Primer Name	Sequence (5'-3')
hACTA2 Fwd	CTGTTCCAGCCATCCTTCAT
hACTA2 Rev	TCATGATGCTGTTGTAGGTGGT
hCOL1A1 Fwd	ATGTTCAGCTTTGTGGACCTC
hCOL1A1 Rev	CTGTACGCAGGTGATTGGTG
hIGF1 Fwd	TGTGGAGACAGGGGCTTTTA
hIGF1 Rev	ATCCACGATGCCTGTCTGA
hIGF1R Fwd	GAGAATTTCCTTCACAATTCCATC
hIGF1R Rev	CACTTGCATGACGTCTCTCC
hIGF2 Fwd	CAAACCGAGCTGGGCG
hIGF2 Rev	CACAGAGAAGCGGAGGGA

Table 1. Cont.

Primer Name	Sequence (5'-3')
hIGF2R Fwd	TCTCCAGTGGACTGCCAAGT
hIGF2R Rev	GTGCTTAGGCCAGTCAGGTC
hIGFBP1 Fwd	AATGGATTTTATCACAGCAGACAG
hIGFBP1 Rev	GGTAGACGCACCAGCAGAGT
hIGFBP2 Fwd	AAGGGTGGCAAGCATCAC
hIGFBP2 Rev	CTGGTCCAGTTCCTGTTGG
hIGFBP3 Fwd	AACGCTAGTGCCGTCAGC
hIGFBP3 Rev	CGGTCTTCCTCCGACTCAC
hIGFBP4 Fwd	CCTCTACATCATCCCCATCC
hIGFBP4 Rev	GGTCCACACACCAGCACTT
hIGFBP5 Fwd	AGAGCTACCGCGAGCAAGT
hIGFBP5 Rev	GTAGGTCTCCTCGGCCATCT
hIGFBP6 Fwd	TGACCATCGAGGCTTCTACC
hIGFBP6 Rev	CATCCGATCCACACACCA
hINSRA Fwd	TTTTCGTCCCCAGGCCATC
hINSRB Fwd	CCCCAGAAAAACCTCTTCAGG
hINSR Rev	GTCACATTCCCAACATCGCC
hPBGD Fwd	TGTCTGGTAACGGCAATGCG
hPBGD Rev	CCCACGCGAATCACTCTCAT
hPLIN2 Fwd	TCAGCTCCATTCTACTGTTCACC
hPLIN2 Rev	CCTGAATTTTCTGATTGGCAC
hPPARG Fwd	TTGCTGTCATTATTCTCAGTGGA
hPPARG Rev	GAGGACTCAGGGTGGTTCAG
mCol1a1 Fwd	CCAAGAAGACATCCCTGAAGTCA
mCol1a1 Rev	TGCACGTCATCGCACACA
mHprt Fwd	CCTAAGATGAGCGCAAGTTGAA
mHprt Rev	CCACAGGACTAGAACACCTGCTAA
mIgf1 Fwd	AGCAGCCTTCCAACTCAATTAT
mIgf1 Rev	GAAGACGACATGATGTGTATCTTTATC
mIgf1r Fwd	AGAATTTCCTTCACAATTCCATC
mIgf1r Rev	CACTTGCATGACGTCTCTCC
mIgf2 Fwd	CGCTTCAGTTTGTCTGTTCG
mIgf2 Rev	GCAGCACTCTTCCACGATG
mIgf2r Fwd	CCTTCTCTAGTGGATTGTCAAGTG
migf2r Rev	AGGGCGCTCAAGTCATACTC
mIgfbp1 Fwd	TGGTCAGGGAGCCTGTGTA
mIgfbp1 Rev	ACAGCAGCCTTTGCCTCTT
mIgfbp2 Fwd	GCGGGTACCTGTGAAAAGAG
mIgfbp2 Rev	CCTCAGAGTGGTCGTCATCA
mIgfbp3 Fwd	GACGACGTACATTGCCTCAG
mIgfbp3 Rev	GACGACGTACATTGCCTCAG
mIgfbp4 Fwd	GACACCTCGGGAGGAACC
mIgfbp4 Rev	AAGAGGTCTTCGTGGGTACG
mIgfbp5 Fwd	GGCGAGCAAACCAAGATAGA
mIgfbp5 Rev	AGGTCTCTTCAGCCATCTCG
mIgfbp6 Fwd	GGGCTCTATGTGCCAAACTG
mIgfbp6 Rev	CCTGCGAGGAACGACACT
mInsr Fwd	TCTTTCTTCAGGAAGCTACATCTG
mInsr Rev	TGTCCAAGGCATAAAAAGAATAGTT

h: human; m: mouse.

2.6. Histology, Immunohistochemistry and Fluorescent Staining

Formalin-fixed, paraffin-embedded mouse and human lung tissues were subjected to immunohistochemistry as we previously described [17,22,23] using antibodies against IGF1 (Abcam, Berlin, Germany) (1:500), IGF1R (Sigma-Aldrich; 1:75) and TTF1 (Abcam; 1:100) and ZytoChem Plus AP Kit (Zytomed Systems, Berlin, Germany). Hematoxylin/eosin and Masson Goldner stains were carried out according to standard procedures. LipidTOX staining was carried out as previously described [18] and imaged using EVOS Cell Imaging System (Thermo Fisher Scientific).

2.7. Western Blotting

Western blots were carried out according to standard procedures. Antibodies against PAI-1 (R&D Systems) and mature COL1A1 (Meridian Life Science, Luckenwalde, Germany) were used.

2.8. Figure Assembly and Statistical Analysis

Quantitative data were assembled and analyzed using GraphPad Prism 9 (GraphPad Software, San Diego, CA, USA). The normality test was carried out whenever the number of biological samples allowed. Outliers in the data from human-derived lung material were detected using the ROUT method. For comparing two groups, t-test or Mann–Whitney test was carried out. One-way ANOVA was used to compare more than two groups. The number of biological samples (depicted as *n*) is shown in the corresponding figure legends. Figures were assembled using Adobe Illustrator (Adobe, San Jose, CA, USA).

3. Results

3.1. Transcriptional Profile of IGF Signaling Components during Embryonic Lung Development

To explore the expression pattern of IGF signaling components during embryonic lung development, embryos were collected from timed pregnant mice and RNA was isolated from lung homogenates and subjected to qPCR at multiple developmental stages (E14.5: Pseudoglandular stage; E16.5: End of pseudoglandular stage-beginning of canalicular stage; E18.5: Saccular stage) (Figure 1). These timepoints were chosen because various epithelial and mesenchymal cell lineages such as alveolar epithelial cells and lipofibroblasts start to emerge around E16.5 [21,24–26]. The results revealed that *Igf1* and *Igf2*, encoding the main IGF ligands, showed a decline from E14.5 to E18.5 (Figure 1a,b). On the other hand, the expression levels of IGF receptors, *Igf1r* and *Igf2r*, showed a 1.77- and a 2.57-fold increase, respectively (Figure 1c,d). *Insr*, encoding the insulin receptor gene, showed a similar upregulation at E18.5 (Figure 1e). Analysis of the expression levels of *Igfbp* genes showed a mixed pattern (Figure 1f–j). *Igfbp1/4/6* showed significant upregulation at E18.5 compared with E14.5 and E16.5. Conversely, *Igfbp2* showed significant downregulation at E18.5, while *Igfbp5* showed significant downregulation at E16.5 and E18.5 compared with E14.5.

The data described in Figure 1a–j reflect gene expression in whole-lung homogenates containing a mixture of endoderm- and mesoderm-derived cells such as epithelial, endothelial and mesenchymal cells. In order to investigate the expression pattern of these genes exclusively in mesenchymal cells, cell suspensions were prepared and subjected to differential adhesion as previously described [21]. Mesenchymal cells were allowed to grow for 24 h (Figure 1k). While *Igf1* showed gradual upregulation from E14.5 to E18.5 (around 6-fold increase at E18.5 compared with E14.5) (Figure 1l), *Igf1r* showed an opposite pattern where its expression levels decreased by 1.9 folds at E16.5 and 3.7 folds at E18.5 (Figure 1m). The expression pattern of *Igfbp* genes was very similar in cultured mesenchymal cells and lung homogenates (Figure 1n–r vs. Figure 1f–j). Immunohistochemistry on E18.5 lung sections showed that IGF1 immunoreactivity could be detected in both the epithelium and the mesenchyme, although the signal was stronger in the epithelium (Figure 1s). In agreement with the qPCR data, IGF1R was detected in epithelial cells rather than mesenchymal cells at this stage (Figure 1t). Collectively, these data indicate that *Igf1* is upregulated while *Igf1r* is downregulated in the lung mesenchyme during last gestation. Moreover, *Igfbp1/4/6* are upregulated while *Igfbp2* is downregulated in this lung compartment.

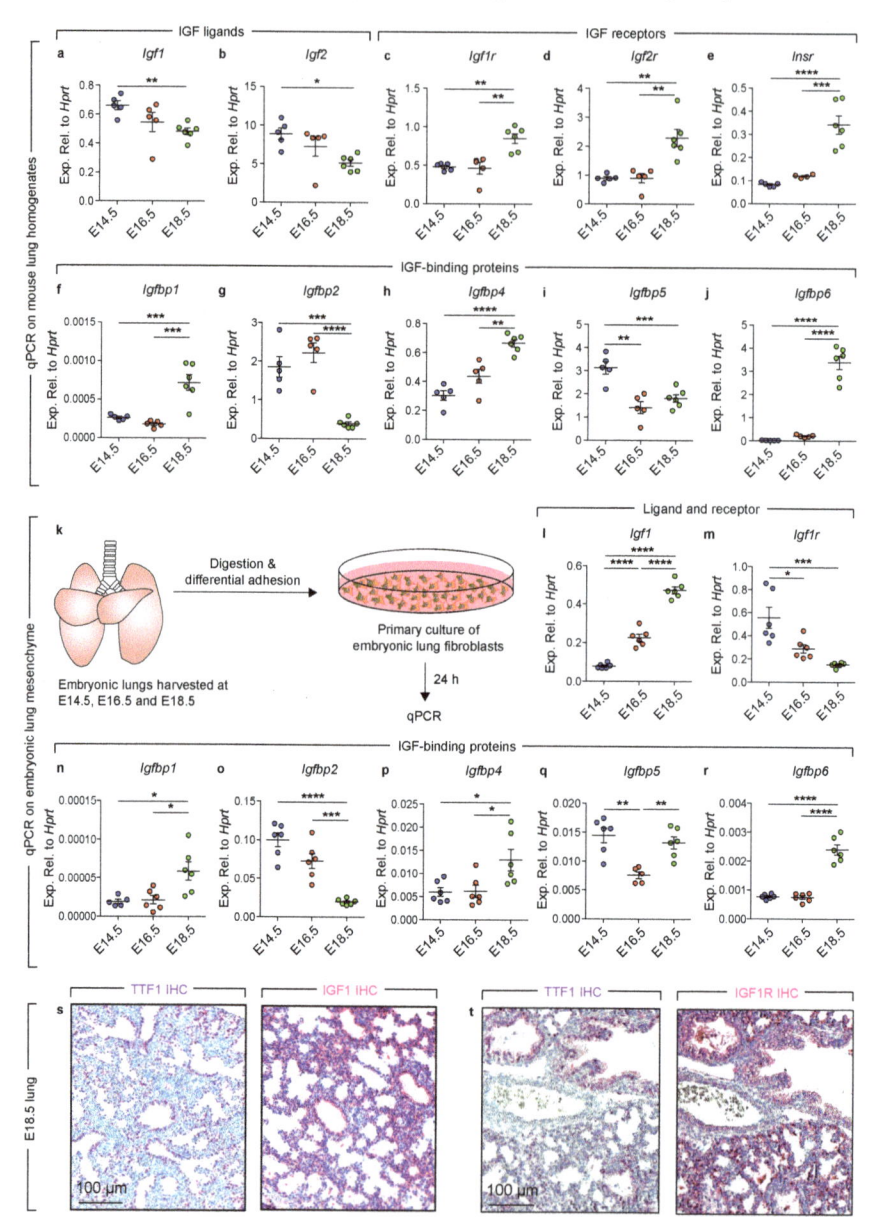

Figure 1. Expression profile of IGF signaling components during lung development. (**a–j**) qPCR on lung homogenates at the indicated developmental stages; (**k**) Scheme for experimental design; (**l–r**) qPCR on primary mesenchymal cells at the indicated developmental stages. (**s**) Immunohistochemistry for TTF1 and IGF1 on E18.5 mouse lungs. (**t**) Immunohistochemistry for TTF1 and IGF1R on E18.5 mouse lungs. One-way ANOVA was used to compare the means. (**a–j**) E14.5: $n = 5$, E16.5: $n = 5$, E18.5: $n = 6$; (**l–r**) E14.5: $n = 5–6$, E16.5: $n = 5–6$, E18.5: $n = 6$. * $p < 0.05$, ** $p < 0.01$, *** $p < 0.001$, **** $p < 0.0001$.

3.2. Increased Igf1 Expression during Fibrosis Development in Bleomycin-Induced Lung Injury

The expression levels of IGF signaling components were also examined in lung homogenates from bleomycin-treated mice at day 7 (end of acute lung injury/inflammatory phase—beginning of fibrotic phase) and day 14 (peak of fibrosis) and were compared with saline controls. Firstly, histological analysis using hematoxylin/eosin and Masson Goldner stains confirmed the presence of fibrosis at day 14 (Figure 2a,b). At the transcriptional level, *Col1a1* showed significant upregulation at days 7 and 14 (Figure 2d). Such upregulation was also confirmed by western blotting (Figure 2c). *Igf1* appeared to mimic *Col1a1* expression pattern where it showed significant upregulation, while *Igf2* did not show significant alterations (Figure 2e,f).

Analysis of genes encoding IGF receptors did not show significant changes in bleomycin-treated lungs (Figure 2g–i). During the course of injury, *Igfbp4* showed transient upregulation at day 7 before normalizing at day 14 (Figure 2k), while *Igfbp6* showed significant downregulation at day 14 (Figure 2m). On the other hand, *Igfbp2/5* did not show significant changes (Figure 2j,l). The upregulation of *Igf1* at the transcriptional level was also reflected at the protein level by immunohistochemistry, where IGF1 immunoreactivity was observed in areas of collagen deposition as well as in epithelial cells (Figure 2n,o). Finally, immunohistochemistry for IGF1R showed a strong signal in epithelial cells (AT2 and bronchial epithelium) in both saline and bleomycin-treated lungs (Figure 2p).

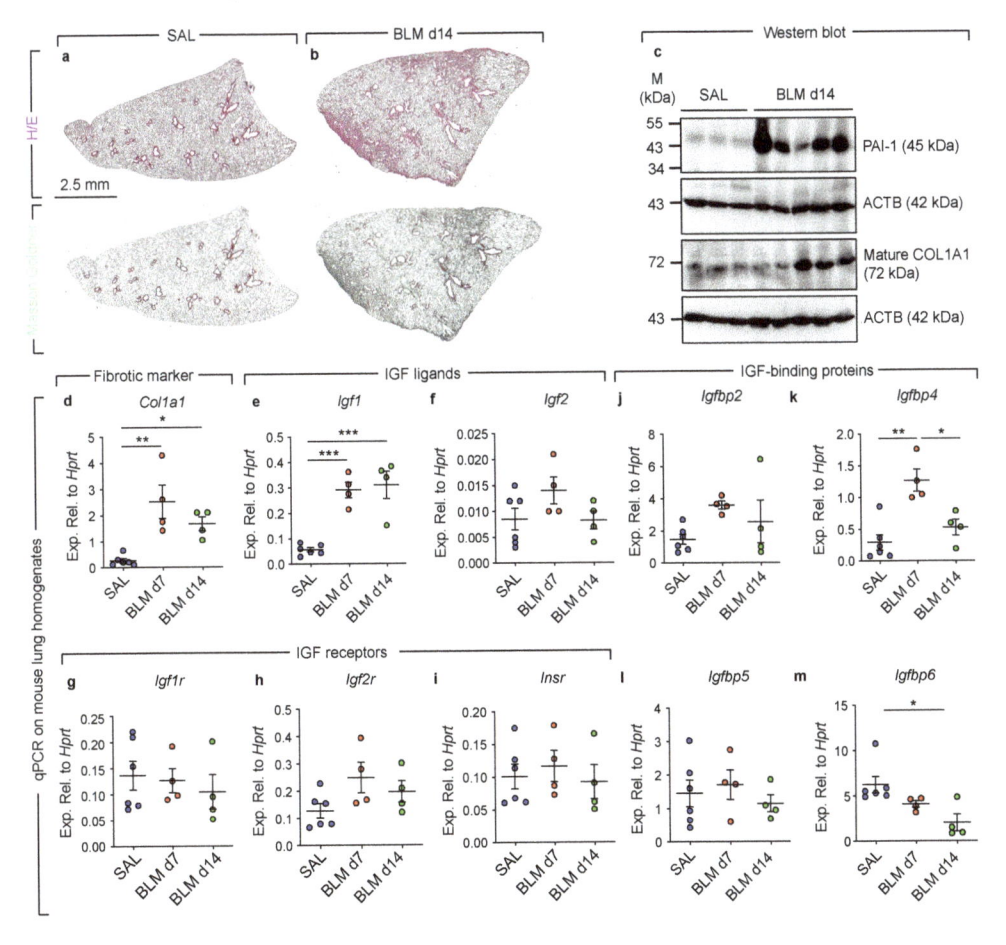

Figure 2. *Cont.*

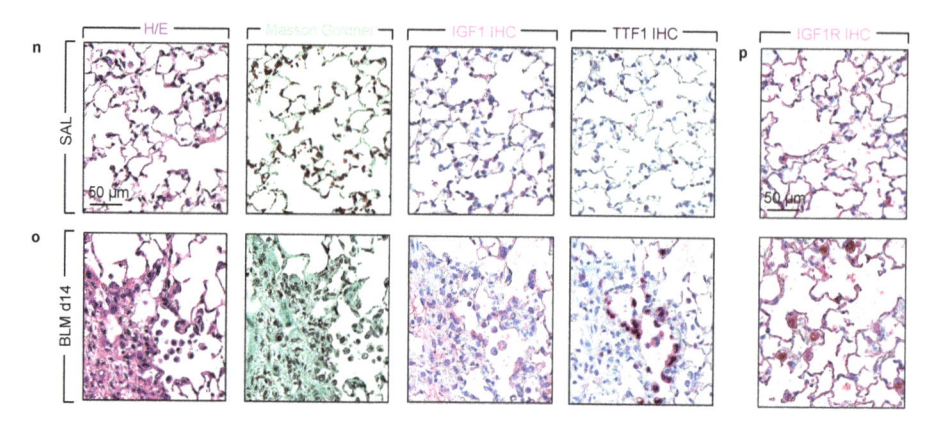

Figure 2. Alteration of IGF signaling in the bleomycin model of lung fibrosis. (**a,b**) Hematoxylin/eosin and Masson Goldner staining showing clear fibrosis in bleomycin-treated mouse lungs compared with saline-treated controls. (**c**) Western blot for PAI-1, COL1A1 and ACTB. (**d–m**) qPCR on lung homogenates at the indicated timepoints. (**n,o**) Hematoxylin/eosin stain, Masson Goldner stain, IGF1 immunohistochemistry and TTF1 immunohistochemistry on saline- and bleomycin-treated mouse lungs. (**p**) IGF1R immunohistochemistry on saline- and bleomycin-treated mouse lungs. One-way ANOVA was used to compare the means. SAL: $n = 6$, BLM d7: $n = 4$, BLM d14: $n = 4$. * $p < 0.05$, ** $p < 0.01$, *** $p < 0.001$. SAL: Saline; BLM: Bleomycin; IHC: Immunohistochemistry.

3.3. IGF1 Expression Is Elevated in IPF Lungs

Lung homogenates from donors and IPF patients were subjected to gene expression analysis. *IGF1* showed a strong 9.9-fold upregulation (Figure 3a) while *IGF1R* showed a 3-fold downregulation in IPF samples compared with donors (Figure 3b).

INSRA/B showed significant downregulation in IPF samples compared with donors (Figure 3d,e). While *IGF2* transcripts could not be detected in human lung tissues, *IGF2R* showed significant downregulation in IPF lungs compared with donor lungs (Figure 3c). No significant changes were observed in the expression levels of *IGFBP1/3* while *IGFBP2/4/5/6* showed significant upregulation in IPF lungs compared with donor lungs (3.9, 4.8, 5.6 and 6.4 folds, respectively) (Figure 3f–k). Finally, immunohistochemistry showed significant upregulation of IGF1 in IPF lung explants compared with donors, where IGF1 immunoreactivity was robust in alveolar and bronchiolar epithelial cells as well as in areas of dense fibrosis (Figure 3l). In contrast, IGF1 immunoreactivity was sparse in any cells of normal donor lungs (Figure 3l). Immunohistochemistry for IGF1R, on the other hand, showed a strong signal in bronchiolar cells in donor lungs, and the signal was weaker in IPF lungs (Figure 3m).

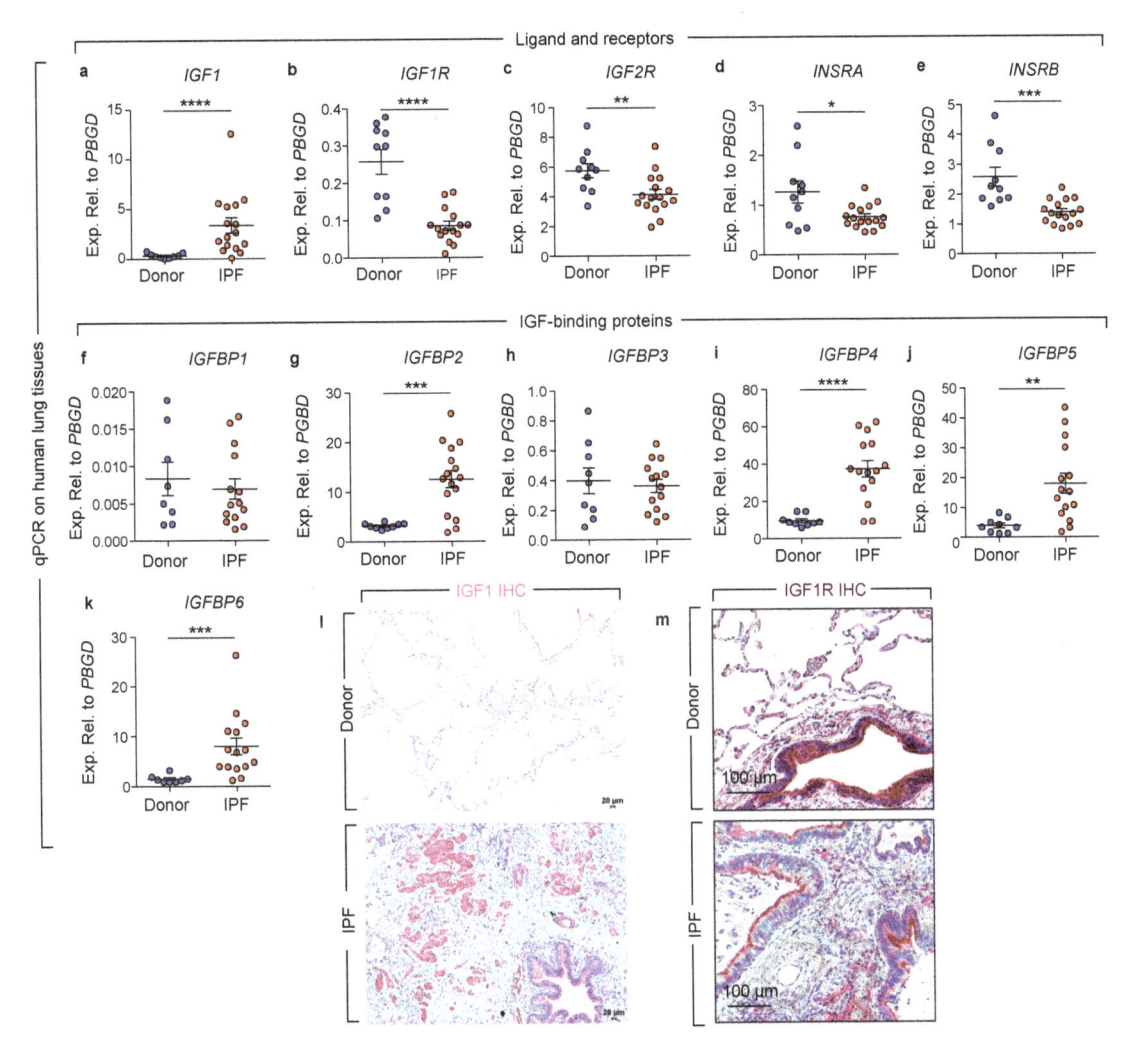

Figure 3. Alteration of IGF1 signaling in idiopathic pulmonary fibrosis. (**a–k**) qPCR on homogenates of lung explants derived from donor or IPF patients; (**l,m**) Immunohistochemistry for IGF1 and IGF1R on donor and IPF lung sections. *t*-test (**b–e,g–j**) or Mann–Whitney test (**a,f,k**) was performed to compare the groups. Donor: $n = 8\text{–}10$, IPF: $n = 14\text{–}16$. * $p < 0.05$, ** $p < 0.01$, *** $p < 0.001$, **** $p < 0.0001$. IHC: Immunohistochemistry.

3.4. Treatment of Human Lung Fibroblasts with Recombinant IGF1 Leads to Loss of Lipid Droplets

Due to the link between IGF1 signaling and lung fibrosis, we decided to investigate whether treatment with recombinant human IGF1 (rhIGF1) affects the expression levels of lipofibroblast and myofibroblast markers using primary cultures of human IPF lung fibroblasts (Figure 4). Given the impact of matrix stiffness on myofibroblast differentiation [27–29], we opted to use two culture conditions: Cells cultured on uncoated plates (plastic) and cells cultured on a 16 kPa matrix that mimics the pathophysiological setting linked to the induction of alpha smooth muscle actin (ACTA2) expression in fibrotic tissue (estimated around 20 kPa) [28,30] (Figure 4a). Treatment of cells cultured on uncoated plates with rhIGF1 did not lead to significant alteration in the expression levels of *ACTA2*, *COL1A1* or *PLIN2* (Figure 4b–d). However, it led to significant upregulation of *PPARG*

(Figure 4e). On the other hand, treatment of cells cultured on coated plates with rhIGF1 led to upregulation of the myofibroblast markers *ACTA2* (trend) and *COL1A1* (significant) in parallel to significant upregulation of *PPARG* (Figure 4f,g,i). The expression levels of *PLIN2* were not significantly changed in response to rhIGF1 treatment (Figure 4h). To confirm whether the lipogenic properties were significantly influenced by rhIGF1 treatment, cells cultured on uncoated plates were stained with the neutral lipid dye, LipidTOX (Figure 4j–m). Quantification did not show induction of adipogenesis but rather showed significant loss of lipid droplets in response to rhIGF1 treatment (Figure 4n).

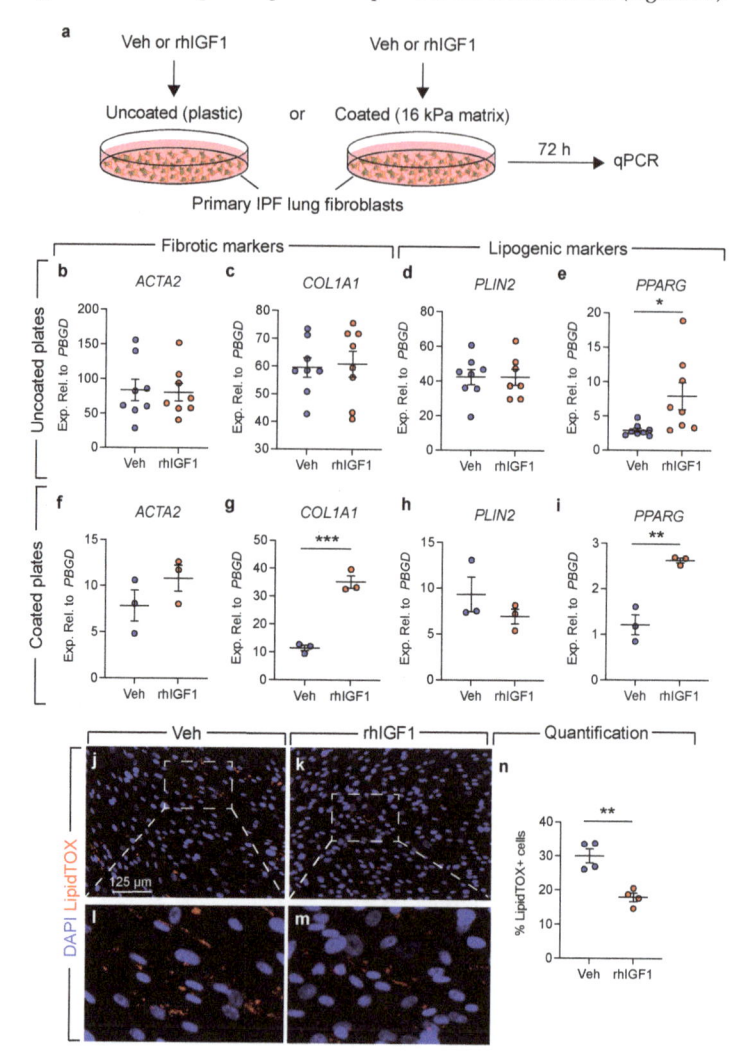

Figure 4. Effect of recombinant IGF1 treatment on primary human lung fibroblasts. (**a**) Scheme for experimental design. (**b–e**) qPCR on primary IPF lung fibroblasts cultured on uncoated plates and treated with vehicle or recombinant human IGF1. (**f–i**) Similar analysis using coated plates. (**j–m**) Neutral lipid stain on primary IPF lung fibroblasts cultured on uncoated plates. Nuclei are stained with DAPI. (**n**) Quantification of LipidTOX staining. rhIGF1: Recombinant human IGF1; Veh: Vehicle. t-test was used to compare the means. (**b–e**) Veh: $n = 8$, rhIGF1: $n = 7$–8; (**f–i**) $n = 3$ per group; (**n**) $n = 4$ per group. * $p < 0.05$, ** $p < 0.01$, *** $p < 0.001$.

4. Discussion

IGF signaling is involved in many developmental and pathological processes, but its regulation remains poorly understood. IGF1/ IGF2, their receptors, insulin signaling components and several IGFBPs contribute to the complexity of this signaling pathway. In this work, we report the transcriptional profile of IGF signaling components during embryonic murine lung development, murine lung fibrosis and human IPF.

A link between IGF signaling and alveolar fibroblast subsets has already been discussed. For instance, a previous study suggested that *Igf1r* is downregulated in lipofibroblasts rather than non-lipofibroblasts after alveolarization, an event that correlates with apoptosis of these cells, thus hinting to a possible role for IGF1R signaling in lipofibroblast survival [31]. Our gene expression analysis showed that *Igf1* is significantly upregulated in mesenchymal cells while *Igf1r* is significantly downregulated during late gestation. Based on available single-cell RNA-seq data [32], myofibroblasts and smooth muscle cells are the main source of *Igf1* at E16.5 while *Igf1r* is more ubiquitously expressed. The significant increase in *Igf1* expression at E18.5 might be due to the increasing number of myofibroblast progenitors that are required for postnatal septation [33]. Interestingly, a previous study showed that in newborn lungs, platelet-derived growth factor receptor alpha-positive (PDGFRα+) alveolar fibroblasts (typically refer to myofibroblasts at this developmental stage) secrete IGF1, which acts on innate lymphoid cell (ILC) progenitors to promote their proliferation [34].

Interestingly, we could detect *Igf1* and *Igf1r*, but not *Igf2* or *Igf2r*, transcripts in our primary cultures of murine lung fibroblasts at various developmental stages. So far, the literature has mainly focused on the role of the IGF1/IGF1R axis in disease and repair. Nevertheless, recent work suggests that like IGF1, IGF2 exerts profibrotic effects and promotes myofibroblast differentiation [35]. It is important to mention that IGF1/2 are often bound to IGFBPs, which regulate the bioavailability of these ligands and suppress or promote IGF signaling in a tissue- and cell-context-dependent manner [36]. The similar expression patterns of *Igfbp1*, *Igfbp4* and *Igfbp6* between E14.5 and E18.5 suggest that they might play similar roles during this period of lung development. On the other hand, it was reported that increased levels of *Igfbp2* result in proliferation arrest of epithelial cells in the lung [37]. This might explain the reduced levels of *Igfbp2* in lung homogenates at late stages (between E16.5 and E18.5), as this coincides with the expansion of alveolar epithelial progenitors.

IGF signaling is involved in controlling glucose and lipid metabolism and is therefore altered in diabetes mellitus. Serum levels of IGF1 were reported to be elevated in type II diabetes mellitus (T2DM) [38]. Whether such dysregulation in the abundance of IGF1 is a cause or consequence of diabetes remains unclear. Metabolic alterations have also been reported in patients suffering from IPF [39,40], and T2DM might be risk factor for IPF [41,42]. Among the metabolic pathways affected in IPF lungs are sphingolipids, arginine, energy (including glucose, fatty acid and citric acid metabolism), bile acid, heme and glutamate/aspartate [39]. Some of these pathways, particularly those related to glucose and fatty acid metabolism can be regulated by IGF1 signaling and might therefore be relevant for IGF1 research in the context of IPF.

We and others have already shown a potent antifibrotic effect for the antidiabetic compound metformin in the lung [18,43–45]. We have shown that metformin, as well as the PPARγ agonist rosiglitazone, accelerate the resolution of pulmonary fibrosis at least partly via inducing the transdifferentiation of collagen-secreting myofibroblasts into pro-alveologenic lipofibroblasts [17,18]. Given the parallels between lipofibroblasts and mature adipocytes, and since insulin signaling is critical for adipogenic differentiation, we tested the possibility that IGF1 plays a similar effect in promoting lipofibroblast formation. Our data, however, do not support this scenario. On the contrary, treatment of primary human IPF lung fibroblasts exacerbated the myofibroblast phenotype and led to the loss of lipid droplets in these cells. These data using human-derived lung samples agree with the gene expression analysis carried out of lung homogenates from bleomycin-challenged mice, where *Igf1* showed a similar expression pattern as *Col1a1* during fibrosis formation. Our data are therefore in line with previous reports showing that blocking IGF1R signaling ameliorates bleomycin-induced pulmonary fibrosis in experimental mice [13]. Our gene expression profiling of IGFBPs in IPF and donor lung explants showed that *IGFBP2,4,5,6* are upregulated while *IGFBP1,3* are unaltered. Some of these IGFBPs have previously been shown to be upregulated in IPF and contribute to ECM protein deposition [46–48]. IGFBP2, in particular, has been proposed as a biomarker for IPF [48].

One last aspect is the effect of matrix stiffness on the phenotype of fibroblasts and whether it modulates the response of these cells to rhIGF1 treatment, particularly in terms of myogenic versus lipogenic differentiation. It has been shown that mouse lung fibroblasts grown on soft substrate (<0.1 kPa), but not stiff substrate, upregulate *Acta2* when treated with recombinant IGF1. The induction of *Col1a1* expression was reported for both conditions (using mouse lung fibroblasts) [28]. Here, we cultured primary human IPF lung fibroblasts on either uncoated plates or 16 kPa substrate. While rhIGF1 showed a clear profibrotic effect on cells cultured on 16 kPa matrix, the corresponding transcriptional changes were not evident in cells grown on uncoated plates. This indicates that a (patho)physiological matrix might be important to "capture" the transcriptomic changes occurring during active myogenic differentiation. One surprising finding was the significant upregulation of *PPARG*, the master regulator of adipogenesis, under both experimental setups. Nevertheless, we could detect significant loss of lipid droplets in cells treated with rhIGF1, which fits with the model of lipogenic-to-myogenic differentiation. Whether IGF1 signaling has a direct impact on lipofibroblasts in vivo warrants further investigation.

In summary, we observed distinct expression patterns for IGF signaling components in different compartments of the lung during murine embryonic development. In the murine model of bleomycin-induced pulmonary fibrosis, we observed upregulation of *Igf1*, transient upregulation of *Igfbp4* and downregulation of *Igfbp6*. The genes encoding IGF1 and several IGFBPs are upregulated in IPF while those encoding IGF and insulin receptors are downregulated. Finally, our data using primary cultures of IPF lung fibroblasts confirm the profibrotic effect of IGF1, and hint to a possible impact on lipofibroblasts in lung fibrosis.

Author Contributions: Conceptualization, E.E.A.; investigation, V.K., A.K., G.K., M.K., M.M.B., I.A. and E.E.A.; methodology, V.K., A.K., G.K., M.K., M.M.B., I.A., A.I.V.-A., M.W. and E.E.A.; resources, A.I.V.-A., C.R., A.G., W.S., S.H. and E.E.A.; data curation, V.K., A.K., G.K., M.K., M.M.B. and E.E.A.; supervision, E.E.A.; funding acquisition, S.H. and E.E.A.; writing—original draft preparation, V.K. and E.E.A.; writing—review and editing, V.K., A.K., M.K., C.R., S.H. and E.E.A. All authors have read and agreed to the published version of the manuscript.

Funding: This work was funded by the Institute for Lung Health (ILH) and the German Research Foundation (DFG; KFO309 P7/8, SFB TR84 B2/9, SFB1021 C5, SFB CRC1213-project A04 and EL 931/4-1).

Institutional Review Board Statement: The part of the study involving human samples was conducted according to the guidelines of the Declaration of Helsinki and approved by the Ethics Committee of the University of Giessen. Animal experiments were approved by the local authorities.

Informed Consent Statement: For the experiments involving human-derived lung material, written consent was obtained from each patient.

Data Availability Statement: There are no deposited or supplementary data associated with this work. The data presented in this study are available in the article.

Acknowledgments: The authors acknowledge the excellence cluster Cardio-Pulmonary Institute (CPI, EXC 2026, Project ID: 390649896) and the German Center for Lung Research (DZL). The authors also acknowledge Saverio Bellusci for providing the embryonic lung tissues used for RNA extraction or primary culture. We finally thank Yelda Pakize Kina, Hannah Hofmann and Ewa Bieniek for their technical assistance.

Conflicts of Interest: The authors declare no conflict of interest.

References

1. Liu, J.P.; Baker, J.; Perkins, A.S.; Robertson, E.J.; Efstratiadis, A. Mice Carrying Null Mutations of the Genes Encoding Insulin-like Growth Factor I (Igf-1) and Type 1 IGF Receptor (Igf1r). *Cell* **1993**, *75*, 59–72. [CrossRef]
2. Keselman, A.C.; Martin, A.; Scaglia, P.A.; Sanguineti, N.M.; Armando, R.; Gutiérrez, M.; Braslavsky, D.; Ballerini, M.G.; Ropelato, M.G.; Ramirez, L.; et al. A Homozygous Mutation in the Highly Conserved Tyr60 of the Mature IGF1 Peptide Broadens the Spectrum of IGF1 Deficiency. *Eur. J. Endocrinol.* **2019**, *181*, K43–K53. [CrossRef]
3. Giabicani, E.; Willems, M.; Steunou, V.; Chantot-Bastaraud, S.; Thibaud, N.; Abi Habib, W.; Azzi, S.; Lam, B.; Bérard, L.; Bony-Trifunovic, H.; et al. Increasing Knowledge in IGF1R Defects: Lessons from 35 New Patients. *J. Med. Genet.* **2020**, *57*, 160–168. [CrossRef] [PubMed]
4. Walenkamp, M.J.E.; Losekoot, M.; Wit, J.M. Molecular IGF-1 and IGF-1 Receptor Defects: From Genetics to Clinical Management. *Endocr. Dev.* **2013**, *24*, 128–137. [CrossRef]
5. Yen, Y.-C.; Hsiao, J.-R.; Jiang, S.S.; Chang, J.S.; Wang, S.-H.; Shen, Y.-Y.; Chen, C.-H.; Chang, I.-S.; Chang, J.-Y.; Chen, Y.-W. Insulin-like Growth Factor-Independent Insulin-like Growth Factor Binding Protein 3 Promotes Cell Migration and Lymph Node Metastasis of Oral Squamous Cell Carcinoma Cells by Requirement of Integrin B1. *Oncotarget* **2015**, *6*, 41837–41855. [CrossRef]
6. Leroith, D.; Scheinman, E.J.; Bitton-Worms, K. The Role of Insulin and Insulin-like Growth Factors in the Increased Risk of Cancer in Diabetes. *Rambam Maimonides Med. J.* **2011**, *2*, e0043. [CrossRef]
7. Pais, R.S.; Moreno-Barriuso, N.; Hernández-Porras, I.; López, I.P.; De Las Rivas, J.; Pichel, J.G. Transcriptome Analysis in Prenatal IGF1-Deficient Mice Identifies Molecular Pathways and Target Genes Involved in Distal Lung Differentiation. *PLoS ONE* **2013**, *8*, e83028. [CrossRef] [PubMed]
8. Epaud, R.; Aubey, F.; Xu, J.; Chaker, Z.; Clemessy, M.; Dautin, A.; Ahamed, K.; Bonora, M.; Hoyeau, N.; Fléjou, J.-F.; et al. Knockout of Insulin-Like Growth Factor-1 Receptor Impairs Distal Lung Morphogenesis. *PLoS ONE* **2012**, *7*, e48071. [CrossRef] [PubMed]
9. Silva, D.; Venihaki, M.; Guo, W.H.; Lopez, M.F. Igf2 Deficiency Results in Delayed Lung Development at the End of Gestation. *Endocrinology* **2006**, *147*, 5584–5591. [CrossRef]
10. Ahamed, K.; Epaud, R.; Holzenberger, M.; Bonora, M.; Flejou, J.-F.; Puard, J.; Clement, A.; Henrion-Caude, A. Deficiency in Type 1 Insulin-like Growth Factor Receptor in Mice Protects against Oxygen-Induced Lung Injury. *Respir. Res.* **2005**, *6*, 31. [CrossRef]
11. López, I.P.; Piñeiro-Hermida, S.; Pais, R.S.; Torrens, R.; Hoeflich, A.; Pichel, J.G. Involvement of Igf1r in Bronchiolar Epithelial Regeneration: Role during Repair Kinetics after Selective Club Cell Ablation. *PLoS ONE* **2016**, *11*, e0166388. [CrossRef] [PubMed]
12. Sun, M.; Ramchandran, R.; Chen, J.; Yang, Q.; Raj, J.U. Smooth Muscle Insulin-Like Growth Factor-1 Mediates Hypoxia-Induced Pulmonary Hypertension in Neonatal Mice. *Am. J. Respir. Cell Mol. Biol.* **2016**, *55*, 779–791. [CrossRef]
13. Choi, J.-E.; Lee, S.; Sunde, D.A.; Huizar, I.; Haugk, K.L.; Thannickal, V.J.; Vittal, R.; Plymate, S.R.; Schnapp, L.M. Insulin-like Growth Factor-I Receptor Blockade Improves Outcome in Mouse Model of Lung Injury. *Am. J. Respir. Crit. Care Med.* **2009**, *179*, 212–219. [CrossRef] [PubMed]
14. Rehan, V.K.; Torday, J.S. The Lung Alveolar Lipofibroblast: An Evolutionary Strategy Against Neonatal Hyperoxic Lung Injury. *Antioxid. Redox Signal.* **2014**, *21*, 1893–1904. [CrossRef]
15. Barkauskas, C.E.; Cronce, M.J.; Rackley, C.R.; Bowie, E.J.; Keene, D.R.; Stripp, B.R.; Randell, S.H.; Noble, P.W.; Hogan, B.L.M. Type 2 Alveolar Cells Are Stem Cells in Adult Lung. *J. Clin. Investig.* **2013**, *123*, 3025–3036. [CrossRef] [PubMed]
16. Taghizadeh, S.; Heiner, M.; Vazquez-Armendariz, A.I.; Wilhelm, J.; Herold, S.; Chen, C.; Zhang, J.S.; Bellusci, S. Characterization in Mice of the Resident Mesenchymal Niche Maintaining AT2 Stem Cell Proliferation in Homeostasis and Disease. *Stem Cells* **2021**, *39*, 1382–1394. [CrossRef] [PubMed]
17. El Agha, E.; Moiseenko, A.; Kheirollahi, V.; De Langhe, S.; Crnkovic, S.; Kwapiszewska, G.; Szibor, M.; Kosanovic, D.; Schwind, F.; Schermuly, R.T.; et al. Two-Way Conversion between Lipogenic and Myogenic Fibroblastic Phenotypes Marks the Progression and Resolution of Lung Fibrosis. *Cell Stem Cell* **2017**, *20*, 261–273.e3. [CrossRef]
18. Kheirollahi, V.; Wasnick, R.M.; Biasin, V.; Vazquez-Armendariz, A.I.; Chu, X.; Moiseenko, A.; Weiss, A.; Wilhelm, J.; Zhang, J.-S.; Kwapiszewska, G.; et al. Metformin Induces Lipogenic Differentiation in Myofibroblasts to Reverse Lung Fibrosis. *Nat. Commun.* **2019**, *10*, 2987. [CrossRef]
19. El Agha, E.; Kramann, R.; Schneider, R.K.; Li, X.; Seeger, W.; Humphreys, B.D.; Bellusci, S. Mesenchymal Stem Cells in Fibrotic Disease. *Cell Stem Cell* **2017**, *21*, 166–177. [CrossRef]
20. Rosen, E.D. The Transcriptional Basis of Adipocyte Development. *Prostaglandins Leukot. Essent. Fat. Acids* **2005**, *73*, 31–34. [CrossRef]
21. Al Alam, D.; El Agha, E.; Sakurai, R.; Kheirollahi, V.; Moiseenko, A.; Danopoulos, S.; Shrestha, A.; Schmoldt, C.; Quantius, J.; Herold, S.; et al. Evidence for the Involvement of Fibroblast Growth Factor 10 in Lipofibroblast Formation during Embryonic Lung Development. *Development* **2015**, *142*, 4139–4150. [CrossRef] [PubMed]
22. El Agha, E.; Schwind, F.; Ruppert, C.; Günther, A.; Bellusci, S.; Schermuly, R.T.; Kosanovic, D. Is the Fibroblast Growth Factor Signaling Pathway a Victim of Receptor Tyrosine Kinase Inhibition in Pulmonary Parenchymal and Vascular Remodeling? *Am. J. Physiol. Lung Cell. Mol. Physiol.* **2018**, *315*, L248–L252. [CrossRef] [PubMed]
23. MacKenzie, B.; Korfei, M.; Henneke, I.; Sibinska, Z.; Tian, X.; Hezel, S.; Dilai, S.; Wasnick, R.; Schneider, B.; Wilhelm, J.; et al. Increased FGF1-FGFRc Expression in Idiopathic Pulmonary Fibrosis. *Respir. Res.* **2015**, *16*, 83. [CrossRef] [PubMed]

24. El Agha, E.; Bellusci, S. Walking along the Fibroblast Growth Factor 10 Route: A Key Pathway to Understand the Control and Regulation of Epithelial and Mesenchymal Cell-Lineage Formation during Lung Development and Repair after Injury. *Scientifica* **2014**, *2014*, 538379. [CrossRef]
25. Volckaert, T.; De Langhe, S.P. Wnt and FGF Mediated Epithelial-Mesenchymal Crosstalk during Lung Development. *Dev. Dyn.* **2015**, *244*, 342–366. [CrossRef]
26. Kina, Y.P.; Khadim, A.; Seeger, W.; El Agha, E. The Lung Vasculature: A Driver or Passenger in Lung Branching Morphogenesis? *Front. Cell Dev. Biol.* **2021**, *8*, 623868. [CrossRef]
27. Chen, H.; Qu, J.; Huang, X.; Kurundkar, A.; Zhu, L.; Yang, N.; Venado, A.; Ding, Q.; Liu, G.; Antony, V.B.; et al. Mechanosensing by the A6-Integrin Confers an Invasive Fibroblast Phenotype and Mediates Lung Fibrosis. *Nat. Commun.* **2016**, *7*, 12564. [CrossRef]
28. Hung, C.F.; Rohani, M.G.; Lee, S.; Chen, P.; Schnapp, L.M. Role of IGF-1 Pathway in Lung Fibroblast Activation. *Respir. Res.* **2013**, *14*, 102. [CrossRef]
29. Zhou, Y.; Huang, X.; Hecker, L.; Kurundkar, D.; Kurundkar, A.; Liu, H.; Jin, T.-H.; Desai, L.; Bernard, K.; Thannickal, V.J. Inhibition of Mechanosensitive Signaling in Myofibroblasts Ameliorates Experimental Pulmonary Fibrosis. *J. Clin. Investig.* **2013**, *123*, 1096–1108. [CrossRef]
30. Hinz, B. Tissue Stiffness, Latent TGF-B1 Activation, and Mechanical Signal Transduction: Implications for the Pathogenesis and Treatment of Fibrosis. *Curr. Rheumatol. Rep.* **2009**, *11*, 120. [CrossRef]
31. Srinivasan, S.; Strange, J.; Awonusonu, F.; Bruce, M.C. Insulin-like Growth Factor I Receptor Is Downregulated after Alveolarization in an Apoptotic Fibroblast Subset. *Am. J. Physiol. Lung Cell. Mol. Physiol.* **2002**, *282*, 457–467. [CrossRef] [PubMed]
32. Du, Y.; Kitzmiller, J.A.; Sridharan, A.; Perl, A.K.; Bridges, J.P.; Misra, R.S.; Pryhuber, G.S.; Mariani, T.J.; Bhattacharya, S.; Guo, M.; et al. Lung Gene Expression Analysis (LGEA): An Integrative Web Portal for Comprehensive Gene Expression Data Analysis in Lung Development. *Thorax* **2017**, *72*, 481–484. [CrossRef]
33. Moiseenko, A.; Kheirollahi, V.; Chao, C.-M.; Ahmadvand, N.; Quantius, J.; Wilhelm, J.; Herold, S.; Ahlbrecht, K.; Morty, R.E.; Rizvanov, A.A.; et al. Origin and Characterization of Alpha Smooth Muscle Actin-Positive Cells during Murine Lung Development. *Stem Cells* **2017**, *35*, 1566–1578. [CrossRef] [PubMed]
34. Oherle, K.; Acker, E.; Bonfield, M.; Wang, T.; Gray, J.; Lang, I.; Bridges, J.; Lewkowich, I.; Xu, Y.; Ahlfeld, S.; et al. Insulin-like Growth Factor 1 Supports a Pulmonary Niche That Promotes Type 3 Innate Lymphoid Cell Development in Newborn Lungs. *Immunity* **2020**, *52*, 275–294.e9. [CrossRef]
35. Garrett, S.M.; Hsu, E.; Thomas, J.M.; Pilewski, J.M.; Feghali-Bostwick, C. Insulin-like Growth Factor (IGF)-II- Mediated Fibrosis in Pathogenic Lung Conditions. *PLoS ONE* **2019**, *14*, e0225422. [CrossRef]
36. Allard, J.B.; Duan, C. IGF-Binding Proteins: Why Do They Exist and Why Are There So Many? *Front. Endocrinol.* **2018**, *9*, 117. [CrossRef]
37. Mouhieddine, O.B.; Cazals, V.; Kuto, E.; Le Bouc, Y.; Clement, A. Glucocorticoid-Induced Growth Arrest of Lung Alveolar Epithelial Cells Is Associated with Increased Production of Insulin-like Growth Factor Binding Protein-2. *Endocrinology* **1996**, *137*, 287–295. [CrossRef]
38. Kim, M.S.; Lee, D.-Y. Insulin-like Growth Factor (IGF)-I and IGF Binding Proteins Axis in Diabetes Mellitus. *Ann. Pediatr. Endocrinol. Metab.* **2015**, *20*, 69–73. [CrossRef] [PubMed]
39. Zhao, Y.D.; Yin, L.; Archer, S.; Lu, C.; Zhao, G.; Yao, Y.; Wu, L.; Hsin, M.; Waddell, T.K.; Keshavjee, S.; et al. Metabolic Heterogeneity of Idiopathic Pulmonary Fibrosis: A Metabolomic Study. *BMJ Open Respir. Res.* **2017**, *4*, e000183. [CrossRef]
40. Yan, F.; Wen, Z.; Wang, R.; Luo, W.; Du, Y.; Wang, W.; Chen, X. Identification of the Lipid Biomarkers from Plasma in Idiopathic Pulmonary Fibrosis by Lipidomics. *BMC Pulm. Med.* **2017**, *17*, 174. [CrossRef]
41. Figueroa, M.C.G.-S.; Carrillo, G.; Pérez-Padilla, R.; Fernández-Plata, M.R.; Buendía-Roldán, I.; Vargas, M.H.; Selman, M. Risk Factors for Idiopathic Pulmonary Fibrosis in a Mexican Population. A Case-Control Study. *Respir. Med.* **2010**, *104*, 305–309. [CrossRef] [PubMed]
42. Wang, D.; Ma, Y.; Tong, X.; Zhang, Y.; Fan, H. Diabetes Mellitus Contributes to Idiopathic Pulmonary Fibrosis: A Review From Clinical Appearance to Possible Pathogenesis. *Front. Public Health* **2020**, *8*, 196. [CrossRef] [PubMed]
43. Rangarajan, S.; Bone, N.B.; Zmijewska, A.A.; Jiang, S.; Park, D.W.; Bernard, K.; Locy, M.L.; Ravi, S.; Deshane, J.; Mannon, R.B.; et al. Metformin Reverses Established Lung Fibrosis in a Bleomycin Model. *Nat. Med.* **2018**, *24*, 1121–1127. [CrossRef]
44. Choi, S.M.; Jang, A.-H.; Kim, H.; Lee, K.H.; Kim, Y.W. Metformin Reduces Bleomycin-Induced Pulmonary Fibrosis in Mice. *J. Korean Med. Sci* **2016**, *31*, 1419–1425. [CrossRef]
45. Sato, N.; Takasaka, N.; Yoshida, M.; Tsubouchi, K.; Minagawa, S.; Araya, J.; Saito, N.; Fujita, Y.; Kurita, Y.; Kobayashi, K.; et al. Metformin Attenuates Lung Fibrosis Development via NOX4 Suppression. *Respir. Res.* **2016**, *17*, 107. [CrossRef] [PubMed]
46. Pilewski, J.M.; Liu, L.; Henry, A.C.; Knauer, A.V.; Feghali-Bostwick, C.A. Insulin-like Growth Factor Binding Proteins 3 and 5 Are Overexpressed in Idiopathic Pulmonary Fibrosis and Contribute to Extracellular Matrix Deposition. *Am. J. Pathol.* **2005**, *166*, 399–407. [CrossRef]
47. Guiot, J.; Bondue, B.; Henket, M.; Corhay, J.L.; Louis, R. Raised Serum Levels of IGFBP-1 and IGFBP-2 in Idiopathic Pulmonary Fibrosis. *BMC Pulm. Med.* **2016**, *16*, 86. [CrossRef]
48. Guiot, J.; Henket, M.; Corhay, J.-L.; Louis, R. Serum IGFBP2 as a Marker of Idiopathic Pulmonary Fibrosis. *Eur. Respir. J.* **2015**, *46*, PA3840.

Article

Differential Discontinuation Profiles between Pirfenidone and Nintedanib in Patients with Idiopathic Pulmonary Fibrosis

Kazutaka Takehara [1,2], Yasuhiko Koga [1,*], Yoshimasa Hachisu [3], Mitsuyoshi Utsugi [4], Yuri Sawada [1], Yasuyuki Saito [5], Seishi Yoshimi [6], Masakiyo Yatomi [1], Yuki Shin [1], Ikuo Wakamatsu [7], Kazue Umetsu [8], Shunichi Kouno [8], Junichi Nakagawa [7], Noriaki Sunaga [1], Toshitaka Maeno [1] and Takeshi Hisada [9]

1. Department of Respiratory Medicine, Gunma University Graduate School of Medicine, 3-39-15, Showa-machi, Maebashi 371-8511, Japan; k-kanplude3@jcom.home.ne.jp (K.T.); g.yr.328@gmail.com (Y.S.); m09702007@gunma-u.ac.jp (M.Y.); shiki0246@gmail.com (Y.S.); nsunaga@gunma-u.ac.jp (N.S.); mutoyu03@gunma-u.ac.jp (T.M.)
2. Department of Respiratory Medicine, Public Tomioka General Hospital, 2073-1, Tomioka 370-2393, Japan
3. Department of Respiratory Medicine, Maebashi Red Cross Hospital, 389-1, Asakura-machi, Maebashi 371-0811, Japan; yhachisu2002@yahoo.co.jp
4. Department of Respiratory Medicine, Kiryu Kosei General Hospital, 6-3, Orihime-machi, Kiryu 376-0024, Japan; mutsugi@gaea.ocn.ne.jp
5. Department of Respiratory Medicine, Isesaki Municipal Hospital, Tsunatorihonchou 12-1, Isesaki 372-0817, Japan; sprq6fc9@road.ocn.ne.jp
6. Department of Respiratory Medicine, Tone Central Hospital, 910-1, Numasu-machi, Numata 378-0012, Japan; s-yoshimi@msi.biglobe.ne.jp
7. Department of Respiratory Medicine, National Hospital Organization Takasaki General Medical Center, 36, Takamatsu-cho, Takasaki 370-0829, Japan; i_18_waka@outlook.jp (I.W.); jnakaga@yahoo.co.jp (J.N.)
8. Department of Respiratory Medicine, Fujioka General Hospital, 813-1, Nakakurisu, Fujioka 375-8503, Japan; emuirakirak@gmail.com (K.U.); contra.since2005@gmail.com (S.K.)
9. Graduate School of Health Sciences, Gunma University, 3-39-22, Showa-machi, Maebashi 371-8514, Japan; hisadat@gunma-u.ac.jp
* Correspondence: ykoga@gunma-u.ac.jp

Abstract: Antifibrotic agents have been widely used in patients with idiopathic pulmonary fibrosis (IPF). Long-term continuation of antifibrotic therapy is required for IPF treatment to prevent disease progression. However, antifibrotic treatment has considerable adverse events, and the continuation of treatment is uncertain in many cases. Therefore, we examined and compared the continuity of treatment between pirfenidone and nintedanib in patients with IPF. We retrospectively enrolled 261 consecutive IPF patients who received antifibrotic treatment from six core facilities in Gunma Prefecture from 2009 to 2018. Among them, 77 patients were excluded if the antifibrotic agent was switched or if the observation period was less than a year. In this study, 134 patients treated with pirfenidone and 50 treated with nintedanib were analyzed. There was no significant difference in patient background, discontinuation rate of antifibrotic treatment over time, and survival rate between the two groups. However, the discontinuation rate due to adverse events within one year of antifibrotic treatment was significantly higher in the nintedanib group than in the pirfenidone group (76% vs. 37%, $p < 0.001$). Furthermore, the discontinuation rate due to adverse events in nintedanib was higher than that of pirfenidone treatment throughout the observation period (70.6% vs. 31.2%, $p = 0.016$). The pirfenidone group tended to be discontinued due to acute exacerbation or transfer to another facility. The results of this study suggest that better management of adverse events with nintedanib leads to more continuous treatment that prevents disease progression and acute exacerbations, thus improving prognosis in patients with IPF.

Keywords: idiopathic pulmonary fibrosis; pirfenidone; nintedanib; discontinuation; body mass index; adverse event; antifibrotic treatment

1. Introduction

Idiopathic pulmonary fibrosis (IPF) is a chronic, progressive, and fatal lung disease of unknown etiology. Environmental and occupational exposures have been suggested to play a role in the pathophysiology of IPF [1,2]. Recently, we reported inhaled silica/silicates in the lungs to be associated with the progression and prognosis in patients with IPF [3]. As an antifibrotic treatment for IPF in Japan, nintedanib became available in 2015, in addition to pirfenidone, which was available since 2008. Pirfenidone has also been reported to be effective in treating familial IPF [4]. However, IPF has an average survival time of 3–5 years and the poorest prognosis among interstitial pneumonias [5].

Pirfenidone was the first approved oral antifibrotic drug. In the CAPACITY trial, pirfenidone decreased the decline in forced vital capacity (FVC) at 72 weeks after treatment [6]. The ASCEND trial evaluated that 52 weeks of treatment reduced the decrease in percent predicted FVC (%FVC) and improved progression-free survival at 52 weeks from baseline [7].

Nintedanib is a multi-intracellular tyrosine kinase inhibitor that targets vascular endothelial growth factor, platelet-derived growth factor, and fibroblast growth factor. The TOMORROW trial showed that compared with placebo, nintedanib treatment resulted in a reduced annual decline in FVC [8]. The INPULSIS trials showed similar favorable results and prolonged the time to the first acute exacerbation [9]. The INPULSIS-ON study showed a long-term safety and toxicity profile [10]. However, the continuity of nintedanib treatment in Asian populations is extremely poor, and its long-term treatment with nintedanib has become a critical issue [11–13]. There still are few reports comparing the drug-related adverse events of these two antifibrotic drugs.

Therefore, in this study, we compared the clinical background, effects, adverse events, and prognosis of IPF upon treatment with pirfenidone and nintedanib and examined their continuity and tolerability.

2. Materials and Methods

2.1. Study Population

We retrospectively recruited 283 patients with interstitial pneumonia (IP), including 261 who were treated with pirfenidone or nintedanib between January 2009 and December 2018 at six regional core facilities in Gunma prefecture, Japan (Figure 1). To ensure data accuracy, we enrolled patients with an observation period of one year or more. A total of 77 patients were excluded for the following reasons: 49, because the observation period was less than one year and 28 because they were treated with pirfenidone and nintedanib in combination or had switched the drugs. This study was conducted in accordance with the tenets of the Declaration of Helsinki and was approved by the Gunma University Hospital Institutional Review Board (approval number: 150021).

2.2. Diagnosis of IPF and Data Collection

The diagnosis of IPF was based on a multidisciplinary discussion according to the official statement of the American Thoracic Society, European Respiratory Society, Japanese Respiratory Society (JRS), and Latin American Thoracic Association [14]. The date of data collection was at treatment initiation. Discontinuation was defined as a permanent termination of antifibrotic treatment.

2.3. Disease Severity

Disease severity was assessed by the gender, age, and physiology (GAP) staging system or the JRS severity staging system. JRS severity was classified as per arterial partial pressure of oxygen (PaO_2) and the 6-min walk test [15]. The stage was defined as stage I, if PaO_2 was more than 80 Torr; stage II, if PaO_2 was more than 70 Torr and not less than 80 Torr; stage III, if PaO_2 was more than 60 Torr and not less than 70 Torr; stage IV, when less than 60 Torr. Stages II or III were changed to III or IV, respectively, if desaturation (< 60 Torr) was obtained during the 6-min walk test.

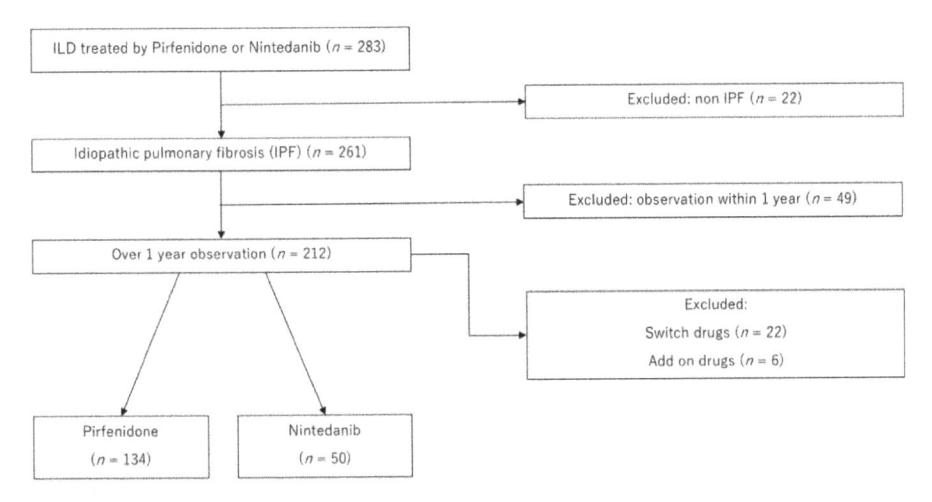

Figure 1. Study population.

2.4. Statistical Analysis

Statistical analyses were performed using the statistical software "EZR" (easy R), which was based on the R and R commander [16,17]. Comparisons of categorical data between the pirfenidone and nintedanib groups were performed using Fisher's exact test. Continuous variables were analyzed using the Mann–Whitney U test and denoted by the median (maximum and minimum) [18,19]. Survival time was analyzed using the Kaplan–Meier method and compared between groups using the log-rank test. Statistical significance was defined as $p < 0.05$.

3. Results

3.1. Clinical Characteristics, Laboratory and Physiological Data, and Prognosis

We enrolled 261 consecutive IPF patients treated with antifibrotic drugs, pirfenidone or nintedanib, between 2009 and 2018. Clinical characteristics and laboratory and physiological data of patients treated with pirfenidone or nintedanib are shown in Table 1.

The median age of patients at the initiation of treatment with pirfenidone or nintedanib was 71 (range, 43–90 years) or 72 (range, 39–87 years) years, respectively. Men accounted for 73.1% and 86.0% of the two treatment groups, respectively. The median %FVC were 74% and 70% and the percent predicted diffusing capacity of carbon monoxide (%DLCO) were 54.4%, and 51.4%, respectively. Serum albumin levels were significantly lower in the pirfenidone than in the nintedanib group (3.8 vs. 4.0 g/dL). The median treatment periods of pirfenidone and nintedanib were 387 and 351 days, respectively. The median annual decline in FVC was 0.100 and 0.180 L, respectively, albeit without statistical significance.

Initial doses of antifibrotic drugs were different between pirfenidone and nintedanib. Pirfenidone was initiated at a lower dose of 600 mg/day for the first 2 weeks; thereafter, doses were sustained, increased or terminated. Nintedanib was administered at a dose of 300 mg/day according to the Japan Pharmaceutical Reference, then sustained, or reduced by 200 mg/day or terminated. The mean final doses of pirfenidone and nintedanib were 1153 ± 420.6 mg and 249 ± 59.69 mg, respectively.

Table 1. Background and treatment of all patients.

Factor	All Patients (n = 184)	Pirfenidone (n = 134)	Nintedanib (n = 50)	p Value
Characteristics				
Age (years)	71 (39–90)	71 (43–90)	72 (39–87)	0.237
Male (male/female)	141 (76.6)	98/36 (73.1%)	43/7 (86%)	0.079
Body mass index (kg/m^2)	22.6 (13.7–36.7)	22.3 (13.7–36.7)	23.1 (14.3–28.1)	0.307
Body surface area (DuBois, m^2)	1.65 (1.18–2.58)	1.63 (1.18–2.16)	1.66 (1.23–2.58)	0.232
Physiologic Marker before Treatment				
FVC (L)	2.20 (0.62–4.56)	2.17 (0.62–4.56)	2.31 (1.03–4.16)	0.838
%FVC (%)	71.8 (27.4–124.9)	74.0 (27.4–124.9)	70.0 (31.0–116.5)	0.761
%DLCO (%)	52.6 (31.0–137.4)	54.4 (3.1–137.4)	51.4 (17.1–76.7)	0.138
JRS severity grade (I/II/III/IV/unknown)	23/12/63/61//25	20/7/40/46//21	3/5/23/15//4	0.104
GAP staging system (−2~0/1/2/3) (4/5/6/7/8//unknown)	6/8/26/29 28/19/6/4/1//57	6/5/20/21 20/12/3/3/0//44	0/3/6/8 8/7/3/1/1//13	0.624
Serological Marker				
Albumin (g/dL)	3.9 (2.1–4.7)	3.8 (2.1–4.6)	4.0 (2.6–4.7)	0.018 *
CRP (mg/dL)	0.26 (0.00–21.87)	0.29 (0.00–21.87)	0.25 (0.03–2.67)	0.280
KL-6 (U/mL)	1260.0 (223.0–9370.0)	1253.0 (303.0–9370.0)	1305.0 (223.0–8593.0)	0.762
SP-D (ng/mL)	237.0 (20.6–1100.0)	237.0 (29.5–1100.0)	259.5 (20.6–728.0)	0.544
Treatment Period and Disease Progress				
Final amount (mg)		1153 ± 420.6	249 ± 59.69	
Observation periods (days)	390 (2–2575)	389 (2–2575)	395 (5–1172)	0.758
Administration period (days)	378 (2–2575)	387 (2–2575)	351 (5–1172)	0.651
FVC decline per a year (L)	0.110 (−3.26–8.21)	0.100(−3.26–8.21)	0.180 (−0.70–1.26)	0.573

FVC, forced vital capacity; %FVC, % predicted forced vital capacity; %DLCO, % predicted diffusing capacity for carbon monoxide. Values are median (minimum-maximum) or number (percentage). The nominal variables were analyzed using Fisher's exact test, and continuous variables were analyzed using the Mann-Whitney U test. * $p < 0.05$.

3.2. Discontinuation Rates over Time

Since we frequently experienced adverse events interrupting antifibrotic treatment, the rate of discontinuation of each agent within one, two, or three years was compared. Discontinuation rates within one year were 48.5% and 50.0% in the pirfenidone and nintedanib groups, respectively (Figure 2). There was no significant difference in the discontinuation rates between the two drugs throughout the study period.

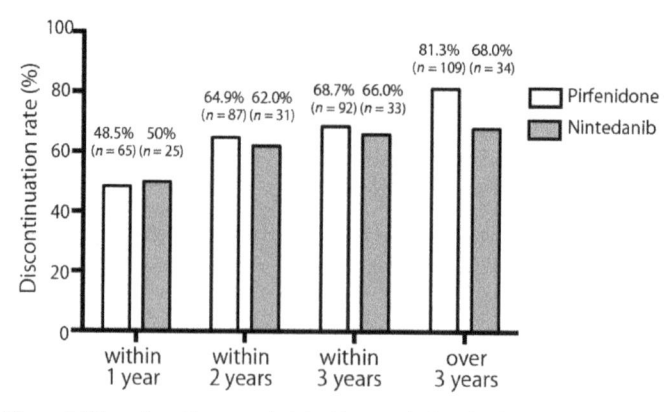

Figure 2. Discontinuation rate of pirfenidone and nintedanib over time.

The discontinuation rate of both drugs within one year after initiation was approximately 50%. The increase in the interruption rate of both drugs over time was gradual over time. The number of cases (n) is the cumulative number.

3.3. Discontinuation Reasons

The reasons for the discontinuation of the two drugs were compared. Over the entire treatment period, the discontinuation rate due to adverse events was significantly higher in the nintedanib group than in the pirfenidone group (70.6 vs. 31.2%, $p = 0.016$). Compared with the pirfenidone group, diarrhea and liver dysfunction were the more common reasons for discontinuation in the nintedanib group (Table 2, Supplementary Figure S1).

Table 2. Discontinuation reasons during the whole period.

	Pirfenidone (n = 109)	Nintedanib (n = 34)	p Value
Acute exacerbation	23 (21.1%)	8 (23.5%)	0.819
Disease progression	15 (13.8%)	3 (8.8%)	0.766
Hospital transfer	15 (13.8%)	1 (2.9%)	0.199
Lung cancer	5 (4.6%)	2 (5.9%)	0.674
Adverse effects	34 (31.2%)	24 (70.6%)	0.016 *
Photosensitivity	2 (1.8%)	0 (0.0%)	1.000
Anorexia/ Nausea	16 (14.7%)	6 (17.6%)	0.790
Diarrhea	2 (1.8%)	5 (14.7%)	0.013 *
Liver disorder	0 (0.0%)	9 (26.5%)	<0.001 **
Cardiac disease	1 (0.9%)	0 (0.0%)	1.000
Thrombosis	0 (0.0%)	0 (0.0%)	1.000
Other adverse effects	13 (11.9%)	10 (29.4%)	0.072
Other reasons except the above	9 (8.2%)	0 (0.0%)	0.209
Unknown	11 (10.1%)	2 (5.9%)	0.734

Nominal variables were analyzed using Fisher's exact test. * $p < 0.05$, ** $p < 0.01$.

Next, the discontinuation rate due to adverse events over time was compared between the two groups. Discontinuation due to adverse events decreased over time in the pirfenidone and nintedanib groups, while the discontinuation rate due to adverse events exceeded 50% within one and 1–2 years in the nintedanib group (Figure 3A). Since half of the patients discontinued antifibrotic drugs within a year, we compared the reasons for discontinuation of both drugs within the first year. The discontinuation rate due to adverse events within the first year was significantly higher in the nintedanib group than in the pirfenidone group (76.9% vs. 36.9%, $p = 0.001$) (Figure 3A,B). However, there was no significant difference in the discontinuation rates between the two groups for other reasons, acute exacerbation, or disease progression (Table 2, Supplementary Figure S1). Interestingly, the pirfenidone group showed a decrease in the rate of adverse events resulting in discontinuation over time, while the nintedanib group showed a high rate of adverse events resulting in discontinuation even after 1 year of treatment. In addition, the rate of discontinuation due to adverse events was higher in the nintedanib group than in the pirfenidone group. Specifically, patients treated with nintedanib had experienced multiple adverse events, such as liver dysfunction and diarrhea, causing discontinuation.

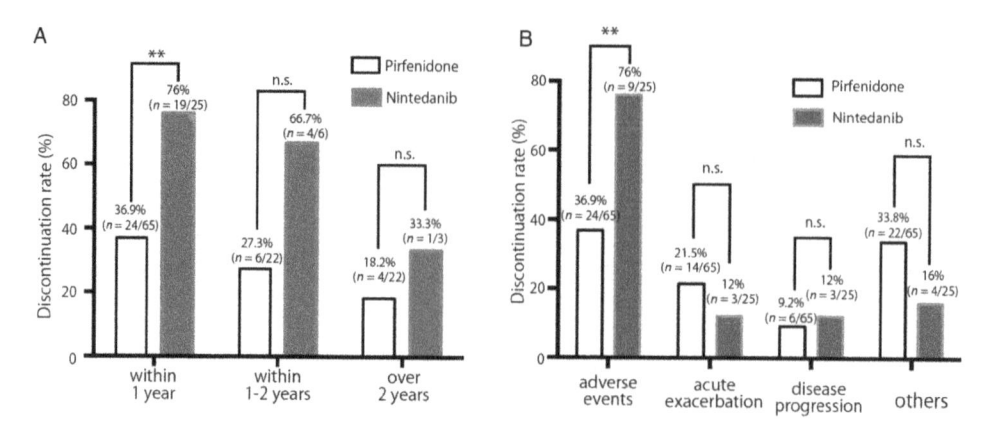

Figure 3. Comparison of (**A**) discontinuation rates due to adverse events over time and (**B**) discontinuation profiles within a year in the pirfenidone and nintedanib treatment. ** $p < 0.01$.

(A) The adverse event discontinuation rate for pirfenidone was less than 50% from the first year, while nintedanib was still above 50% after the first year. The discontinuation rate of nintedanib due to adverse events in the first year was significantly higher than that of pirfenidone in the first year.

(B) Comparison of first-year causes leading to discontinuation of pirfenidone and nintedanib. A comparison of reasons for discontinuation in the first year showed that nintedanib had fewer acute exacerbations and significantly more adverse events than pirfenidone. ** $p < 0.01$.

3.4. Survival Time

The survival time after antifibrotic treatment is shown in Figure 4. The median survival times in the pirfenidone and nintedanib groups were 19 months and 20 months, respectively. Kaplan–Meier survival analysis showed that there was no significant difference in survival periods between the pirfenidone and nintedanib groups.

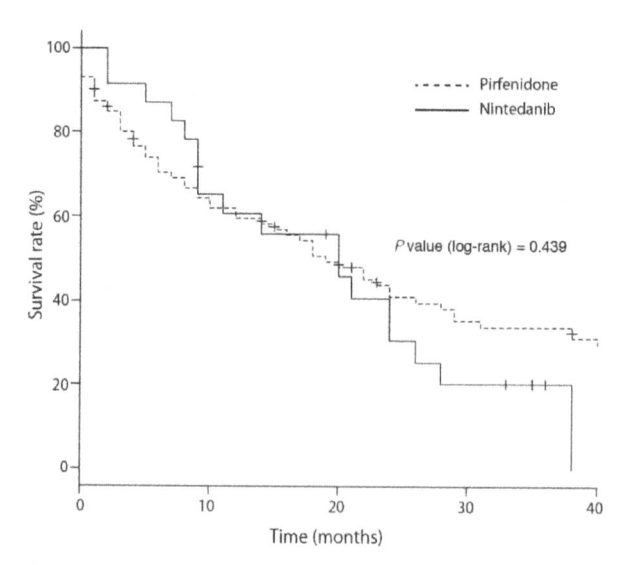

Figure 4. Kaplan-Meier survival analysis between pirfenidone and nintedanib treatment in patients with idiopathic pulmonary fibrosis.

Kaplan-Meier survival analysis did not show a significant difference between pirfenidone- and nintedanib-treated patients with idiopathic pulmonary fibrosis. (19 months for pirfenidone (95% confidence interval, 12–28) vs. 20 months for nintedanib (95% confidence interval, 9–26), respectively; $p = 0.439$). Chi-square tests of 1-year ($p = 0.603$) and 2-year ($p = 0.611$) survival rates also showed no significant difference between the pirfenidone and nintedanib groups.

4. Discussion

The rate of discontinuation due to adverse events was as high as 50% even after 1 year or more of nintedanib treatment, exceeding that of the pirfenidone treatment, throughout the observation period. Notably, there was no significant difference in the interruption rate of both drugs over time. To the best of our knowledge, this is the first study to compare the discontinuation profiles of the two key antifibrotic drugs, pirfenidone and nintedanib.

4.1. Discontinuation of Pirfenidone

In a post-marketing surveillance study including 1371 patients in Japan, only 48% of patients treated with pirfenidone had a longer therapy duration of over one year [20]. In our study, the most common reasons for discontinuation of pirfenidone were acute exacerbations, disease progression, or hospital transfers, caused by IPF progression. Prevention or interventions for these events are difficult in patients with IPF. Similarly, patients with advanced IPF were associated with the discontinuation of pirfenidone within one year [21,22].

4.2. Discontinuation of Nintedanib

In the INPULSIS study, the interruption rate due to adverse events was as low as 10%, and the same result was obtained with INPULSIS-ON [9,10]. However, reports limited to Asian populations showed that the discontinuation rate of nintedanib was approximately 50% [11]. According to a study limited to Japanese patients, 40% were forced to discontinue nintedanib at a regular dose (300 mg/day) within six months [23]. Another study demonstrated a similar rate of discontinuation of nintedanib [13]. A key insight from our study is that attention should be paid to the occurrence of adverse events not only at the beginning, but also during treatment with nintedanib.

The overall discontinuation rates for pirfenidone and nintedanib were 81.3% ($n = 109/134$) and 68% ($n = 34/50$), respectively. In the analysis of reasons for discontinuation, the overall discontinuation rates due to adverse events of pirfenidone and nintedanib were 25.3% (34/134) and 48% ($n = 24/50$), respectively. Furthermore, the overall discontinuation rate due to disease progression or hospital transfer was 27.5% ($n = 30/134$) for pirfenidone, while it was 8% ($n = 4/50$) for nintedanib. This appears to have resulted in a discrepancy in the difference between the overall discontinuation rate and the adverse event-related discontinuation rate between the two drugs.

4.3. Risk Factors of Nintedanib Adverse Events

In recent years, countermeasures against adverse events have been reported. Kato et al. reported that a low body mass index (BMI) of 21.6 or less was a risk factor for diarrhea in patients treated with nintedanib [24]. It has been reported that the use of two or more intestinal regulators aided longer treatment with nintedanib [25], while diarrhea caused by nintedanib is suppressed not only by the use of antidiarrheal medication [26] but by dose reduction as well [25]. Poor performance status tends to cause nausea with the annual decline in FVC being poor; thus, the average survival time is poor in patients with nausea symptoms [24]. Since the introduction of nintedanib at 300 mg/day is likely to cause nausea, a reduced starting dose of 200 mg/day was suggested for cases of poor performance status.

Liver dysfunction caused by nintedanib was more likely to occur in patients with low body surface area and BMI and is often ameliorated by the termination of nintedanib [27].

Approximately half of the patients continue nintedanib with liver dysfunction by dose reduction [12,27]. In the INPULSIS-ON trial, dose reduction due to adverse events did not affect the annual rate of FVC decline [10]. Therefore, it is important to reduce the dose, if necessary. Additionally, patients with low body surface area and BMI may also consider a 200 mg/day dose at the start of nintedanib administration. Regarding the start of dose reduction of nintedanib (200 mg/day) in Japanese patients, there was less early discontinuation, liver dysfunction, and gastrointestinal adverse events than the start of regular dose (300 mg/day), and there was no significant difference in the decrease in annual decline in FVC [23].

4.4. Discontinuation of Nintedanib in Asian Population

A subgroup analysis of the INPULSIS trial reported that Japanese patients had a higher frequency of adverse events leading to discontinuation than the overall population [28]. In the report, the BMI of Japanese patients was 24.4, despite the BMI of the overall population being 28.1, showing a tendency of lower BMI in Japanese patients. Ikeda et al. suggested that a relatively smaller physique was associated with an increased incidence of severe adverse events, causing termination of nintedanib treatment [27]. Kato et al. reported that patients with a median BMI of 22.8 treated with nintedanib had a one-year discontinuation rate of 51% [13]. Combining the insights of these studies with ours, there seem to be many reasons for discontinuing nintedanib treatment following adverse events, for which a lower BMI is considerably associated.

Antifibrotic drug therapy that considers personalized differences such as racial and physical, has aided the longer-term and continuous treatment, leading to better management of IPF. Since nintedanib is often discontinued due to adverse events, paying attention to adverse events such as diarrhea and liver dysfunction at the initiation of nintedanib treatment may lead to tolerability and longer antifibrotic therapy, thus improving prognosis.

4.5. Limitations

This study had several limitations. First, this was a retrospective design. Prospective studies are required to evaluate the significance of managing adverse events, thus reducing the discontinuation of antifibrotic treatment. Second, the number of patients included was small, and fewer patients were treated with nintedanib than with pirfenidone. However, the baseline characteristics in our study were similar to those reported in previous studies [11,13,21]. In this study, there was no difference in the antifibrotic effect on annual declining FVC, treatment duration, discontinuation rate over time, and median survival time between pirfenidone and nintedanib. These results were consistent with those of previous real-world studies showing similar effects on the decline of annual FVC or survival time [29–31]. Third, during the post-marketing surveillance period, all institutions registered unified adverse events; however, one of the limitations of this study is that the subsequent registration of adverse events was entrusted to the medical record description at the discretion of the attending physician. It is necessary to unify them and examine the effect of side-effects prospectively, for better management. Fourth, the reasons for discontinuation of the antifibrotic treatment varied. The transfer was due to the progression of the disease in this study. IPF end-of-life care has many problems as it is not covered by hospice treatment health insurances such as cancer end-of-life care. In Japan, most IPF patients die in regional core hospitals, but some IPF patients are transferred from core hospitals to non-acute hospitals and meet their demise. According to a study on end-of-life care for IPF in Japan, hospice mortality rates were 36.4% and 0.6% for lung cancer and IPF, respectively [32]. In our study, antifibrotic treatment was discontinued due to transfer to another hospital as expensive nintedanib-based treatments were not covered by Japanese health insurance at the hospital where the terminal treatment of IPF was performed. Therefore, in Japan, after transfer from a core hospital to a non-acute hospital, patients may obtain informed consent and discontinue antifibrotic treatment. Furthermore, acute exacerbations were considered a reason for discontinuation apart from other adverse events. Acute exacerbations are a fatal, unlike other adverse events. Several studies have also focused on the incidence of acute exacerbations during antifibrotic treatment, and our study also analyzed the incidence of acute exacerbations, distinct from other adverse events. Case fatality rates for acute exacerbations were 18/34 (52.9%) and 3/12 (25%) ($p = 0.356$) in the pirfenidone and nintedanib groups, respectively. IPF treatment may be discontinued for various reasons and is a clinical issue for future IPF treatment.

5. Conclusions

There was no significant difference in the effect on annual FVC reduction, duration of oral administration, discontinuation rate, and median survival time between pirfenidone and nintedanib treatment. Treatment with nintedanib was frequently discontinued because of adverse events during the treatment period, unlike pirfenidone, which is often discontinued due to progression of IPF or acute exacerbations. Paying attention to the initial dose of nintedanib adjusted to the differences in physique and careful management of adverse events throughout the treatment may contribute to the longer nintedanib treatment with superior prognostic effects in patients with IPF.

Supplementary Materials: The following supporting information can be downloaded at: https://www.mdpi.com/article/10.3390/cells11010143/s1, Figure S1: Comparison of discontinuation reasons during the whole period between pirfenidone and nintedanib.

Author Contributions: Conceptualization, K.T. and Y.K.; Data curation, K.T., Y.K., Y.H., M.U., Y.S. (Yuri Sawada), Y.S. (Yasuyuki Saito), S.Y., M.Y., Y.S. (Yuki Shin), I.W., K.U., S.K., J.N., N.S. and T.M.; Formal analysis, K.T.; Funding acquisition, Y.K.; Investigation, K.T.; Methodology, K.T.; Project administration, Y.K.; Supervision, Y.K. and T.H.; Validation, Y.K.; Writing—original draft, K.T. and Y.K.; Writing—review & editing, K.T. and Y.K. All authors have read and agreed to the published version of the manuscript.

Funding: This work was supported by Grants-in-Aid for Scientific Research (JSPS KAKENHI) (No.20K12493 for Y.K.).

Institutional Review Board Statement: The study was conducted according to the guidelines of the Declaration of Helsinki, and approved by the ethical committee of the Gunma University School of Medicine (HS2019-021).

Informed Consent Statement: Informed consent was waived because of the retrospective nature of the study and the analysis used anonymous clinical data.

Data Availability Statement: Datasets are freely available upon request.

Acknowledgments: We thank N. Fukuda for her paperwork to prepare the manuscript.

Conflicts of Interest: The authors declare no conflict of interest.

References

1. Trethewey, S.P.; Walters, G.I. The Role of Occupational and Environmental Exposures in the Pathogenesis of Idiopathic Pulmonary Fibrosis: A Narrative Literature Review. *Medicina* **2018**, *54*, 108. [CrossRef] [PubMed]
2. Sack, C.; Raghu, G. Idiopathic pulmonary fibrosis: Unmasking cryptogenic environmental factors. *Eur. Respir. J.* **2019**, *53*, 1801699. [CrossRef] [PubMed]
3. Koga, Y.; Satoh, T.; Kaira, K.; Hachisu, Y.; Ishii, Y.; Yajima, T.; Hisada, T.; Yokoo, H.; Dobashi, K. Progression of Idiopathic Pulmonary Fibrosis Is Associated with Silica/Silicate Inhalation. *Environ. Sci. Technol. Let.* **2021**, *8*, 903–910. [CrossRef]
4. Koga, Y.; Hachisu, Y.; Tsurumaki, H.; Yatomi, M.; Kaira, K.; Ohta, S.; Ono, J.; Izuhara, K.; Dobashi, K.; Hisada, T. Pirfenidone Improves Familial Idiopathic Pulmonary Fibrosis without Affecting Serum Periostin Levels. *Medicina* **2019**, *55*, 161. [CrossRef]
5. Fernandez Perez, E.R.; Daniels, C.E.; Schroeder, D.R.; St Sauver, J.; Hartman, T.E.; Bartholmai, B.J.; Yi, E.S.; Ryu, J.H. Incidence, prevalence, and clinical course of idiopathic pulmonary fibrosis: A population-based study. *Chest* **2010**, *137*, 129–137. [CrossRef]
6. Noble, P.W.; Albera, C.; Bradford, W.Z.; Costabel, U.; Glassberg, M.K.; Kardatzke, D.; King, T.E., Jr.; Lancaster, L.; Sahn, S.A.; Szwarcberg, J.; et al. Pirfenidone in patients with idiopathic pulmonary fibrosis (CAPACITY): Two randomised trials. *Lancet* **2011**, *377*, 1760–1769. [CrossRef]

7. King, T.E., Jr.; Bradford, W.Z.; Castro-Bernardini, S.; Fagan, E.A.; Glaspole, I.; Glassberg, M.K.; Gorina, E.; Hopkins, P.M.; Kardatzke, D.; Lancaster, L.; et al. A phase 3 trial of pirfenidone in patients with idiopathic pulmonary fibrosis. *N. Engl. J. Med.* **2014**, *370*, 2083–2092. [CrossRef]
8. Richeldi, L.; Costabel, U.; Selman, M.; Kim, D.S.; Hansell, D.M.; Nicholson, A.G.; Brown, K.K.; Flaherty, K.R.; Noble, P.W.; Raghu, G.; et al. Efficacy of a tyrosine kinase inhibitor in idiopathic pulmonary fibrosis. *N. Engl. J. Med.* **2011**, *365*, 1079–1087. [CrossRef]
9. Richeldi, L.; du Bois, R.M.; Raghu, G.; Azuma, A.; Brown, K.K.; Costabel, U.; Cottin, V.; Flaherty, K.R.; Hansell, D.M.; Inoue, Y.; et al. Efficacy and safety of nintedanib in idiopathic pulmonary fibrosis. *N. Engl. J. Med.* **2014**, *370*, 2071–2082. [CrossRef]
10. Crestani, B.; Huggins, J.T.; Kaye, M.; Costabel, U.; Glaspole, I.; Ogura, T.; Song, J.W.; Stansen, W.; Quaresma, M.; Stowasser, S.; et al. Long-term safety and tolerability of nintedanib in patients with idiopathic pulmonary fibrosis: Results from the open-label extension study, INPULSIS-ON. *Lancet Respir. Med.* **2019**, *7*, 60–68. [CrossRef]
11. Song, J.W.; Ogura, T.; Inoue, Y.; Xu, Z.; Quaresma, M.; Stowasser, S.; Stansen, W.; Crestani, B. Long-term treatment with nintedanib in Asian patients with idiopathic pulmonary fibrosis: Results from INPULSIS(R)-ON. *Respirology* **2020**, *25*, 410–416. [CrossRef] [PubMed]
12. Ikeda, S.; Sekine, A.; Baba, T.; Yamakawa, H.; Morita, M.; Kitamura, H.; Ogura, T. Hepatotoxicity of nintedanib in patients with idiopathic pulmonary fibrosis: A single-center experience. *Respir. Investig.* **2017**, *55*, 51–54. [CrossRef] [PubMed]
13. Kato, M.; Sasaki, S.; Tateyama, M.; Arai, Y.; Motomura, H.; Sumiyoshi, I.; Ochi, Y.; Watanabe, J.; Ihara, H.; Togo, S.; et al. Clinical Significance of Continuable Treatment with Nintedanib Over 12 Months for Idiopathic Pulmonary Fibrosis in a Real-World Setting. *Drug Des. Devel. Ther.* **2021**, *15*, 223–230. [CrossRef] [PubMed]
14. Raghu, G.; Remy-Jardin, M.; Myers, J.L.; Richeldi, L.; Ryerson, C.J.; Lederer, D.J.; Behr, J.; Cottin, V.; Danoff, S.K.; Morell, F.; et al. Diagnosis of Idiopathic Pulmonary Fibrosis. An Official ATS/ERS/JRS/ALAT Clinical Practice Guideline. *Am. J. Respir. Crit. Care Med.* **2018**, *198*, e44–e68. [CrossRef] [PubMed]
15. Kondoh, S.; Chiba, H.; Nishikiori, H.; Umeda, Y.; Kuronuma, K.; Otsuka, M.; Yamada, G.; Ohnishi, H.; Mori, M.; Kondoh, Y.; et al. Validation of the Japanese disease severity classification and the GAP model in Japanese patients with idiopathic pulmonary fibrosis. *Respir. Investig.* **2016**, *54*, 327–333. [CrossRef]
16. Kanda, Y. Investigation of the freely available easy-to-use software 'EZR' for medical statistics. *Bone Marrow. Transpl.* **2013**, *48*, 452–458. [CrossRef] [PubMed]
17. Hachisu, Y.; Murata, K.; Takei, K.; Tsuchiya, T.; Tsurumaki, H.; Koga, Y.; Horie, T.; Takise, A.; Hisada, T. Prognostic nutritional index as a predictor of mortality in nontuberculous mycobacterial lung disease. *J. Thorac. Dis.* **2020**, *12*, 3101–3109. [CrossRef]
18. Hachisu, Y.; Koga, Y.; Kasama, S.; Kaira, K.; Yatomi, M.; Aoki-Saito, H.; Tsurumaki, H.; Kamide, Y.; Sunaga, N.; Maeno, T.; et al. Treatment with Tumor Necrosis Factor-alpha Inhibitors, History of Allergy, and Hypercalcemia Are Risk Factors of Immune Reconstitution Inflammatory Syndrome in HIV-Negative Pulmonary Tuberculosis Patients. *J. Clin. Med.* **2019**, *9*, 96. [CrossRef]
19. Hachisu, Y.; Murata, K.; Takei, K.; Tsuchiya, T.; Tsurumaki, H.; Koga, Y.; Horie, T.; Takise, A.; Hisada, T. Possible Serological Markers to Predict Mortality in Acute Exacerbation of Idiopathic Pulmonary Fibrosis. *Medicina* **2019**, *55*, 132. [CrossRef]
20. Ogura, T.; Azuma, A.; Inoue, Y.; Taniguchi, H.; Chida, K.; Bando, M.; Niimi, Y.; Kakutani, S.; Suga, M.; Sugiyama, Y.; et al. All-case post-marketing surveillance of 1371 patients treated with pirfenidone for idiopathic pulmonary fibrosis. *Respir. Investig.* **2015**, *53*, 232–241. [CrossRef]
21. Ogawa, K.; Miyamoto, A.; Hanada, S.; Takahashi, Y.; Murase, K.; Mochizuki, S.; Uruga, H.; Takaya, H.; Morokawa, N.; Kishi, K. The Efficacy and Safety of Long-term Pirfenidone Therapy in Patients with Idiopathic Pulmonary Fibrosis. *Intern. Med.* **2018**, *57*, 2813–2818. [CrossRef]
22. Barratt, S.L.; Mulholland, S.; Al Jbour, K.; Steer, H.; Gutsche, M.; Foley, N.; Srivastava, R.; Sharp, C.; Adamali, H.I. South-West of England's Experience of the Safety and Tolerability Pirfenidone and Nintedanib for the Treatment of Idiopathic Pulmonary Fibrosis (IPF). *Front. Pharm.* **2018**, *9*, 1480. [CrossRef]
23. Ikeda, S.; Sekine, A.; Baba, T.; Katano, T.; Tabata, E.; Shintani, R.; Yamakawa, H.; Niwa, T.; Oda, T.; Okuda, R.; et al. Low starting-dosage of nintedanib for the reduction of early termination. *Respir. Investig.* **2019**, *57*, 282–285. [CrossRef]
24. Kato, M.; Sasaki, S.; Nakamura, T.; Kurokawa, K.; Yamada, T.; Ochi, Y.; Ihara, H.; Takahashi, F.; Takahashi, K. Gastrointestinal adverse effects of nintedanib and the associated risk factors in patients with idiopathic pulmonary fibrosis. *Sci. Rep.* **2019**, *9*, 12062. [CrossRef]
25. Hirasawa, Y.; Abe, M.; Terada, J.; Sakayori, M.; Suzuki, K.; Yoshioka, K.; Kawasaki, T.; Tsushima, K.; Tatsumi, K. Tolerability of nintedanib-related diarrhea in patients with idiopathic pulmonary fibrosis. *Pulm. Pharm.* **2020**, *62*, 101917. [CrossRef]
26. Mazzei, M.E.; Richeldi, L.; Collard, H.R. Nintedanib in the treatment of idiopathic pulmonary fibrosis. *Ther. Adv. Respir. Dis.* **2015**, *9*, 121–129. [CrossRef]
27. Ikeda, S.; Sekine, A.; Baba, T.; Yamanaka, Y.; Sadoyama, S.; Yamakawa, H.; Oda, T.; Okuda, R.; Kitamura, H.; Okudela, K.; et al. Low body surface area predicts hepatotoxicity of nintedanib in patients with idiopathic pulmonary fibrosis. *Sci. Rep.* **2017**, *7*, 10811. [CrossRef] [PubMed]
28. Azuma, A.; Taniguchi, H.; Inoue, Y.; Kondoh, Y.; Ogura, T.; Homma, S.; Fujimoto, T.; Sakamoto, W.; Sugiyama, Y.; Nukiwa, T. Nintedanib in Japanese patients with idiopathic pulmonary fibrosis: A subgroup analysis of the INPULSIS(R) randomized trials. *Respirology* **2017**, *22*, 750–757. [CrossRef]

29. Bargagli, E.; Piccioli, C.; Rosi, E.; Torricelli, E.; Turi, L.; Piccioli, E.; Pistolesi, M.; Ferrari, K.; Voltolini, L. Pirfenidone and Nintedanib in idiopathic pulmonary fibrosis: Real-life experience in an Italian referral centre. *Pulmonology* **2019**, *25*, 149–153. [CrossRef] [PubMed]
30. Cerri, S.; Monari, M.; Guerrieri, A.; Donatelli, P.; Bassi, I.; Garuti, M.; Luppi, F.; Betti, S.; Bandelli, G.; Carpano, M.; et al. Real-life comparison of pirfenidone and nintedanib in patients with idiopathic pulmonary fibrosis: A 24-month assessment. *Respir. Med.* **2019**, *159*, 105803. [CrossRef] [PubMed]
31. Cameli, P.; Refini, R.M.; Bergantini, L.; d'Alessandro, M.; Alonzi, V.; Magnoni, C.; Rottoli, P.; Sestini, P.; Bargagli, E. Long-Term Follow-Up of Patients With Idiopathic Pulmonary Fibrosis Treated With Pirfenidone or Nintedanib: A Real-Life Comparison Study. *Front. Mol. Biosci.* **2020**, *7*, 581828. [CrossRef] [PubMed]
32. Koyauchi, T.; Suzuki, Y.; Sato, K.; Hozumi, H.; Karayama, M.; Furuhashi, K.; Fujisawa, T.; Enomoto, N.; Nakamura, Y.; Inui, N.; et al. Quality of dying and death in patients with interstitial lung disease compared with lung cancer: An observational study. *Thorax* **2021**, *76*, 248–255. [CrossRef] [PubMed]

Review

Targeting Histone Deacetylases in Idiopathic Pulmonary Fibrosis: A Future Therapeutic Option

Martina Korfei [1,2,*], Poornima Mahavadi [1,2] and Andreas Guenther [1,2,3,4,†]

1. Biomedical Research Center Seltersberg (BFS), Justus Liebig University Giessen, D-35392 Giessen, Germany; poornima.mahavadi@innere.med.uni-giessen.de (P.M.); andreas.guenther@innere.med.uni-giessen.de (A.G.)
2. Department of Internal Medicine, Universities of Giessen and Marburg Lung Center (UGMLC), Member of the German Center for Lung Research (DZL), D-35392 Giessen, Germany
3. Lung Clinic, Evangelisches Krankenhaus Mittelhessen, D-35398 Giessen, Germany
4. European IPF Registry and Biobank, D-35392 Giessen, Germany
* Correspondence: martina.korfei@innere.med.uni-giessen.de; Tel.: +49-641-9942425; Fax: +49-641-9942429
† Member of the Cardiopulmonary Institute (CPI), D-35392 Giessen, Germany.

Abstract: Idiopathic pulmonary fibrosis (IPF) is a progressive and fatal lung disease with limited therapeutic options, and there is a huge unmet need for new therapies. A growing body of evidence suggests that the histone deacetylase (HDAC) family of transcriptional corepressors has emerged as crucial mediators of IPF pathogenesis. HDACs deacetylate histones and result in chromatin condensation and epigenetic repression of gene transcription. HDACs also catalyse the deacetylation of many non-histone proteins, including transcription factors, thus also leading to changes in the transcriptome and cellular signalling. Increased HDAC expression is associated with cell proliferation, cell growth and anti-apoptosis and is, thus, a salient feature of many cancers. In IPF, induction and abnormal upregulation of Class I and Class II HDAC enzymes in myofibroblast foci, as well as aberrant bronchiolar epithelium, is an eminent observation, whereas type-II alveolar epithelial cells (AECII) of IPF lungs indicate a significant depletion of many HDACs. We thus suggest that the significant imbalance of HDAC activity in IPF lungs, with a "cancer-like" increase in fibroblastic and bronchial cells versus a lack in AECII, promotes and perpetuates fibrosis. This review focuses on the mechanisms by which Class I and Class II HDACs mediate fibrogenesis and on the mechanisms by which various HDAC inhibitors reverse the deregulated epigenetic responses in IPF, supporting HDAC inhibition as promising IPF therapy.

Keywords: idiopathic pulmonary fibrosis (IPF); histone deacetylase (HDAC); histone acetylation; non-histone protein acetylation; fibroblast-to-myofibroblast differentiation (FMD); type-II alveolar epithelial cell (AECII); bronchiolar basal cells; bronchiolization; Class I-HDAC-inhibitor; (pan-)HDAC-inhibitor

1. Introduction

1.1. Pathomechanisms of Idiopathic Pulmonary Fibrosis

Idiopathic pulmonary fibrosis (IPF) is a devastating interstitial lung disease of unknown origin with a poor prognosis. It predominantly affects individuals aged 60 to 75 years old, with a median mortality rate of 3–5 years after diagnosis, which is comparable to or even worse than many cancers [1,2]. Although pirfenidone (Esbriet®) and nintedanib (Ofev®) have recently been approved as IPF therapies, which are effective in reducing the rate of lung function decline, neither is curative for the disease [3–5]. IPF still has a high mortality rate, and there is an unmet medical need for an improved drug or for a cure.

The current pathogenic model of IPF suggests that lung fibrosis develops as a result of unremitting insults in combination with genetic- and ageing-related risk factors to type-I/-II alveolar epithelial cells (AECI/II), which consecutively trigger an aberrant wound healing response through the activation of fibroblasts and myofibroblasts and the replacement of injured alveolar epithelium with fibrotic scar tissue due to a decreased renewal capacity of the alveolar epithelium [6–8]. The so-called fibroblast foci, subepithelially located, represent the active sites of fibrosis and consist of apoptosis-resistant myofibroblasts and the extracellular matrix (ECM) they produce, resulting in persistent collagen deposition, progressive scarring and overall lung tissue stiffness [6,9]. Another prominent hallmark of IPF is the bronchiolisation of distal alveoli, involving structures that are composed of "proliferative" bronchiolar basal cells and mucin-producing airway secretory cells [10–12]. In addition, it has been widely observed that airway epithelium consisting of p63$^+$ cytokeratin-5/KRT5$^+$ positive basal cell sheets (underneath luminal-ciliated bronchial cells) overlie the fibroblast foci, indicating that the integrity of the alveolar epithelium is severely disrupted in IPF [10,13]. In agreement, death of AECII is a prominent feature in IPF [8,14–17] and has been linked to endoplasmic reticulum (ER) stress as a variety of studies have documented the induction of the unfolded protein response (UPR) and markers of pro-apoptotic ER stress in the AECII of patients with sporadic and familial IPF [18–21].

1.1.1. Genetic Factors Affecting IPF-Epithelial Cells

Compelling evidence indicates that genetic susceptibility plays a part in AECII ER stress and the development of IPF. Among the stimuli and triggering conditions capable of inducing the UPR and ER stress in AECII are the discovered (heterozygous) mutations in the surfactant protein (SP)-C (*SFTPC*)- and SP-A2 (*SFTPA2*) genes in familial IPF, which cause misfolded SP-C and SP-A2 proteins, respectively [22–25]. In experimental models with transgenic mice that conditionally overexpress the mutation *SFTPC*^{C121G} in AECII, ER stress severely increased after the induction of mutant SP-C^{C121G} protein expression, which resulted in AECII apoptosis and the development of spontaneous lung fibrosis in mice [26], suggesting that AECII ER stress indeed precedes the development of fibrosis in human IPF. Importantly, ER stress and apoptosis do not seem to differ in extent between *SFTPC/A2*-associated familial IPF and sporadic IPF cases in the absence of gene mutations [19]. In addition, mutations in six genes linked to telomere function have been found in familial IPF (telomerase reverse transcriptase, *TERT* [27,28]; telomerase RNA component, *TR* [27,28]; dyskerin, *DKC1* [29]; telomere interacting factor 2, *TINF2* [30]; regulator of telomere elongation helicase, *RTEL1* [31]; and poly(A)-specific ribonuclease deadenylation nuclease, *PARN* [31]), which implicate telomere shortening and DNA-damage responses in IPF pathogenesis and which are also strongly suggested to induce AECII apoptosis [27–29,31]. It was shown that systemic telomere attrition in AECII, but not fibroblasts, led to lung remodelling and fibrosis in a mouse model [32]. However, it is currently unclear which role ER stress may play under these conditions and *vice versa*; it is currently unknown why AECII ER stress is a prominent characteristic of sporadic cases of IPF [18], which comprise ~85% of the total IPF population [33]. Importantly, premature telomere shortening has also been observed in the AECII of sporadic IPF patients [34]. Moreover, some of these abovementioned mutations have been reported not only in familial IPF but also in sporadic IPF cases [34], suggesting a similarity between these two types of IPF and that sporadic IPF is also a disease with a genetic predisposition. In agreement, genome-wide association studies have found that a single-nucleotide polymorphism (SNP) in the promoter region of the mucin 5B gene is the strongest risk factor for familial and sporadic IPF described so far as this gain-of-function *MUC5B* promoter variant rs35705950 was similarly present in subjects with familial and sporadic IPF [35,36], accounting for 30–35% of the risk of developing IPF [35]. Interestingly, the rs35705950 variant not only predisposes to IPF but has also been associated with improved survival compared with patients without this variant, although this latter association remains somewhat controversial because this gain-of-function variant was shown to result in increased mucin 5B expression and impaired mucuciliary clearance in the bronchial cells of IPF subjects (as well as healthy subjects) carrying this variant, suggesting that bronchial cell defects can affect the onset of disease [37]. Moreover, further research by the same group revealed that *MUC5B* was even found to be co-expressed with *SFTPC* expression in the columnar epithelial cells of abnormal bronchiolar structures as well as the AECII of IPF patients with the rs35705950 variant, but also in normal bronchioles and AECII of healthy subjects with this variant [38]. It was also demonstrated that transgenic mice overexpressing Muc5b in the distal lung indicated greater and more aggravated lung fibrosis than wild-type mice following bleomycin treatment [38]. With this conflicting background, the functional and pathomechanistic consequences of the *MUC5B* rs35705950 T/G polymorphism in IPF need further investigation.

1.1.2. The Core in IPF: Disturbed AECII–Mesenchymal Communication and AECII/Fibroblast Apoptosis Imbalance

Considering IPF as an alveolar epithelium-driven disease, the molecular mechanisms leading to fibrotic remodelling and the aberrant epithelial repair, including the abnormal bronchiolisation process in response to the causal AECII injury and death, are still incompletely resolved. Following injury, AECII proliferates and differentiates into AECI for the repair of alveolar structure [38]. In IPF, however, AECII differentiates and features an abnormally activated phenotype, characterised as cells undergoing hyperplasia, senescence and apoptosis, which contribute as paracrine factors to fibroblast proliferation and their transformation into myofibroblasts through the production and release of profibrotic cytokines and growth factors (amongst them, transforming growth factor beta (TGF-β), connective tissue growth factor (CTGF), platelet-derived growth factor (PDGF), tumour necrosis factor-alpha (TNF-α), and endothelin-1) or other mediators [39–42]. Targeted AECII damage in transgenic mice was also shown to induce plasminogen activator inhibitor 1 (PAI-1) overexpression in AECII and lung macrophages, which resulted in the development of fatal lung fibrosis. [43]. Another study revealed that the uptake of apoptotic AECII by alveolar macrophages contributed to fibrosis through the increased expression and secretion of TGF-β by such activated macrophages [44]. Aside from AECII and macrophages, TGF-β and the abovementioned profibrotic molecules are excessively found in fibroblast foci and continuously promote AECII apoptosis via autocrine and paracrine mechanisms [41,45,46]. Myofibroblasts have been shown to upregulate NADPH oxidase 4 (NOX4) to produce high levels of extracellular H_2O_2 in response to TGF-β (or other growth factors), which promote damage to AECII while increasing fibroblast proliferation, fibroblast-to-myofibroblast differentiation (FMD) and resistance to apoptosis in fibroblasts and myofibroblasts [47,48]. Other factors promoting the proliferation and anti-apoptosis of fibrotic fibroblasts/myofibroblasts include the increased expression of inhibitors of apoptosis in myofibroblasts, such as surviving [49], cellular FLICE-like inhibitory protein (c-FLIP) [50,51], phosphatidylinositol-3-kinase-gamma (PI3K-γ) [52], secreted protein acidic and rich in cysteine (SPARC) [53], and X-linked inhibitor of apoptosis (XIAP) [54].

1.1.3. Key Fibrotic Pathways behind IPF

TGF-β has been regarded as a central factor in fibroblast activation, driving the development of lung fibrosis and IPF progression through the activation of numerous profibrotic and survival-related signalling cascades [55]. TGF-β interacts with its receptors (TGF-βRs) on the surface of fibroblasts, and, in the canonical pathway, it phosphorylates mothers against decapentaplegic homolog (SMAD)2 and 3, which then heterodimerise with SMAD4 to form SMAD2/4 and SMAD3/4 complexes that translocate to the nucleus to activate profibrotic- and proliferation-related genes [55]. In the non-canonical (SMAD-independent) activation pathways, tyrosine-protein kinase ABL1 [56], Janus kinases (JAK) [57,58], PI3K [52,59], and mitogen-activated protein kinases (MAPKs) [60] have been shown to be directly activated by TGF-β, mediating persistent activation of fibroblastic cell populations in IPF.

The contribution of the PI3K/protein kinase B (PKB/AKT) signalling pathway to both fibroblast proliferation and differentiation into myofibroblasts is prominent as fibroblasts isolated from IPF patients have been demonstrated to display pathological activation of AKT [61] and pan-inhibition of upstream class I PI3Ks by the small molecule LY294002-abrogated TGF-β-induced proliferative effects as well as α-SMA expression and collagen production in lung fibroblasts in vitro and bleomycin-induced lung fibrosis in rats in vivo [62,63]. The catalytic subunit of PI3K occurs in four isoforms (α, β, γ, and δ), which are ubiquitously expressed and found in lung fibroblasts [59]. Interestingly, selective suppression of PI3K-α or PI3K-γ by *small interfering* (si)RNAs was able to elicit significant antifibrotic effects in TGF-β-stimulated human lung fibroblasts, comparable to that induced by pan-PI3K inhibition, confirming a crucial role of these both isoforms in fibrotic lung fibroblasts [62]. Moreover, PI3K-γ has been found to be significantly overexpressed in fibroblast foci and bronchiolar basal cells in IPF lungs and co-localised with cell markers for proliferation and survival [52]. Subsequent research revealed that targeting PI3K-γ activity genetically or pharmacologically (by the small molecule AS-252424 or AS-605240) was able to significantly dampen fibrogenesis in IPF-fibroblast cultures alone and prevent bleomycin-induced lung fibrosis in rats in vivo [52,64]. These findings are important, considering that in cancer, the activation of the PI3K-γ pathway is involved in the lack of regulation of cell proliferation [65]. Moreover, other studies indicate that the increase of AECII apoptosis in IPF is closely related to pathological PI3K/AKT activation, which causes the release of H_2O_2 and subsequent damage to adjacent AECIIs [66,67].

Several studies also indicate a significant role of phosphorylated, activated signal transducer and activator of transcription 3 (STAT3), which can be induced by TGF-β, PDGF, as well as the IL-6 family of cytokines in IPF fibroblasts [68–70]. In response to such ligands, STAT3 becomes specifically phosphorylated at tyrosine 705 (Tyr705) by growth factor/cytokine receptor-associated JAK2 kinase, translocates to the nucleus and serves as a potent transcription factor for surviving [71] and the genes involved in myofibroblast differentiation [70]. In IPF fibroblasts, active p-STAT3 was shown to confer resistance to FasL-induced apoptosis [72]. It could also be demonstrated that C-188-9, a small molecule STAT3 inhibitor that targets the Tyr705 peptide binding pocket, decreased FMD induced by TGF-β in cultured lung fibroblasts as well as significantly reduced experimental pulmonary fibrosis in mice [69]. Similarly, selective JAK2 tyrosine kinase inhibition by fedratinib attenuated TGF-β- and IL-6-induced myofibroblast activation regulated by JAK2/p-STAT3 as well as reduced bleomycin-induced lung fibrosis in mice in vivo [70]. Interestingly, it was shown that STAT3 phosphorylation participates in both lung epithelial damage and fibroblast-to-myofibroblast transformation [69]. Studies also revealed that JAK2/STAT3 signalling undergoes hyperactivation in IPF patients [73].

Enhanced activation of the coagulation cascade, including the significant overexpression of several zymogens in the alveolar compartment, as well as fibroblast foci, has also been demonstrated in the setting of pulmonary fibrosis and IPF [74]. In addition to fibrin deposition in the lungs, it has been shown that this cascade is also closely related to ECM generation as locally produced and circulation-derived FII (thrombin) and/or FXa were shown to induce profibrotic effects via the proteolytic activation of protease-activated receptor-1 (PAR1) and the subsequent differentiation of fibroblasts into myofibroblast [75,76]. Thrombin was also shown to induce CTGF expression in human lung fibroblasts through the activation of the c-Src/JAK2/STAT3 signalling pathway [77]. *Vice versa*, in AECII, thrombin induced cell death through the induction of pro-apoptotic ER stress [78]. In aggregate, in IPF, the dysregulated crosstalk and the abnormally increased profibrotic mediators between AECII and fibroblasts lead to AECII apoptosis, fibroblast anti-apoptosis, excessive ECM deposition and aberrant bronchiolar tissue generation.

1.1.4. Deregulation of microRNAs in IPF

The deregulation of microRNAs (miRNAs) in pulmonary fibrosis has also received much attention as it contributes to the evolution and progression of the disease [79]. miRNAs are non-coding RNAs, 18–22 nucleotides in length, that repress gene expression by decreasing stability or inhibiting the translation of target messenger RNAs. Various miRNA microarray analyses showed that the expression of profibrotic miR-21 and miR-199a-5p was increased in the lungs of IPF patients as well as bleomycin-injured mice, while the expression of anti-fibrotic miR-26a, let-7d, miR-9-5p, miR-29 and miR-200 was decreased [79–81].

SMAD7, which is known to inhibit TGF-β/SMAD2/3 signalling, is a direct target of miR-21, and the upregulation of miR-21 promoted cell proliferation and collagen synthesis in lung fibroblasts [82,83]. The upregulation of miR-199a-5p during the fibrotic response to epithelial injury mediated TGF-β induced fibroblast activation through the degradation of the anti-fibrotic mediator caveolin-1 [84]. Among the anti-fibrotic miRNAs downregulated in lung fibrosis, miR-26a was shown to inhibit myofibroblast differentiation and experimental lung fibrosis through its ability to downregulate the expression of its target CTGF [85], and forced expression of miR-9-5p was demonstrated to suppress FMD and lung fibrosis development through downregulating Nox4 and TGF-βRII [86]. Similarly, miR-29 was reported as a main negative regulator of ECM production [87]. Decreased expression of let-7d and miR-200 has been associated with the abnormally activated phenotype of AECII in IPF [81,88], whereas the overexpression of miR-200 family members was recently demonstrated to reduce senescence in primary IPF-AECII in vitro and restore their ability to transdifferentiate into AECI [89]. Moreover, antagomirs for the augmentation of miR-323a-3p, which is also found downregulated in the epithelial cells of IPF lungs, were shown to lower epithelial caspase-3 expression and TGF-β signalling and suppress murine lung fibrosis after bleomycin injury [90]. Taken together, cell-specific deregulation of miRNAs significantly contributes to AEC/fibroblast apoptosis imbalance and the production of profibrotic mediators in IPF.

1.2. Treatment of Idiopathic Pulmonary Fibrosis

1.2.1. Established Therapies for IPF

At present, the FDA-approved drugs nintedanib (Ofev®, Boehringer Ingelheim, Ingelheim, Germany) and pirfenidone (Esbriet®, Roche, Basel, Switzerland) are widely used for IPF therapy [91,92]. Nintedanib is a small molecule nonreceptor and receptor tyrosine kinase inhibitor. Nintedanib can block activation of platelet-derived growth factor receptor (PDGFR), fibroblast growth factor receptor (FGFR), vascular endothelial growth factor receptor (VEGFR) and Src family kinases involved in fibroblast proliferation, migration, and transformation [93]. The antifibrotic property of pirfenidone is demonstrated by its ability to inhibit the direct production of profibrotic growth factors and cytokines, such as TGF-β, interleukin-1β (IL-1β), and TNF-α [94–97], as well as the synthesis of procollagens I and II [98,99]. Pirfenidone has also been reported to attenuate experimental lung fibrosis through the reduction of reactive oxygen species (ROS) generation by downregulating Nox4 expression and improving the expression of antioxidant enzymes such as superoxide dismutase (SOD), catalase and glutathione peroxidase (GPx1) [100,101].

The efficacy and safety of nintedanib and pirfenidone have been demonstrated in several large phase 3, randomised, controlled clinical trials in patients with IPF [3,4,102,103]. It has also recently been proven that combining both drugs indicates controllable safety and tolerability in patients [104], but the efficacy is still under evaluation in trials. Whether the combination of pirfenidone and nintedanib may enhance efficacy is questionable. It has been reported that both drugs simply mitigate symptoms and retard progression but fail to significantly prolong survival [5]. Thus, IPF research is increasingly focused on developing new molecular targets and treatment options.

1.2.2. Therapeutic Targets Proposed for IPF Treatment

Agents that inhibit the activation of TGF-β signalling are currently under study. The integrin alpha-V:beta-6 (αvβ6 integrin) is known as a key driver of TGF-β activation [105], and it is significantly upregulated in IPF-lung tissue and localised to damaged epithelial sites [106]. The development of a monoclonal antibody against αvβ6 integrin (clinically known as BG00011) has completed a phase 2 trial for IPF (clinicaltrials.gov (accessed on 20 January 2022) identifier NCT01371305). BG00011 was shown to suppress TGF-β activation in IPF patients, as evidenced by a reduction of p-SMAD2 signalling and TGF-β dependent gene expression in the BAL cells of patients. However, BG00011 was withdrawn due to safety concerns [107]. In contrast to BG00011, the small molecule αvβ6 integrin-inhibitor GSK3008348 developed by GlaxoSmithKline represents a therapeutic agent for inhaled delivery to IPF patients. It was found to efficiently degrade αvβ6 integrin in IPF tissues and isolate epithelial cells from IPF patients [108]. Although a phase 1 first-time-in-humans clinical trial (NCT02612051) revealed that inhaled GSK3008348 was safe and well-tolerated [108], the study also recently underwent early termination. Currently, a phase 2a randomised, double-blind, dose-ranging, placebo-controlled study of a dual selective inhibitor of the integrins αVβ1/αVβ6 (clinically known as PLN-74809) in IPF is ongoing (NCT04396756). Another approach to target TGF-β signalling is via gene silencing, as exemplified by TRK-250, a single-stranded oligonucleotide that produces siRNA targeting human *TGFB* mRNA. A phase 1 study of this inhaled nucleic acid medication is currently in progress (NCT03727802).

As described above, the PI3K/AKT pathway has been demonstrated to offer a reasonable target for the treatment of IPF [59]. Despite the evident antifibrotic effects of the specific PI3K/AKT inhibitor LY294002 in preclinical models of lung fibrosis [62,63], clinical trials with this drug have yet not been initiated. Further, there has been no new progress in the use of other pan- or isoform-specific PI3K inhibitors in the clinical treatment of IPF.

Because the JAK2/STAT3 signalling pathway is crucially involved in IPF [58,70,73], inhibitors targeting this pathway have been proposed to treat the disease. However, there are no clinical trials that study STAT3 inhibition in IPF patients. Further, the clinical use of JAK inhibitors is only described in myelofibrosis and autoimmune-disorder-associated interstitial lung disease (ILD) [109,110], and there is still a lack of studies on idiopathic ILDs. The abovementioned JAK2 inhibitor fedratinib [70], sold under the brand name Inrebic, is an approved anti-cancer medication used to treat myelofibrosis and other myeloproliferative diseases [109]. Baricitinib (Olumiant), a small molecule JAK1/JAK2 inhibitor, is approved for the treatment of rheumatoid arthritis (RA) and has been proven to reduce lung fibrosis and inflammation in patients with RA-associated ILD (RA-ILD) [110]. The JAK1/2/3 inhibitor tofacitinib (Xeljanz) is another approved therapy for RA [111]. Ruxolitinib (Jakafi) is another JAK1/JAK2 inhibitor approved for the treatment of intermediate and high-risk myelofibrosis [112]. This drug has also been shown to significantly ameliorate bleomycin-induced lung fibrosis in mice [113]. Tocilizumab (Actemra), a humanised monoclonal antibody against the interleukin-6 receptor, acts as an indirect JAK/STAT inhibitor through the inhibition of IL-6/JAK/STAT signalling and is used for the treatment of moderate-to-severe RA [114]. Tocilizumab was also granted emergency use authorization (EUA) for the treatment of Coronavirus Disease 2019 (COVID-19) in the United States in June 2021 [115].

Despite their significant therapeutic effects on myofibroblast activation in preclinical models of lung fibrosis [70,73,113], JAK inhibitors have yet not been evaluated for the treatment of IPF, presumably due to toxicities related to their immunosuppressive effects, including infectious events [116].

1.2.3. Senotherapies for IPF

Very recently, senolytics have been suggested as IPF therapy [117]. AECII senescence is a hallmark in IPF that is suspected of driving lung fibrosis as a paracrine factor through the senescence-associated secretory phenotype (SASP), involving the release of multiple profibrotic cytokines and ROS molecules [7,118,119]. A recent study demonstrated that the combination of quercetin, a natural compound with antioxidant properties, and the tyrosine kinase inhibitor dasatinib attenuated progressive lung fibrosis in a transgenic mouse model with conditional p53/p21-induced AECII senescence through the ablation of senescent AECII [120]. In addition, this senolytic cocktail was also shown to attenuate bleomycin-induced lung fibrosis in mice [121]. Importantly, quercetin is also described as a potent inhibitor of NOX4 [122], which is found upregulated in fibroblast foci as well as in the AECII of IPF lungs [47,48], and the full deficiency of *Nox4* has been shown to protect mice against bleomycin-induced AECII apoptosis and lung fibrosis [123]. Moreover, another study suggested that quercetin abrogates the resistance to apoptosis in IPF fibroblasts via the up-regulation of FAS and caveolin-1 and the inhibition of AKT phosphorylation [124].

Based on the therapeutic effects of the senolytic drug combination quercetin and dasatanib in preclinical data, a first-in-humans, small scale, pilot clinical trial for this senolytic cocktail has been undertaken in stable IPF patients, which was generally well-tolerated in patients. Although the effects of both senolytics on circulating SASP-factors were inconclusive, patients showed improved physical function [125]. However, evaluation of drug combination quercetin and dasatanib in larger randomised controlled trials for IPF has yet not been initiated. It should also be noted that each quercetin and dasatanib act on a myriad of pathways and mechanisms implicated in diverse biological processes, which makes it difficult to decipher how they eliminate or otherwise impact senescent cells. Thus, it is difficult to attribute any therapeutic or detrimental effects they may have on senescent cells. Further, senescent cells per se appear to be heterogeneous collections of cells with fewer shared core properties than anticipated; additionally, the composition of the SASP varies by cell type and senescence-inducing stressor [126]. It is not 100% clear if every type of senescence is actually targeted by quercetin and dasatanib. Further, dasatanib, known as the approved therapy for chronic myelogenous leukemia (CML), reveals major known adverse effects, such as pleural effusion and pulmonary arterial hypertension (PAH) [127]. We thus suggest that the use of senolytics as a therapeutic option for the treatment of IPF should be reconsidered.

1.2.4. Current Therapies for IPF in Development

Current IPF therapies in (advanced) development include mainly molecules that are directed against several growth factors and cytokines or other molecular targets known to play a role in the proliferation, activation, differentiation or inappropriate survival of fibroblasts.

Lysophosphatidic acid (LPA) has been identified as a key fibroblast chemokine in experimental lung fibrosis and is believed to increase fibroblast recruitment and the apoptosis resistance of fibroblasts through the activation of the LPA_1 receptor [128]. In line, LPA_1 receptor knockout mice are protected from bleomycin-induced lung fibrosis [129]. Increased LPA levels have also been seen in the BALF from patients with IPF [130]. The LPA_1 receptor antagonist, BMS-986278, has shown promise in pre-clinical and phase 1 studies [131,132] and is currently in phase 2 clinical trials, with study arms for both IPF and PF-ILD subjects (NCT0438681).

Pamrevlumab, a human recombinant monoclonal antibody against CTGF, which plays an important role in fibrosis, has been shown in the phase 2 trial PRAISE to significantly reduce the decline of FVC and progression of IPF. Pamrevlumab was well tolerated, with no significant differences from placebo in the adverse event profile [133].

Pentraxin-2 (PTX2) is a serum amyloid reported to have an antifibrotic and anti-inflammatory effect by inhibiting the differentiation of monocytes into profibrotic macrophages and fibrocytes [134]. It also inhibits the direct production of TGF-β [135]. PTX2 levels are significantly lower in lung tissue, BALF and serum of IPF-patients than in healthy subjects [135,136]. The results of a second randomised, double-blind placebo-controlled phase 2 study (PRM-151-202) of IPF patients receiving recombinant human pentraxin-2 in intravenous infusions in comparison with placebo showed a significantly slower decline in pulmonary function and improved physical capacity in the PRM-151 group. The infusions were well tolerated and had increased circulating levels of PTX2 [137]. The phase 3 efficacy and safety study of PRM-151 (NCT04552899) is underway, with an estimated completion date of December 2023.

Galectin-3 is another potential target under investigation as antifibrotic therapy in IPF. Galectin-3 is a profibrotic β-galactosidase-binding protein that is elevated in the BALF and serum of patients with IPF [138]. The profibrotic function of Galectin-3 is multifactorial due to its ability to cross-link and promote signalling via multiple cell surface receptors, including integrins and growth factor receptors, such as TGF-β, VEGF and PDGF receptors [139,140]. A phase 1/2 clinical trial with TD139, an inhaled small-molecule galectin-3 inhibitor, has revealed promising results in IPF patients and healthy subjects as

TD139 was well-tolerated and patients showed reduced serum levels of biomarkers of IPF progression, including PDGF and the chemokine CCL18, compared to placebo [140].

1.2.5. Past Treatment Strategies Not Recommended Anymore

Medications examined in multiple clinical studies in the past, such as anticoagulation (warfarin) [141], N-acetylcysteine in combination with either azathioprine–prednisone (PANTHER trial) [142] or pirfenidone (PANORAMA study) [143], endothelin receptor antagonists (BUILD trials, ARTEMIS-IPF trial) [144,145], phosphodiesterase inhibitors (sildenafil) [146], imatinib [147], cyclophosphamide [148], interferon gamma-1b (INSPIRE) [149], and simtuzumab (monoclonal antibody against lysyl oxidase homolog 2 [LOXL2]) [150], are not recommended anymore as IPF therapies because they are ineffective or harmful.

In conclusion, there is yet no available curative treatment for IPF. Further, it is unpredictable if therapies employing antagonists directed against individual profibrotic molecules (mentioned in Section 1.2.4.) will help to cure IPF. Therefore, there is still an unmet medical need for novel drugs or for a cure.

1.3. Similarities between IPF and Cancer: Histone Deacetylases as Novel Therapeutic Targets in IPF

Although main molecular pathways responsible for fibroblast activation and disease progression can be blocked by the established therapies nintedanib or pirfenidone, no cure of IPF can be achieved with these drugs, presumably due to the non-targetable irreversible "endless healing" process in IPF, which is self-perpetuating, as increased lung tissue stiffness and epithelial damage further recruits and activates myofibroblasts without any exogenous stimulus [151,152]. Further, the salient features of the progressive fibrotic phenotype of IPF fibroblasts include the resistance to apoptosis and the acquired ability of IPF fibroblasts to invade ECM [153] as well as damage the basement membrane underneath the (injured) epithelium [154]. Apoptosis resistance and the invasive phenotype appear durable because they persist in isolated IPF fibroblasts after their removal from patients [155]. In this regard, IPF resembles cancer. However, myofibroblasts within fibroblast foci in IPF are polyclonal and "disease-derived" whereas cancer cells are thought to be monoclonal. Though, IPF shares a series of risk factors (ageing, smoking and environmental exposures), pathogenic pathways (PI3K-γ/AKT, JAK2/STAT3) and biological abnormalities (genetic and epigenetic alterations) with cancer [156]. In particular, there is a growing interest in the epigenetic abnormalities characterizing IPF and cancer. Epigenetic mechanisms lead to changes in gene expression without alterations in the DNA sequence and can be mediated by the expression of non-coding RNAs, DNA methylation and histone modifications. Recent studies show that IPF and (lung) cancer share the deregulation of some miRNAs. As with IPF, the expression of (above-mentioned) miR-200 and let-7d was reported to be downregulated in various cancers [157–159], while miR-21 (targeting SMAD7) was upregulated and allied with high oncogenic property [160,161]. Further, similar to tumour cells, results from our group and other groups suggest that epigenetic histone modifications account for the aggressive phenotype and the persistent activated state of IPF fibroblasts [162–165], which indicated a "cancer-like" upregulation of almost all Class I and Class II histone deacetylase (HDAC) enzymes and (amongst other HDAC-induced activities) [165] the abnormal "malignant" repression of proapoptotic genes [163,164]. HDACs are enzymes that deacetylate chromatin and lead to epigenetic repression of gene transcription, whereas HDAC inhibitors favour chromatin acetylation resulting in active chromatin, facilitating gene transcription [166]. Huang et al. (2013) found that increased HDAC expression was responsible for the downregulation of the apoptosis-mediating surface antigen *FAS* [tumour necrosis factor (TNF) receptor superfamily member 6] in fibrotic fibroblasts, and treatment with HDAC inhibitors increased FAS expression and restored susceptibility to FAS-mediated apoptosis [163]. Similarly, epigenetically repressed expression of the proapoptotic *BAK* (Bcl-2 homologous antagonist/killer) gene in IPF fibroblasts was shown to be reversed in response to HDAC-inhibitor treatment [164]. In addition, defective histone acetylation was shown to be responsible for the diminished expression of the antifibrotic cyclooxygenase (COX)-2 enzyme in IPF fibroblasts, which could be restored by HDAC-inhibitor treatment [162]. Interestingly, and *vice versa*, treatment of IPF fibroblasts with HDAC inhibitors resulted in the reduction of profibrotic genes, such as *COL3A1*, in association with marked chromatin alterations [164,165,167]. Further, many scientific groups have demonstrated that various HDAC inhibitors targeting global HDAC activity or single HDAC enzymes decreased lung fibrosis and ECM deposition in bleomycin-treated mice [164,168–171]. Of note, HDAC inhibitors have been known for a long time as successful anticancer agents as they specifically induce cell cycle arrest and apoptosis in "abnormal" cancer cells, whereas normal healthy cells are relatively resistant to HDAC-inhibitor-induced cell death [172,173]. Moreover, the abovementioned preclinical studies in lung fibrosis reveal that HDAC inhibitors may also offer a new therapeutic strategy in IPF by blocking fibrotic remodelling through (i) suppression of profibrotic gene expression, (ii) restoration of antifibrotic genes and (iii) increasing myofibroblast susceptibility to apoptosis.

Importantly, similar to myofibroblasts, the very same Class-I and Class-II HDACs were also found to be upregulated in abnormal "proliferative" KRT5$^+$ bronchiolar basal cells covering fibroblast foci, distal airspaces and honeycomb cysts in IPF lungs, whereas proSP-C$^+$ AECII revealed a marked lack of many HDAC enzymes, suggesting that HDACs may govern the aberrant bronchiolization process of distal alveoli in IPF as well [165,174]. In agreement, Prasse et al. (2019) observed that airway/bronchiolar basal cells are increased in bronchoalveolar lavage (BAL) fluids of IPF patients and that this signature was associated with a lower survival rate [175]. Moreover, bronchial epithelium in IPF has been recognised to contribute to fibrogenesis, as it indicates the abnormal production of profibrotic growth factors, especially insulin growth factor-1 (IGF-1), TGF-β and PDGF [10].

Taken together, we suggest that in IPF, repetitive AEC injury in a (genetically susceptible) ageing individual leads to abnormal HDAC overexpression and HDAC-mediated epigenetic reprogramming in lung fibroblasts as well as bronchiolar basal cells, resulting in excessive production of profibrotic mediators, persistent AECII injury, progressive bronchiolisation, and the ongoing activation and persistence of lung fibroblasts/myofibroblasts. We thus believe that HDACs offer novel molecular targets for IPF therapy, and HDAC inhibitors may be promising therapeutic agents for the treatment of IPF. In the following chapters, the different HDAC classes, their inhibitors, and the role of HDAC enzymes in the pathogenesis of pulmonary fibrosis are described.

1.4. The HDAC Family/HDAC Classes and Their Function—Lessons from Cancer Research

The HDAC enzymes can be grouped into four distinct groups based on function, DNA sequence and domain organisation, and, to date, there are 18 members [176]. Class I HDACs comprise HDAC1, -2, -3 and -8, and these are widely expressed and are found mainly in the nucleus of cells. Class II HDACs are subdivided according to the presence of one or two catalytical domains. HDAC4, -5, -7 and -9 harbour one catalytically active site and are grouped into Class IIA in contrast to Class IIB, comprising HDAC6 and -10, containing two catalytic domains. In contrast to Class I HDACs, the Class IIA HDACs show a more restricted pattern of expression and are located mainly in the cell cytoplasm but can shuttle into the nucleus in a signal-dependent manner, indicating that they are unique signal transducers able to transduce signals from the cytoplasm to chromatin in the nucleus. Once inside the nucleus, Class IIA HDACs interact with myocyte enhancer factor 2 (MEF2) and other transcription factors, mainly acting as transcriptional corepressors. The Class IIB member HDAC6 is mainly cytoplasmic, and HDAC10 is pancellular. Class IV contains only one member, HDAC11, which is found in the nucleus and shares homology with Class I as well as Class II HDACs [176]. Whereas Class I, II and IV HDACs require zinc dications (Zn^{2+}) for catalysis, the Class III deacetylases, the sirtuins 1–7 (*SIRT1–7*), use oxidised nicotinamide adenine dinucleotide (NAD^+) as a co-factor [176,177].

The first identified substrates of HDACs were the histones. HDACs deacetylate the ε-amino group of lysines located at the N-terminal tail of histones, which leads through chromatin compaction to a repressive chromatin formation (heterochromatin) and the suppression of gene expression [166,176,177]. In contrast, histone acetyltransferases (HATs), such as p300, counteract histone deacetylation through the introduction of acetyl groups from acyl-CoA to histone N-terminal tails, which generates an open and relaxed chromatin structure (euchromatin), enabling transcription factors to access DNA and to activate their target genes [178]. In this regard, acetylated histones also serve as binding sites for bromodomain-containing proteins (BRDPs) to recruit macromolecular transcriptional complexes at gene promoter regions [179]. Therefore, HATs generally have the opposite function to HDACs, and the balance between the actions of these enzyme families serves as a critical regulatory mechanism for gene expression.

Further, a continuously growing number of non-histone substrates of HDACs and HATS have been described [180,181]. Many of these proteins are signal transducers (e.g., SMADs) or transcription factors (TFs), such as p53, Sp-1, AP-1, erythroid differentiation factor GATA1, runt-related transcription factors (RUNXs), nuclear factor NF-kappa-B (NF-κB) and STATs (e.g., STAT3), and, therefore, changes in the transcriptome/cellular signalling due to altered acetylation status of such TFs as a result of imbalanced HDAC/HAT activity can be the consequence of direct modulation of TF activities. For example, HDAC1 and HDAC2 catalyze the deacetylation of lysine residues (K320, K373, K382) of the tumour suppressor p53, resulting in the impaired DNA binding of p53 and the inhibition of its proapoptotic transcriptional activity, such as the activation of *CIP1* (p21 or cyclin-dependent kinase inhibitor 1), *PIG3* (=*TP53I3*, p53-induced gene 3) and the caspase 9-activating gene *NOXA* (=*PMAIP1*, phorbol-12-myristate-13-acetate-induced protein 1) [182,183]. "Non-TF substrates" of HDACs are peroxiredoxin (PRDX)1 and 2, β-catenin, heat shock protein 90 (HSP90), cortactin, and α-tubulin, which are all deacetylated by the cytoplasmic and cytoskeleton-associated HDAC6 [184–187]. The deacetylation of HSP90 by HDAC6 has been associated with the stabilisation of several HSP90 oncogenic client proteins, such as AKT, hypoxia-inducible factor 1-alpha (HIF1-α), surviving and TERT, and is thus linked to carcinogenesis [186,188]. In addition, HDAC6 plays a vital role in the proteolysis pathway of misfolded proteins as it deacetylates α-tubulin for induction of aggresome formation, in which (cytotoxic) ubiquitylated protein aggregates are sequestered for lysosomal degradation and autophagic clearance, thereby attenuating ER stress [187]. HDAC6-dependent autophagy is considered to confer malignancy and aggressiveness to cancer cells and is linked to resistance to proteasome inhibitors (e.g., bortezomib) in patients with various cancers [189]. In addition, HDAC6 is implicated in metastasis formation through the induction of TGF-β-dependent epithelial–mesenchymal transition (EMT) [190,191]. HDAC6 is also involved in anti-apoptosis by deacetylating the Ku70 protein, which then forms a complex with BAX, a proapoptotic protein, allowing the inhibition of apoptosis [192]. In aggregate, overexpression of HDAC6 gives rise to cancer.

Importantly, in the vast majority, upregulation of HDAC enzymes is associated with cell proliferation, migration, cell growth, transformation and anti-apoptosis. Thus, HDAC overexpression is a common and salient feature of various cancers [166,193,194]. The Class I HDACs, especially HDAC2, epigenetically silence pro-apoptotic genes *CIP1*/p21, *PUMA* (p53 upregulated modulator of apoptosis), APAF1 (apoptotic protease-activating factor 1) and *GADD45A*/*DDIT1* (growth arrest and DNA damage-inducible protein GADD45 alpha) [182,195,196]. In addition, Class I HDACs contribute to adenocarcinoma metastasis through the induction of EMT via loss of E-cadherin expression due to epigenetic silencing by a transcriptional repressor complex containing the TF Snail (zinc finger protein SNAI1) acting in concert with HDAC1 and HDAC2 [197]. Moreover, HDAC2 supports its own expression in cancers via repressing the degradation of its transcription factor β-catenin and also promotes the expression of the proto-oncogene c-Myc [182]. Overexpression of HDAC3 is also correlated with poor prognosis in various cancers as it participates in *CIP1*/p21 repression together with HDAC1 and -2 through histone deacetylation at the proximal *CIP1* promoter or via p53 deacetylation and inhibition [198,199]. Similarly, Class IIA HDACs also promote tumorigenesis: HDAC4 promotes the growth of colon cancer cells or the progression of epithelial ovarian cancer via epigenetic CIP1/p21 repression by acting as a corepressor in a complex with HDAC3 [200,201] and mediates cisplatin resistance in various cancer cells through the dysregulation of autophagy and apoptosis pathways [202,203]. HDAC5 promotes the migration and invasion of hepatocellular carcinoma via increasing the transcription of hypoxia-inducible factor-1α (HIF1-α) under hypoxic conditions [204]. Further, HDAC5 displays a significant upregulation in lung cancer and increases the proliferation and invasion of lung cancer cells through the upregulation of DLL4 (Delta-like protein 4), Notch-1 (Neurogenic locus notch homolog protein 1) and Twist-1 (Twist-related protein 1) [205]. HDAC7 has been shown to protect from apoptosis by inhibiting c-Jun expression [206] and contributes to carcinogenesis by transcriptional activation of c-Myc [207]. HDAC7 also inhibits the expression of the tumour suppressor gene *JUP* (Junction plakoglobin) to promote lung cancer cell growth and metastasis [208]. Further, HDAC7 levels are increased in RAS-transformed cells, in which this protein favours the proliferation and growth of cancer stem-like cells and the invasive features of such cells [209].

Of note, HDAC1, -2, -3, -4, -5, -6 and -7 appear to be most crucial for the proliferation, aggressiveness and apoptosis resistance of cancer cells, and high expression levels of these HDACs in tumours are associated with a poor prognosis for the cancer patients [182,192,204,210–212]. In contrast, the depletion of many HDACs is associated with growth arrest and apoptosis. Targeted disruption of both *Hdac1* alleles in mice has been shown to result in embryonic lethality due to severe proliferation defects and retardation in development, which was correlated with increased expression of cyclin-dependent kinase inhibitors p21^{Cip1} and p27^{Kip1} [213]. Regarding the loss of HDAC2, there are contrasting reports in the literature. One study found that homozygous $Hdac2^{(-/-)}$ mice died within the first 24 h after birth from severe cardiac malformations [214], whereas another reported that mice harbouring a *lacZ* insertion in *Hdac2* (gene-trap method) indicated partial perinatal lethality, and surviving mice with null mutation were generally indistinguishable from wild-type mice by 2 months of age [215].

The phenotypes of other (germline) full knockout of HDAC enzymes *Hdac3*, *Hdac4*, *Hdac7* and *Hdac8* are lethal, whereas $Hdac5^{(-/-)}$ and $Hdac9^{(-/-)}$ knockout mice are viable but with cardiac defects [177]. $Hdac6^{(-/-)}$ and $Hdac11^{(-/-)}$ mice are viable with no obvious phenotype [216,217]. Although α-tubulin is dramatically hyperacetylated in multiple tissues of $Hdac6^{(-/-)}$ mice, the normal phenotype of these mice indicates that this is not detrimental to normal development [216]. The knockout phenotype of *Hdac10* is yet not determined, and little is known about the functions of HDAC10 [177].

The Class III HDACs are represented by the mammalian sirtuin protein family and comprise seven members (sirtuins1–7, *SIRT1–7*) of HDAC enzymes that differ in subcellular localisation and enzymatic activity and which require NAD$^+$ for their catalytic activity. Gene products of *SIRT1* and *SIRT2* are found in the nucleus and cytoplasm, whereas *SIRT6* and *SIRT7* encode nuclear proteins, while gene products of *SIRT3*, *SIRT4* and *SIRT5* are localised in mitochondria [218]. The dependence of sirtuins on NAD$^+$ links their enzymatic activity directly to the energy status of the cell, such as the cellular NAD$^+$:NADH ratio and the absolute levels of nicotinamide, which is generated through NAD$^+$ hydrolysis during lysine deacetylation and is an inhibitor of sirtuin activity itself [219]. Sirtuins are best known for their role in ageing and have been shown to prolong the mean and maximal life spans in many species across all taxonomic groups (yeast, worms, flies, mice, primates) in response to caloric restriction or activation with molecules, such as resveratrol, a potent inducer of *SIRT1*/*Sirt1* expression [218,220,221].

Because sirtuins are structurally and mechanistically distinct from Classes I, IIA, IIB and IV of histone deacetylases and are not inhibited by the widely used Zn^{2+}-dependent HDAC inhibitors, they will not be covered in this review.

1.5. Histone Deacetylase Inhibitors

Several natural and synthetic compounds are currently known to inhibit HDACs. Since HDAC inhibitors do not inhibit all HDAC enzymes to the same extent, these agents can be grouped into pan-, Class II- and Class I-specific inhibitors [222]. Hydroxamic acids, for example, TSA (trichostatin A, which occurs naturally), belinostat, SAHA (suberoylanilide hydroxamic acid, also known as vorinostat) and LBH589 (panobinostat) are pan-HDAC inhibitors targeting (all) Class I, Class II and Class IV HDACs [222]. The related, hydroxamic acid-based pan-HDAC-inhibitor SB939 (pracrinostat) selectively inhibits Class I, II, IV HDACs except HDAC6 [223]. In contrast, the short-chain fatty acid valproic acid (VPA), the benzamide MS-275 (entinostat), and the bicyclic tetrapeptides FK228 (romidepsin) and spiruchostatin A are rather Class I-specific HDAC inhibitors [222]. The short-chain fatty acids sodium butyrate (natural compound) and 4-phenyl-butyrate (4-PBA, synthetic compound) have been reported to inhibit Class I and Class IIA HDACs (but not Class IIB HDACs) in relatively high, millimolar working concentrations [224]. The synthetic compounds TMP269, MC1575 and MC1568 have been described as specific inhibitors for Class IIA HDACs [225,226].

Importantly, the above-listed Class I and pan-HDAC inhibitors have been reported as successful anticancer agents as they induce cell-cycle arrest, differentiation and/or apoptosis in cancer cells by increasing the acetylation status of the chromatin and various non-histone proteins, such as p53, leading to their stabilization and activation. Moreover, it has been reported that both HDAC inhibitor types possess the ability to selectively induce apoptosis in "abnormal" tumour cells, whereas normal cells are relatively resistant to HDAC-inhibitor-induced cell death [172,173]. In contrast, much less is yet clear about the effects of Class IIA HDAC inhibitors in cancer cells, which still require further investigation in preclinical studies.

Importantly, HDAC inhibitors SAHA, pracrinostat, belinostat and romidepsin are FDA-approved drugs for some T-cell lymphomas [222,223,227,228], with panobinostat for multiple myeloma [229]. Pracrinostat has also been approved in 2014 as an orphan drug for acute myelocytic leukaemia (AML) [223]. Valproic acid has been in medical use since 1962 for the treatment of epilepsy and bipolar disorder, and it is marketed under the brand names Depakene and Epival (both Abbott Laboratories) [230]. It has also been tested in clinical trials as an anticancer agent and has demonstrated a promising clinical response [231]. 4-PBA, though not in oncology, was approved by the FDA in 1996 for the treatment of urea cycle disorders [224] and is now being investigated for therapy in some types of cancer [232]. In addition, a new clinical-stage HDAC inhibitor, CG-745, specific for Class I HDACs and Class IIB HDAC6, has recently been granted an orphan drug designation by the FDA for the treatment of patients with pancreatic cancer [233]. All these encouraging results justify that more and more HDAC inhibitors are currently being investigated in a number of clinical trials as part of mono- or combination therapies for the treatment of various cancers. Class I, II, IV and pan-HDAC inhibitors chelate the Zn^{2+} cation within the enzyme active site, resulting in the inhibition of HDAC activity. Importantly, the Class III HDACs sirtuins1–7, which contain a NAD^+-dependent catalytic domain, are insensitive to these agents [172,177,222].

Due to the broad activity of classical Class I and pan-HDAC inhibitors across HDAC isoforms, the development of second-generation HDAC inhibitors has been focused on improving the selectivity of HDAC inhibitors, resulting in the discovery of a series of isoform-specific HDAC inhibitors. Until now, most of the agents developed and reported in existing articles have selectivity for HDAC3 [234], HDAC6 [174,189,235,236] and HDAC8 [171,237] and are currently being evaluated in preclinical studies. At present, only the HDAC6 inhibitor ACY-1215 (Ricolinostat) has been tested in a phase 2 clinical trial as a treatment strategy for relapsed/refractory lymphoid malignancies (NCT02091063) [238].

In contrast to Class I, II, and IV HDAC inhibitors, much less is known about sirtuin inhibitors. The protein-deacetylating activities of both sirtuin-1 and sirtuin-2 can be inhibited simultaneously by the small molecules tenovin-1/-6 or sirtinol (with no effects on other sirtuins and Zn^{2+}-dependent HDACs), which are currently being targeted as potential therapeutic agents for cancer since they induce p53-dependent proapoptotic activity in malignant cells while having no effect on normal cells [239,240]. The indole compound selisistat (EX527) is a potent and selective sirtuin-1 inhibitor [240]. Surprisingly, until now, no clinical trials are underway to evaluate the efficacy of Class III HDAC inhibitors in cancer. Because the Zn^{2+}-dependent HDACs (Classes I, IIA, IIB and IV) are recognised as "classical HDACs" and common targets for therapy, the Class III sirtuins and their inhibitors are not in the scope of this review.

2. Imbalanced Histone Deacetylase (HDAC) Activities in Idiopathic Pulmonary Fibrosis: Effects and Therapeutic Correction

Increased activity and overexpression of histone deacetylases (HDACs) have been described for a long time in various pathological conditions such as cancer, cardiac hypertrophy and hypertension [166,193,241,242]. Upregulated HDAC activities are also observed in fibrotic diseases involving the heart, liver, kidneys and lungs; and experimental studies performed on animal models have shown that HDAC inhibitors can ameliorate various forms of fibrosis [164,168–170,243–245].

In IPF, where persistent fibroblast activation underlies progressive fibrotic disease, HDAC-mediated gene repression of antifibrotic molecules and proapoptotic factors appears to be a critical event [162–164,246]. We have recently reported that lung fibroblasts from patients with IPF exhibit a profibrotic phenotype with "cancer-like features" due to the abnormal overexpression of all Class I and Class II HDAC enzymes, which appeared responsible for their aberrant activation and persistence in IPF, presumably as the result of changes in expression profiles and cellular signalling due to alterations in the acetylation status of the chromatin and various non-histone proteins [165]. In accordance, it could be demonstrated that the pan-HDAC inhibitor panobinostat (LBH589), an FDA-approved drug for the treatment of multiple myeloma since 2015 [229], reduced proliferation, collagen-I biosynthesis, and anti-apoptotic genes in IPF fibroblasts in vitro, with concomitant induction of $p21^{Cip1}$ and ER stress-mediated apoptosis [165]. In addition, panobinostat also restored and enhanced the expression of antifibrotic genes silenced in IPF fibroblasts [162,247]. These processes were accompanied by massive chromatin and α-tubulin acetylation, confirming efficient Class I/IIA/IIB HDAC inhibition through panobinostat [165]. In addition, Jones and coworkers (2019) identified the pan-HDAC inhibitor pracrinostat, approved in 2014 as an orphan drug for AML, as a potent attenuator of lung fibroblast activation in IPF patient-derived fibroblasts [246]. Sanders and coworkers (2014) demonstrated the inactivation of IPF fibroblasts as well as the amelioration of experimental pulmonary fibrosis in response to global HDAC inhibition by SAHA [164]. The "older" pan-HDAC inhibitor SAHA was the first FDA-approved HDAC-inhibiting drug for the treatment of cancers, and it has been in clinical use since 2006 [222]. Table 1 summarises the broad therapeutic effects of various pan-HDAC inhibitors on preclinical models of lung fibrosis/IPF, which will be outlined in the following chapters of this article.

Table 1. Pan-HDAC-inhibitors for treatment of pulmonary fibrosis/IPF.

Study	Lung Fibrosis Model	HDAC Inhibiton	Effect/Involved Molecules
Coward et al. (2009) [162]	TGF-β-treated IPF fibroblasts	*Panobinostat (LBH589)* pan-HDAC	H3 and H4 acetylation at *COX2* promoter, derepression of *COX2* expression
Huang et al. (2013) [163]	Lung fibroblasts of bleomycin mice, Primary IPF fibroblasts	*Trichostatin A (TSA), vorinostat (SAHA)* pan-HDAC	H3 acetylation at the *Fas/FAS* promoter, derepression of *Fas/FAS* expression
Sanders et al. (2014) [164]	Primary IPF fibroblasts, Bleomycin mouse model	*Vorinostat (SAHA)* pan-HDAC	In vitro: proliferation H3 and H4 acetylation, H3K9Ac ↑ *BAK* ↑ *BID* ↑ *BCL2L1* ↓ In vivo: ameliorated lung fibrosis H3K9Ac ↑, *Bak* ↑ *Bcl2l1* ↓

Table 1. Cont.

Study	Lung Fibrosis Model	HDAC Inhibiton	Effect/Involved Molecules
Korfei et al. (2015) [165]	Primary IPF fibroblasts	Panobinostat (LBH589) pan-HDAC	Tubulin acetylation ↑, H3K27 acetylation, *CIP1*/p21 ↑, CHOP ↑, proliferation (*CCND1*) ↓, FMD (*ACTA2*, *COL1A1*, *COL1A3*, *FN*) ↓, surviving ↓ BCL-XL ↓
Zhang et al. (2013) [167]	Primary IPF fibroblasts, Bleomycin mouse model	Vorinostat (SAHA) pan-HDAC	In vitro: H3 and H4 acetylation, *COL3A1* (mRNA and protein) ↓ In vivo: ameliorated lung fibrosis, collagen-III ↓
Ota et al. (2015) [168]	TGF-β-stimulated A549 cells, Bleomycin mouse model	Trichostatin A (TSA)	In vitro: EMT ↓ restoration of *CDH1* expression. In vivo: Partial attenuation of fibrosis, restoration of AECII-*Sftpc* expression
Kim et al. (2019) [233]	Bleomycin mouse model, PHMG induced lung fibrosis	CG-745 Class I-HDAC + HDAC6	Abrogation of bleomycin-fibrosis, H3 acetylation, Pai-1 ↓ α-Sma ↓ collagen-I ↓ BALF: Tnf-α ↓ Il-6 ↓ Attenuation of PHMG-fibrosis
Jones et al. (2019) [246]	TGF-β-treated primary IPF fibroblasts	Pracrinostat pan-HDAC, except HDAC6	H3 acetylation at *PGC1A* promoter, derepression of *PGC1A* expression, HDAC7 signalling ↓, *ACTA2* ↓ *TNC* ↓ *IL6* ↓ *PDGFA* ↓ Inhibition of FMD
Coward et al. (2010) [247]	TGF-β-treated primary IPF fibroblasts	Panobinostat (LBH589) pan-HDAC	H3 and H4 acetylation at *CXCL10* promoter, reduction of repressive H3K9Me3 at *CXCL10* promoter, derepression of *CXCL10* expression
Sanders et al. (2011) [248]	Fibrotic rat Thy1 (-) lung fibroblasts	Trichostatin A (TSA)	H3 and H4 acetylation, derepression of *Thy1* (*CD90*) expression
Korfei et al. (2018) [249]	Primary IPF fibroblasts	Panobinostat (LBH589) pan-HDAC	Tubulin acetylation ↑, H3K27Ac ↑ STAT3-pTyr705 ↓, proliferation ↓, FMD ↓ ECM (pro-collagen-I) ↓ HDAC1 ↓ HDAC2 ↓ HDAC7 (mRNA and protein) ↓
Guo et al. (2009) [250]	TGF-β-treated human normal lung fibroblasts	Trichostatin A (TSA) pan-HDAC	HDAC4 signalling ↓ *ACTA2* ↓ *COL1A1* ↓ *CTGF* ↑ (!) Inhibition of FMD, α-SMA ↓ AKT phosphorylation ↓
Ye et al. (2014) [251]	Bleomycin rat model	Trichostatin A (TSA) pan-HDAC	Reduction of lung fibrosis, HDAC2 (mRNA and protein) ↓
Rao et al. (2016) [252]	TGF-β-treated normal human lung fibroblasts (HFL1), paraquat-induced lung fibrosis in rats	Vorinostat (SAHA) pan-HDAC	In vitro and in vivo: SMAD7 acetylation and stabilization, SMAD3 dephosphorylation, FMD ↓ attenuation of lung fibrosis
Glenisson et al. (2007) [253]	TGF-β-treated primary normal skin fibroblasts (human)	Trichostatin A (TSA) pan-HDAC	HDAC4 signalling ↓ *ACTA2*/α-SMA ↓ Inhibition of FMD
Kabel et al. (2016) [254]	Bleomycin rat model	4-phenyl-butyrate (4-PBA) Class I- and Class IIA-HDAC	attenuation of lung fibrosis, oxidative stress ↓ BALF: IL6 ↓ TGF-β ↓ TNF-α ↓

Table 1. Cont.

Study	Lung Fibrosis Model	HDAC Inhibiton	Effect/Involved Molecules
Jiang et al. (2018) [255]	A549 cells overexpressing mutant SP-A^{G231V} or SP-A^{F198S}	(4-PBA) Class I- and Class IIA-HDAC	GRP78 ↑ suppressed protein aggregation, improved secretion
Zhao et al. (2015) [256]	Bleomycin mouse model	(4-PBA) Class I- and Class IIA-HDAC	ER stress ↓ EMT ↓ NK-κB (p65) ↓ cytokines ↓ α-SMA ↓ Col1a1 ↓ Col1a2 ↓ alleviation of lung fibrosis

Definition of abbreviations: IPF: idiopathic pulmonary fibrosis; EMT: epithelial–mesenchymal transition; ECM: extracellular matrix; FMD: fibroblast-to-myofibroblast differentiation; H3/H4: histone H3/H4; Ac: acetylation; BALF: bronchoalveolar lavage fluid; PHMG: polyhexamethylene guanidine; ↑: upregulation; ↓: downregulation.

The reported evidence that alterations of protein function or chromatin accessibility through imbalanced deacetylation/acetylation are obviously key in the pathogenesis of IPF has led to the initiation of research studies to identify the exact targets and direct effects of HDAC enzymes in the setting of pulmonary fibrosis. Chromatin immunoprecipitation (ChIP) studies examining histone modifications have identified that several important anti-fibrotic genes are silenced in fibrotic and IPF fibroblasts, including *CAV1* (encoding caveolin 1) [257], *CXCL10* (encoding CXC motif chemokine 10) [247], *THY1* (encoding the anti-fibrotic receptor Thy1 membrane glycoprotein, also known as CD90) [248], *NFE2L2* (encoding the antioxidant transcription factor nuclear factor erythroid-derived 2-related factor-2, also known as NRF2) [258], *PPARG* (encoding the peroxisome proliferator-activated receptor-gamma, PPARγ) [171], *PGC1A* (encoding the PPARγ coactivator 1-alpha, PGC1-α) [246], and *COX2* (encoding cyclooxygenase-2) [162], all of which were restored upon HDAC-inhibitor treatment.

The aberrant HDAC-mediated silencing of *COX2* results in the loss of its metabolite prostaglandin E2, an autocrine anti-fibrotic mediator that controls fibroblast cellular overactivation while promoting the survival of AECII. Of note, the fibroblasts isolated from IPF patient lungs indicate reduced levels of COX2 or NRF2 even after 6 or more passages [162,258,259], hinting at the involvement of epigenetic repression mechanisms and that HDAC-mediated gene repression of antifibrotic molecules precedes growth-factor-induced profibrotic gene expression in IPF. In agreement with the increased apoptosis resistance and persistence of lung fibroblasts in IPF, proapoptotic genes *BAK* and *FAS* are also epigenetically repressed in IPF fibroblasts [163,164]. Importantly, in addition to reduced histone H3 acetylation, the promoters of *BAK* and *FAS* exhibited an increased level of trimethylated lysine 9 on histone H3 (H3K9me3), a repressive chromatin marker [163,164], indicating the close crosstalk between histone deacetylation with histone hypermethylation changes at specific histone residues [260]. In particular, histone modifications H3K9me3 and H3K27me3 are associated with decreased gene expression and linked to the increased recruitment of HDACs at promoters [260]. HDAC inhibitors have also been demonstrated to reverse repressive histone hypermethylation as ChIP assays revealed that SAHA treatment of IPF fibroblasts resulted in an enrichment of the pro-apoptotic *BAK* gene with acetylated lysine 9 on histone H3 (H3K9Ac), an active chromatin mark, and the depletion of *BAK* with H3K9Me3, thereby corresponding to increased *BAK* expression in the "corrected" IPF fibroblasts [164].

On the other side, increased expression of anti-apoptotic proteins surviving and the BCL-XL in IPF fibroblasts becomes paradoxically downregulated in response to pan-HDAC inhibitors known to increase general histone acetylation. Similarly, genes involved in myofibroblast differentiation, such as *ACTA2*, *COL1A1*, *COL3A1* and *FN*, are suppressed in primary IPF fibroblasts in response to panobinostat or SAHA [164,165,249]. Jones et al., observed that TGF-β induced-expression of *ACTA2*, *TNC*, *IL6*, *IL11* and *PDGFA* was abrogated in IPF fibroblasts upon treatment with pracrinostat [246]. In agreement with these findings, it could be demonstrated that panobinostat abrogated STAT3-phosphorylation at tyrosine 705 (Tyr705) and its fibrotic action in IPF fibroblasts, thus offering a plausible explanation for the reduction of survival- and ECM-associated genes in response to global HDAC inhibition and evidence for the involvement of HDACs in increased expression of such profibrotic genes [249]. Various reports from the cancer field suspect that Class I HDAC activity and increased deacetylation of STAT3 appear to be required for its phosphorylation at Tyr705 and nuclear translocation as HDAC1, -2 and -3 have been reported to reduce STAT3 acetylation [261,262] and as selective inhibition of Class I HDACs was sufficient in efficiently suppressing STAT3-pTyr705 phosphorylation and its signalling in a variety of malignant cells [262–264]. Similarly, Class I HDACs were demonstrated to be required for the activation of the extracellular signal-regulated kinase-1 (ERK/MAPK3) and PI3K pathways by TGF-β in lung fibroblasts and, thus, for the subsequent ECM gene induction dependent on these non-SMAD signalling pathways [265].

Further, Class IIA HDAC4, which is prominently upregulated in IPF versus normal fibroblasts, was shown to form a protein complex with some cytoplasmic protein phosphatases (PP) in response to TGF-β to prevent the dephosphorylation and inhibition of AKT in fibrotic lung fibroblasts for inducing and maintaining AKT-mediated profibrotic gene expression [250]. Similarly, TGF-β induced expression of ECM genes has been suspected to require Class IIB HDAC6 function in AKT activation as well, as selective HDAC6 inhibition was shown to disrupt TGF-β-elicited AKT signalling in fibrotic lung fibroblasts [235]. Together, these data suggest that HDACs also mediate profibrotic signalling in fibrotic/IPF-fibroblasts through interaction with various non-histone protein targets, which is reversed by HDAC inhibition. On the other side, it must not be excluded that HDACs mediate profibrotic gene expression due to epigenetic silencing of repressors of profibrotic genes. Importantly, temporal gene expression analyses of TGF-β-treated primary lung fibroblasts done by Jones and coworkers (2019) have revealed that TGF-β-mediated HDAC signalling repressed antifibrotic genes prior to the upregulation of profibrotic genes [246].

Interestingly, similar to IPF fibroblasts/myofibroblasts, Class I and Class II HDACs were also found to be upregulated in abnormal, "proliferating" $KRT5^+$ bronchiolar basal cells at sites of aberrant re-epithelialization and co-localised with the expression of p-STAT3 and surviving [165,249]. The crucial intrinsic activity of HDACs in cell proliferation, cell migration and anti-apoptosis suggests a strong contribution of these enzymes in the "re-programming" and abnormal activation of such cells in the progressive bronchiolisation of damaged alveolar epithelium and the fibrosing process in IPF [165,174]. Further studies proved the eminent profibrotic effect of airway/bronchiolar basal cells derived from IPF patients [174,266], which, interestingly, could be largely abrogated by the selective inhibition of HDAC6 [174].

Importantly, in contrast to myofibroblasts and basal cells, expression of many HDACs appeared to be sparse or even absent in IPF-AECII undergoing proapoptotic ER stress [165], which is in agreement with the degradation and depletion of many HDAC enzymes under conditions of severe ER/oxidative stress or apoptosis [267–271].

Taken together, IPF appears to be characterised by a significant imbalance of HDAC activities, with an abnormal increase of HDAC expression in fibroblasts/myofibroblasts and bronchiolar basal cells but a lack of HDAC expression in AECII due to irremediable ER stress and apoptosis. The consequent (differentially) deregulated acetylation status of histone tails and non-histone proteins/TF substrates in fibroblast populations and basal cells versus the AECII of IPF lungs may lead ultimately to altered chromatin transcription profiles and shifted cellular signalling and disturbed inter-cellular communication, which contribute to fibrosis (Figure 1). In the following chapters, the pathogenic role of different HDAC classes/HDAC isoforms in IPF and their therapeutic correction in preclinical models are described.

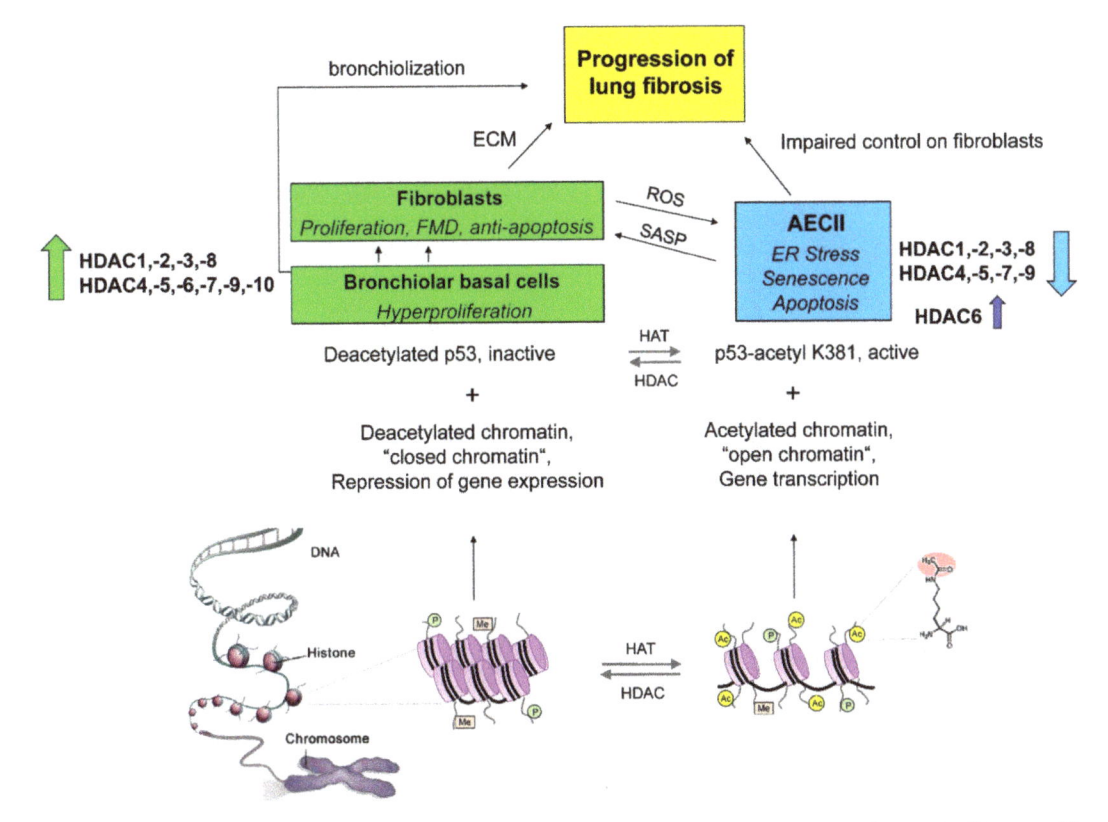

Figure 1. Imbalanced histone deacetylase activities in IPF. IPF is characterised by a significant imbalance of histone deacetylase (HDAC) activities, with an abnormal increase of HDAC expression in fibroblasts/myofibroblasts and bronchiolar basal cells, but a lack of HDAC expression in AECII due to ER stress, senescence and apoptosis. This imbalance contributes and perpetuates the fibrotic process. Abbreviations: ECM: extracellular matrix; FMD: fibroblast-to-myofibroblast differentiation; AECII: type-I/-II alveolar epithelial cell; ROS: reactive oxygen species; SASP: senescence-associated secretory phenotype; HAT: histone acetyltransferase; P = phosphorylation, Me = methylation, Ac = acetylation.

2.1. Class I Histone Deacetylases in IPF: Expression Profile, Function and Preclinical Studies

In our report from 2015, we found all Class I HDAC enzymes significantly upregulated on the proteomic level in IPF lung tissues as well as in primary IPF fibroblast isolations by immunoblotting studies, in comparison to tissues and fibroblast isolates obtained from normal lungs [165], in agreement with other studies [171]. Immunohistochemical studies confirmed strong induction and predominant localisation of HDAC1, -2, -3 and -8 in α-SMA expressing myofibroblasts of fibroblast foci, but also revealed robust expression of all Class I HDACs in abnormal, hyperplastic bronchiolar basal cells at sites of aberrant re-epithelialisation in IPF. In marked contrast, expression of Class I-HDACs was absent in the proSP-C⁺ AECII of IPF lungs [165].

In addition, ciliated bronchial cells of IPF bronchioles also indicated a prominent upregulation of HDAC2 and -3 compared to healthy control lung tissues. This observation appeared to be conceptual since KRT5⁺ expressing basal cells are the progenitors for non-ciliated Club cells and ciliated FOXJ1⁺ bronchial cells, and they are suggested to initiate the progressive bronchiolization process of alveolar spaces in IPF. Further, in agreement with various reports about expression patterns and functions of Class I enzymes, HDAC1, -2, and -3 indicated a dominant nuclear expression in the abovementioned cell types, whereas HDAC8 indicated cytoplasmic as well as nuclear localisation [165]. Further, HDAC2 and HDAC3 have been observed to be upregulated in various rodent models of pulmonary fibrosis [251,272], with predominant localisation in fibrotic lesions and lung fibroblasts [163,258,273].

Abnormal overexpression of Class I HDACs in IPF fibroblasts/myofibroblasts appears to play a crucial role in the fibrotic process, as ChIP studies by Coward and coworkers (2009) revealed that the CoREST (REST corepressor 1) and Sin3a (Sin3 histone deacetylase corepressor complex component SDS3) transcriptional corepressor complexes, which consist of HDAC1 and HDAC2, and the N-CoR (nuclear receptor corepressor 1) complex consisting of HDAC3, were bound to the promoter of the antifibrotic gene COX2 in primary IPF fibroblasts, resulting in the deacetylation of histone H3 and H4 at the COX2 promoter and decreased transcription factor binding, leading to diminished COX2 expression in IPF fibroblasts [162]. Similar observations they made for the CXCL10 gene, which is suppressed in IPF fibroblasts as well due to insufficient histone H3/H4 acetylation and repressive histone H3 hypermethylation at its promoter as a result of decreased recruitment of HATs but increased recruitment of Class I HDAC-containing transcriptional repressor complexes in IPF fibroblasts [247]. In agreement, treatment of IPF fibroblasts with the well-characterised pan-HDAC inhibitor panobinostat resulted in the restoration of COX2 and CXCL10 expression through the creation of an active chromatin structure at their promoters, manifested as the accumulation of acetylated histones H3 and H4 [162,247]. The malignant repression of FAS in fibrotic fibroblasts was also attributed in part to increased HDAC2 expression [163].

Further, profibrotic STAT3-pTyr705 phosphorylation and activation are prominently upregulated in IPF fibroblasts [73,249] and suggested to be promoted by lysine deacetylation of STAT3 through HDAC1, -2 and/or -3 [261,262]. In addition, Class I HDACs have also been reported to be involved in the activation of the upstream JAK2 kinase [264]. In agreement, STAT3-pTyr705 phosphorylation was abrogated in response to panobinostat treatment, resulting in a reduction of cell proliferation, surviving expression and ECM associated genes in IPF fibroblasts [249]. Moreover, panobinostat not only inhibited HDACs, but it also led to significant proteolysis of HDAC1 and HDAC2 and, thus, the efficient inactivation of both HDACs in IPF fibroblasts, whereas the mRNA levels for both enzymes were not affected [249]. The tumour suppressor p53 is another substrate of Class I HDACs, and the enormous loss of HDAC1/2 function in response to panobinostat was associated with the strong upregulation of p21^{CIP1} and other p53 target genes in IPF fibroblasts [165].

Interestingly, SMAD7, which is known to inhibit TGF-β/SMAD2/3 signalling, has also been identified as a non-histone protein target of HDAC1 and is destabilised through deacetylation [274]. In TGF-β-stimulated human lung fibroblasts, HDAC1 was shown to become upregulated, while SMAD7 became downregulated [252]. Further studies revealed that treatment of TGF-β-stimulated lung fibroblasts with the pan-HDAC inhibitor SAHA prevented SMAD7 deacetylation by inhibiting TGF-β-induced HDAC1 activity, resulting in increased SMAD7 expression and decreased SMAD3 phosphorylation with subsequent reduction of profibrotic signalling. SAHA also attenuated paraquat-induced lung fibrosis in rats in vivo through the restoration of Smad7 protein expression and the suppression of the canonical TGF-β pathway [252].

As can be seen, many studies characterizing the function, contribution and therapeutic correction of aberrant Class I HDAC activity in lung fibrosis are based on the use of pan-HDAC inhibitors. In the next two chapters, the therapeutic effects of specific Class I HDAC inhibitors and Class I isoform-selective inhibitors in preclinical models of lung fibrosis are summarised.

2.1.1. Class I HDAC Inhibitors in Preclinical Studies of Lung Fibrosis

The crucial role of Class I HDACs in lung fibrosis is also underscored by the fact that their specific inhibition through spiruchostatin A has been shown to significantly reduce fibroblast proliferation and myofibroblast markers on protein level in TGF-β-stimulated IPF fibroblasts in vitro. Spiruchostatin A also increased histone H3 acetylation and CIP1/p21 expression, suggesting that direct cell-cycle regulation was the mechanism for inhibiting proliferation [275]. The related FDA-approved Class I inhibitor romidepsin indicated the very same effects, in addition to its profound capability in downregulating the protein expression of lysyl oxidase (LOX), an enzyme involved in collagen-crosslinking, in TGF-β-treated IPF fibroblasts. Interestingly, it was also demonstrated that romidepsin exerted minimal effects on primary normal human AECII at doses that markedly suppressed the proliferation of IPF fibroblasts [169]. In vivo, romidepsin inhibited bleomycin-induced lung fibrosis in mice in association with suppression of LOX expression [169].

Interestingly, the weak Class I inhibitor valproic acid (VPA) was also shown to efficiently reduce cell proliferation, surviving expression, collagen-I protein turnover in IPF fibroblasts, and these effects were accompanied by the significant degradation and loss of HDAC2 [165], an effect which has been observed in various cells upon VPA treatment [276]. Although VPA has been shown to selectively inhibit STAT3-pTyr705 phosphorylation in various malignant and non-malignant cells [263,277], this effect, however, has yet not been addressed in fibrotic fibroblasts. In fibrotic A549 cells, VPA was shown to decrease TGF-β induced histone deacetylation and subsequently restored TGF-β downregulated epithelial genes in A549 cells, but only partially inhibited EMT, as many profibrotic genes upregulated by TGF-β were not suppressed by VPA, with the exception of *COL1A1* [278]. Similarly, in IPF fibroblasts, VPA significantly suppressed pro-collagen-I expression but upregulated the α-SMA level [165]. Interestingly, silencing of *HDAC2* by RNA interference (RNAi) was also shown to further increase *ACTA2* expression in TGF-β-stimulated human skin fibroblasts, whereas *HDAC8* silencing significantly suppressed TGF-β-induced *ACTA2* expression in these cells [253]. Depletion of *Hdac3* by RNAi resulted in the downregulation of TGF-β induced disintegrin and metalloproteinase domain-containing protein-12 (*Adam12*) and metalloproteinase inhibitor-1 (*Timp1*) expression in mouse fibroblasts but was strictly dependent on the suppression of TGF-β-activated ERK (MAPK3) and PI3K signalling pathways and, thus, restricted to ECM genes dependent on these Smad-independent signalling pathways as TGF-β-upregulated *Pai1* expression was unaffected [265].

Interestingly, in contrast to in vitro studies, VPA was shown to significantly attenuate EMT and lung fibrosis in bleomycin-treated mice in vivo, which was associated with Smad2/3 deactivation but without Akt cellular signal involvement [170]. In bleomycin-treated rats, it reduced oxidative stress and proinflammatory cytokines in injured lungs, together with significant improvement of the histopathological picture [254]. The failure of VPA to deactivate Akt signalling is presumably due to the fact that VPA specifically inhibits the activities of HDAC1 and HDAC2 [165,222] but not of HDAC3 (involved in mediating TGF-β-induced PI3K signalling [265], as mentioned above). In agreement, the Class I HDAC inhibitor entinostat (MS-275), specific for HDAC1 and HDAC3, also led to the inactivation of the PI3K/Akt pathway in TGF-β-stimulated lung fibroblasts [265]. In addition, entinostat was shown to suppress TGF-β-induced expression of SPARC, a matricellular protein involved in the ECM turnover and apoptosis resistance of myofibroblasts in cultured human lung fibroblasts. In detail, entinostat restored the expression of ARHGEF3 (Rho guanine nucleotide exchange factor 3, also known as XPLN = exchange factor found in platelets and leukemic and neuronal tissues), a negative regulator of *SPARC* expression, as *ARHGEF3* was repressed by TGF-β-induced HDAC1/3 signalling [279]. In summary, all these studies prove the significant antifibrotic efficacy of Class I-selective HDAC inhibitors in preclinical models of lung fibrosis and underscore the crucial role of Class I HDACs in mediating profibrotic signalling in IPF/fibrotic lung fibroblasts.

However, one contrary report also exists by Rubio and coworkers, describing reduced HDAC activity in nuclear extracts of IPF versus normal fibroblasts, despite evidenced upregulation of HDAC1 and HDAC2 in IPF fibroblasts [280]. Hence, HDAC activity was upregulated in the cytosolic fraction of IPF fibroblasts. Subsequent studies revealed that histone acetyltransferase p300 inactivated the nuclear activity of HDAC1 by acetylation, thereby resulting in the disruption of the multicomponent RNA-protein complex "MiCEE", which is considered a repressor of general gene transcription in IPF fibroblasts. Indeed, this could explain the exaggerated expression of ECM genes during fibrogenesis in IPF fibroblasts. In line with this suggestion, inhibition of p300 resulted in reduced ECM production in IPF fibroblasts in vitro and decreased lung fibrosis in bleomycin-treated mice in vivo [280]. Taken together, the results from this very interesting study support a key role of active p300 and Class I HDAC inactivation during IPF and propose p300 inhibition as therapy for IPF, but stands in vast contrast to numerous reports suggesting HDAC inhibitors for targeting increased Class I HDAC activity in fibrotic fibroblasts as a therapeutic option for IPF patients.

The effects of Class I HDAC inhibitors on bronchiolar basal cells and the aberrant bronchiolization process in IPF remain to be determined, which would help to clarify the role of the eminent upregulation of all Class I HDACs in basal cells, Clara cells as well as FOXJ1 expressing the bronchial cells of IPF lungs. Interestingly, COX2 protein expression was also previously observed to be diminished in the bronchiolar epithelial cells of IPF lungs [281], which might be caused by aberrant Class I HDAC-mediated epigenetic repression of *COX2* expression, as observed in IPF fibroblasts.

The effects of Class I HDAC inhibitors and Class I isoform-selective inhibitors on preclinical models of lung fibrosis/IPF are summarised in Table 2.

Table 2. Class I HDAC inhibitors and Class I isoform-selective inhibitors for treatment of pulmonary fibrosis.

Study	Lung Fibrosis Model	HDAC Inhibition	Effect/Involved Molecules
Korfei et al. (2015) [165]	Primary IPF fibroblasts	*Valproic acid (VPA)* HDAC1, -2	H3K27 acetylation, CIP1 ↑, cell proliferation ↓ *BIRC5*/surviving ↓ collagen-I ↓ HDAC2 ↓ HDAC7 ↓
Conforti et al. (2017) [169]	TGF-β-treated primary IPF fibroblasts, Bleomycin mouse model	*Romidepsin (FK228)* HDAC1, -2	In vitro: H3 acetylation, CIP1 ↑ ACTA2 ↓ COL3A1 ↓ LOX ↓ HDAC4 ↓ inhibition of FMD. In vivo: inhibited lung fibrosis, ECM genes ↓ Lox protein ↓
Chen et al. (2021) [170]	TGF-β-treated A549 cells, Bleomycin mouse model	*Valproic acid* HDAC1, -2	In vitro and in vivo: SMAD2/3 deactivation, inhibition of EMT
Barter et al. (2010) [265]	TGF-β-treated embryonic mouse fibroblasts	*Entinostat (MS-275)* HDAC1, -3; HDAC3 siRNA	Inhibition of PI3K and ERK pathways *Adam12* ↓ *Timp1* ↓
Davies et al. (2012) [275]	TGF-β-treated primary IPF fibroblasts	*Spiruchostatin A* HDAC1, -2	H3 acetylation, CIP1 ↑ cell proliferation ↓ inhibition of FMD
Noguchi et al. (2015) [278]	TGF-β-treated A549 cells	*Valproic acid* HDAC1, -2	H3K27 acetylation, partial inhibition of EMT
Kabel et al. (2016) [254]	Bleomycin rat model	*Valproic acid* HDAC1, -2	attenuation of lung fibrosis, oxidative stress ↓ BALF: IL6 ↓ TGF-β ↓ TNF-α ↓
Kamio et al. (2017) [279]	TGF-β-treated normal human lung fibroblasts	*Entinostat (MS-275):* HDAC1, -3	Restoration of *ARHGEF3*/XPLN (negative regulator of *SPARC*) ↑ SPARC ↓
Saito et al. (2019) [171]	TGF-β-treated normal human lung fibroblasts, Bleomycin mouse model	NCC170 HDAC8	In vitro: H3K27 acetylation, restoration of *PPARG* expression, ECM protein production ↓ In vivo: inhibited lung fibrosis
Chen et al. (2021) [258]	Bleomycin mouse model	RGFP966 HDAC3	H3 acetylation at the *Nrf2* promoter, restoration of *Nrf2* expression, E-cadherin expression ↑ ECM proteins ↓
Yuan et al. (2020) [273]	RA-ILD mouse model	HDAC3 siRNA	miR-19a-3p ↑ IL17RA ↓ IL17/IL17RA signalling ↓ Inflammation ↓ attenuation of lung fibrosis

Definition of abbreviations: IPF: idiopathic pulmonary fibrosis; EMT: epithelial–mesenchymal transition; ECM: extracellular matrix; FMD: fibroblast-to-myofibroblast differentiation; H3: histone H3; RA-ILD: rheumatoid arthritis (RA) associated interstitial lung disease (ILD); siRNA: small interfering RNA; BALF: bronchoalveolar lavage fluid; ↑: upregulation; ↓: downregulation.

2.1.2. Class I Isoform-Selective Inhibitors in Preclinical Models of Lung Fibrosis

Recently, published work highlights a crucial role of single Class I HDAC enzymes, in particular HDAC3, in progressive fibrotic lung diseases as the HDAC3-selective inhibitor RGFP966 effectively reduced pulmonary fibrosis in bleomycin-treated wild-type mice and conditional $Hdac3^{(-/-)}$ mice were largely resistant to bleomycin-induced lung fibrosis [258]. HDAC3 was observed to be overexpressed in IPF lungs and to be preferentially upregulated in the fibrotic phase in bleomycin-injured lungs at day 14 and day 21 post-bleomycin and was found to repress *Nrf2* expression in concert with the profibrotic Forkhead box M1 (FOXM1) transcription factor. Conversely, RGFP966 treatment reduced the HDAC3 and FOXM1 bindings and elevated histone H3 acetylation levels at the *Nrf2* promoter, resulting in *Nrf2* derepression and increased Nrf2-induced expression of antioxidants. In addition, this treatment also restored epithelial E-cadherin expression while downregulating profibrotic ECM molecules [258]. Similarly, in IPF, NRF2 is largely absent in myofibroblasts within fibroblast foci [282], while increased HDAC3 expression in these foci is observed [165]. Taken together, aberrant overexpression of HDAC3 and its exerted suppression of NRF2 plays a pivotal role in lung fibrosis, including IPF, which can be attenuated by selective inhibition of HDAC3.

Moreover, HDAC3 has also been reported to negatively regulate miR-19a-3p to increase interleukin 17 receptor A (IL17RA) expression in rheumatoid arthritis (RA)-associated interstitial lung disease (ILD) [273]. Interestingly, both HDAC3 and IL17RA were found to be much more upregulated in the lung tissues of RA-ILD patients than in patients with IPF versus healthy controls. Further analysis revealed a positive correlation of expression between HDAC3 and IL17RA in RA-ILD. Using an RA-ILD mouse model, HDAC3 downregulated miR-19a-3p expression in the lung fibroblasts of these mice, which resulted in increased IL17/IL17RA signalling and ECM protein expression, an effect that was abrogated by overexpression of miR-19a-3p or siRNA-mediated *Il17ra* or *Hdac3* silencing. Of note, delivery of *Hdac3*-targeting siRNA to RA-ILD mice attenuated lung fibrosis in mice in vivo [273].

Similar to the effects of HDAC3 inhibitor, selective inhibition of Hdac8 was also shown to ameliorate bleomycin-induced lung fibrosis in mice through the reduction of ECM synthesis [171]. Interestingly, HDAC8 has been regarded for a long time as a marker for myofibroblasts and smooth muscle cells, where it displays a strong association with α-SMA, and *si*RNA-mediated silencing of *HDAC8* revealed that it is essential for smooth muscle cell contractility [283,284]. HDAC8 expression has been demonstrated to increase in human lung fibroblasts in response to TGF-β, where it deacetylated chromosomes protein-3 (SMC3), a specific substrate of HDAC8, but not of other HDACs in the nucleus, while inducing α-SMA stress fibre formation in the cytoplasm of TGF-β-treated fibroblasts. This process was associated with increased production of ECM proteins and was abrogated by *HDAC8* silencing or inhibition of HDAC8 with NCC170. Further studies revealed that HDAC8 inhibited antifibrotic PPARγ-signalling through the repression of the *PPARG* transcription as HDAC8 was found in ChIP assays to deacetylate histone H3 at *PPARG* gene enhancer regions. *Vice versa*, HDAC8 inhibition ameliorated the TGF-β-induced loss of the active chromatin marker H3K27ac and restored *PPARG* expression. Interestingly, HDAC8 inhibition did not appear to alter the TGF-β-induced phosphorylation of SMAD2, SMAD3 or AKT, suggesting that PPARγ upregulation was at least partially responsible for the suppressive effects of HDAC8 inhibition on TGF-β induced fibroblast-to-myofibroblast transformation [171].

Taken together, these three studies involving animal models of lung fibrosis highlight the obviously potent antifibrotic efficacy of pharmacological inhibition or genetic knockdown of single Class I isoforms to block the evolvement of lung fibrosis (Table 2) and emphasise an underestimated dominant role of HDAC3 and HDAC8 in the pathogenesis of fibrotic lung disease.

2.1.3. Loss of Sin3-HDAC1/HDAC2 Repressor Complex Activity in AECII Results in Alveolar Senescence

The observed eminent lack of Class I HDACs in proSP-C+ expressing AECII in IPF is not only plausible due to increased alveolar ER stress and apoptosis but also considerably mirrored by increased p53-p21CIP1 activation and senescence in IPF-AECII, which has been widely reported by many scientists [17,118–120]. AECII senescence in IPF has been associated with p21-induced cell-cycle arrest and gradual apoptotic cell loss and with the senescence-associated secretory phenotype (SASP) contributing to myofibroblast expansion [17,120]. In addition, ER stress involving Chop has recently been shown to promote AECII senescence and SASP phenotype in two different experimental models of pulmonary fibrosis [285,286].

Moreover, it could be recently demonstrated that the AECII-specific conditional loss of *Sin3a*, a key component of the Sin3-HDAC1/HDAC2 corepressor complex, results in profound AECII senescence and spontaneous progressive lung fibrosis in mutant mice that closely resembles the pathological remodelling seen in IPF [120]. Fibrosis in these mice was diminished either by the selective loss of p53 function in AECII or by the ablation of senescent AEC cells through systemic delivery of senolytic drugs [120]. Previous research by the same group showed that loss of *Sin3a* in mouse early foregut endotherm led to a specific and profound defect in lung development, with complete loss of epithelial cells at later stages, resulting in the death of neonatal pubs at birth due to respiratory insufficiency. Further analyses revealed that embryonic lung epithelial cells adopted a senescence-like state with permanent cell-cycle arrest in the G1 phase before their demise [287]. Similarly, mice with foregut endoderm-specific, global deletion of *Hdac1* and *Hdac2*, but not individual loss of these HDACs, died at birth because of respiratory distress due to loss of Sox2 expression and a block in proximal airway development [288]. Total loss of *Hdac3* in the developing lung epithelium led to the diminished spreading of AECI cells and a disruption of lung sacculation, and newborn mutant mice died shortly after birth [289]. In adult mice, conditional loss of *Hdac1/Hdac2* in the proximal airway epithelium led to increased expression of the cell-cycle regulators Rb1 (retinoblastoma-associated protein), p21^{Cip1}, and p16^{Ink4a} (cyclin-dependent kinase inhibitor 2A), resulting in a loss of cell-cycle progression and defective regeneration of Sox2-expressing airway epithelium after naphthalene injury [288].

In summary, all these data suggest that AECII senescence and apoptosis in IPF are mediated by both ER stress and a lack of Class I HDACs.

2.2. Class IIA Histone Deacetylases in IPF: Expression Profile, Function, and Preclinical Studies

In our report from 2015, we also found all Class IIA HDACs (HDAC4,-5,-7 and -9) significantly upregulated on the proteomic level in IPF lung tissues in comparison to normal lungs. Immunohistochemical analyses showed strong overexpression of all Class IIA enzymes in myofibroblasts within fibroblast foci and abnormal hyperplastic bronchiolar epithelium, including ciliated bronchial cells of IPF lungs. Immunoblot analyses revealed, especially for HDAC4 and HDAC7, a striking upregulation in IPF versus control fibroblasts, which was also evident on the mRNA level in addition to robust *HDAC5* and (Class IV) *HDAC11* upregulation. Further, all Class IIA HDACs indicated a predominant cytoplasmic localisation in myofibroblasts in IPF [165,290], which appeared to be necessary for their profibrotic function. Co-immunoprecipitation studies indicated that HDAC4 interacts directly with α-SMA and appears to be required for a-SMA fibre formation and cell contraction in lung fibroblasts in response to TGF-β stimulation [290]. Further, the translocation of Class IIA HDAC enzymes (HDAC4,-5,-7 and -9) from the nucleus to the cytoplasm is associated with the activation of transcription factors myocyte-enhancer factor-2 (MEF2) and serum response factor (SRF), which activate myogenic genes such as *ACTA2* and which are repressed by nuclear localisation of Class IIA HDACs. The HDAC-mediated repression of MEF2 activity is abrogated by calcium/calmodulin-dependent protein kinase (CaMK) through phosphorylation of HDAC4,-5,-7,-9 "in response to stress stimuli", resulting in consequent dissociation from MEF2 and their nuclear export, enabling MEF2 to stimulate profibrotic and progrowth genes [291–293].

Gene silencing studies using RNAi technology identified HDAC4 as an HDAC that mediates TGF-β-induced differentiation of normal lung/skin fibroblasts into myofibroblasts [250,253]. Additionally, here, the cytoplasmic localisation of HDAC4 was required for the activation of the AKT signalling pathway, which is necessary for the expression of *ACTA2* and other ECM genes in response to TGF-β [250]. As a mechanism, it has been suggested that HDAC4 captures cytoplasmic serine/threonine phosphatases PP1 and PP2A, thereby protecting AKT from being dephosphorylated. Conversely, RNAi-mediated silencing of *HDAC4* as well as pan-HDAC inhibition through TSA led to the disruption of the HDAC4/PP1/PP2A complex and the liberation of PP1 and PP2A, followed by the dephosphorylation and inactivation of AKT, with the consequent blockade of TGF-β-stimulated α-SMA expression [250]. Importantly, abrogation of TGF-β-induced fibroblast-to-myofibroblast transformation by TSA was SMAD2/3-independent [250]. It was also suggested that TGF-β promoted HDAC4 nucleus-to-cytoplasm translocation through increased NOX4-derived ROS production, which leads to cysteine oxidation and intramolecular disulfide bond formation within HDAC4, facilitating its nuclear export and consequent profibrotic effects in the cytoplasm of stimulated lung fibroblasts [290]. Taken together, Class IIA HDAC enzymes such as HDAC4 alter gene expression profiles and cellular signalling not only through histone deacetylation but also through protein–protein interactions in the cytoplasm.

Interestingly, HDAC4 revealed an entirely cytoplasmic expression in KRT5 expressing basal cells of hyperplastic IPF bronchioles or adjacent to fibroblast foci, whereas luminal ciliated bronchial cells in IPF bronchiolar structures indicated a dominant nuclear localisation of HDAC4 [165]. Nuclear functions of HDAC4 include the repression of MEF2 activity and/or p21^{CIP1} expression. ChIP analyses demonstrated that HDAC4 represses p21^{CIP1} expression as a component of the HDAC4–HDAC3–N–CoR corepressor complex bound to the proximal *CIP1* promoter [200,201]. HDAC4 was also suggested to be involved in the repression of *FAS* in fibrotic fibroblasts, together with Class I HDAC2 [163]. In IPF fibroblasts, HDAC4 was observed in both the cytoplasm and the nucleus. In aggregate, HDAC4 appears to manifest its distribution in the cytoplasm and/or nucleus depending on cell type, the stage of cell differentiation, and the physiological condition.

More recently, Class IIA HDAC7 has been identified as a key enzyme facilitating TGF-β-mediated regulation of key pro- and anti-fibrotic genes in IPF. Specific HDAC gene silencing (*HDAC1* through *HDAC11*, except *HDAC6*) by RNAi in TGF-β-stimulated IPF fibroblasts with the use of *ACTA2* transcript levels as a readout parameter revealed that the silencing of *HDAC7* by RNAi was the most effective in reducing TGF-β-induced *ACTA2* expression in primary IPF fibroblasts [246]. Aside from *ACTA2*, the knockdown of *HDAC7* by RNAi resulted in a significant reduction of TGF-β-upregulated profibrotic mediators *NOX4* and *CTGF* in stimulated IPF fibroblasts, while expression of the TGF-β-suppressed antifibrotic gene *PGC1A* was increased. Moreover, silencing of *HDAC7* also led to reduced expression of *HDAC2*, *HDAC6*, *HDAC8* and *HDAC10* but increased *HDAC9* expression, suggesting that HDAC7 affected gene expression profiles through the regulation of the expression of other HDACs in response to TGF-β [246]. Interestingly, RNAi-mediated knockdown of *HDAC7* was also shown to reduce TGF-β induced SMAD2/3 activation, myofibroblast differentiation and ECM production in primary fibroblasts derived from human Peyronie's disease plaque [294]. In TGF-β-treated skin fibroblasts from patients with systemic sclerosis, *HDAC7* silencing resulted in reduced collagen-I and collagen-III production [295]. A recent study showed that HDAC7 was involved in endothelin-1-induced production of CTGF in lung fibroblasts through the formation of a transcriptional complex with p300 and AP-1 and recruitment to the *CTGF* promoter region, resulting in *CTGF* expression. In detail, endothelin-1 promoted HDAC7 translocation from the cytosol to nucleus and HDAC7 initiated AP-1 transcriptional activity (surprisingly) through the recruitment of p300 and consequent p300-mediated AP-1 acetylation. Conversely,

RNAi-mediated silencing of either *HDAC7* or *EP300* suppressed endothelin-1-induced *CTGF* expression [296]. Taken together, these results indicate a crucial role for *HDAC7* in cytokine/growth factor-induced expression of profibrotic molecules during fibrogenesis. Interestingly, pan-HDAC inhibitors such as TSA [295] and panobinostat [165] were observed to result in the profound suppression of HDAC7 on the transcriptomic and proteomic levels in primary IPF fibroblasts. Even the weak Class I inhibitor VPA reduced it significantly on mRNA and protein levels [165].

In contrast to HDAC4 and HDAC7, much less is known about the role and functions of HDAC5 and HDAC9 in lung fibrosis. Interestingly, silencing of *HDAC5* by RNAi was shown to further increase *ACTA2* expression in TGF-β-stimulated IPF fibroblasts, whereas *HDAC9* silencing decreased TGF-β-induced *ACTA2* expression in these cells [246]. Other studies showed that overexpression of HDAC9 and of its alternatively spliced isoform histone deacetylase-related protein (HDRP) in normal lung fibroblasts led to myofibroblast transformation and increased apoptosis resistance of transgenic fibroblasts [297], and HDRP was found in IHC studies to be significantly overexpressed in the myofibroblast foci of IPF lungs [165].

However, the role of the eminent upregulation of all four Class IIA HDACs in bronchiolar basal cells in IPF remains elusive and needs further investigation.

Interestingly, in contrast to Class I, HDAC inhibitors targeting specifically Class IIA HDACs (e.g., TMP269, MC1575 and MC1568) are poorly described in the literature, and there is yet no report about the use of Class IIA HDAC-inhibitors in the preclinical models of lung fibrosis. A study by Mannaerts et al. (2013) demonstrated that Class IIA HDAC inhibition by MC1568 blocked the activation of primary mouse hepatic stellate cells (HSC), as shown by the reduced expression of ECM genes *Col1a1*, *Col3a1*, *Acta2* and *Lox* [298]. Interestingly, this effect was mediated by the upregulation of miR-29 expression, which is an antifibrotic miRNA known to downregulate ECM molecules [87]. Moreover, knockdown of *Hdac4* by siRNA also resulted in significant miR-29 upregulation, *Col1a1* downregulation and partial inhibition of HSC activation [298]. In aggregate, this study revealed that HDAC4 regulates miR-29 expression, which represents a function of nuclear HDAC4 in fibrotic mesenchymal cells.

Due to a lack of studies about the use of Class IIA HDAC-inhibitors in preclinical models of lung fibrosis, published studies about the function, contribution and therapeutic correction of increased HDAC4 and -7 activity in fibrotic lung fibroblasts are yet based on single-gene silencing experiments and on the use of pan-HDAC inhibitors, as mentioned above. The effects of gene-targeting siRNAs for *HDAC4* and *HDAC7* are summarised in Table 3.

Table 3. Effects of Class IIA gene targeting siRNAs in fibrotic fibroblasts.

Study	Model	HDAC Inhibiton	Effect/Involved Molecules
Jones et al. (2019) [246]	TGF-β-treated primary IPF fibroblasts	*HDAC7* siRNA	*ACTA2* ↓ *CTGF* ↓ *NOX4* ↓ *HDAC2* ↓ *HDAC6* ↓ *HDAC8* ↓ *HDAC10* ↓ *HDAC9* ↑ Derepression of *PGC1A* expression
Guo et al. (2009) [250]	TGF-β-treated human normal lung fibroblasts	*HDAC4* siRNA	ACTA2 ↓ Inhibition of FMD, AKT phosphorylation ↓
Glenisson et al. (2007) [253]	TGF-β-treated primary normal skin fibroblasts (human)	*HDAC4* siRNA	ACTA2/α-SMA ↓ FMD ↓ Upregulation of TGIF1 and TGIF2 (= Inhibitors of TGF-β signalling)
Kang et al. (2018) [294]	TGF-β-treated fibroblasts isolated from PD plaque	*HDAC7* siRNA	Inhibition of SMAD2/3 activation, FMD ↓ ECM protein production ↓
Hua et al. (2021) [296]	Endothelin-treated human normal lung fibroblasts (WI-38)	*HDAC7* siRNA	Deacetylation of AP-1, AP-1 activity ↓ α-SMA ↓ CTGF ↓

Definition of abbreviations: IPF: idiopathic pulmonary fibrosis; ECM: extracellular matrix; FMD: fibroblast-to-myofibroblast differentiation; PD: Peyronie's disease; siRNA: small interfering RNA; ↑: upregulation; ↓: downregulation.

2.3. Class IIB Histone Deacetylases in IPF: Expression Profile, Function and Preclinical Studies

Immunohistochemical studies on IPF and normal control lung tissues revealed that both Class IIB HDAC enzymes HDAC6 and HDAC10 were found to be robustly upregulated in myofibroblasts within fibroblast foci in IPF. In contrast, expression of HDAC6 and -10 was absent in the interstitium of normal lungs. In accordance, immunoblot analyses of primary fibroblasts confirmed the upregulation of both Class IIB HDACs in IPF fibroblasts, and α-tubulin deacetylation, a surrogate marker for HDAC6 activity, was significantly increased in primary IPF versus normal lung fibroblasts [165]. Increased HDAC6 expression and consecutive α-tubulin-deacetylation have also been encountered in normal lung fibroblasts in response to TGF-β exposure [235], suggesting a crucial role of HDAC6 in TGF-β-dependent fibrogenesis. Other studies have shown that HDAC6 mediates TGF-β-induced EMT via SMAD3 activation in A549 cells, which was accompanied by α-tubulin-deacetylation and mesenchymal stress fibre formation [190,191,299]. Rapid HDAC6-dependent deacetylation of HSP90 was also observed, and a post-translational protein modification of HSP90 was reported to increase HSP90 chaperone function, which led to Notch1 activation during TGF-β-induced EMT [191]. Importantly, silencing of *HDAC6* by siRNA abrogated Notch1 signalling, decreased generation of EMT markers and restored expression of epithelial genes in TGF-β-treated A549 cells, indicating that HDAC6 was required for mediating the TGF-β–Notch1 signalling cascade during EMT [190,191]. Surprisingly, in fibrotic lung fibroblasts, siRNA-mediated silencing of *HDAC6* did not affect TGF-β-induced α-SMA and collagen-I expression. The same result was also observed for *HDAC10* silencing as well as for *HDAC6/HDAC10* double-knockdown [235]. These findings are interesting, as increased tubulin acetylation upon *HDAC6* silencing was observed, an indicator for successful HDAC6 inactivation. Thus, the cellular effects of its marked upregulation upon TGF-β in lung fibroblasts remain elusive and need further investigation. In addition, "HDAC6 gain of function" studies in human lung fibroblasts would help to clarify the role of overexpressed HDAC6 in IPF fibroblasts. This also applies to HDAC10, which has not yet been described much in lung fibrosis.

2.3.1. Peculiar Role of HDAC6 in IPF Epithelial Cells?

As a regulator of microtubule acetylation, HDAC6 is constitutively expressed in ciliated bronchial cells of normal lungs to regulate autophagy and mucociliary clearance [300]. In IPF, HDAC6 was found to be robustly upregulated in abnormal, hyperplastic bronchiolar structures, including airway basal cells (Figure 2) [165,174]. Subsequent loss-of-function studies revealed that HDAC6 appears to be responsible for the hyperproliferative phenotype of basal cells in IPF. It was thus suggested that overexpressed HDAC6 substantially governs the aberrant bronchiolization process in IPF [174].

Further, in contrast to all other HDAC enzymes, HDAC6 appeared to be the only HDAC expressed in IPF–AECII but not in the AECII of normal lungs (Figure 2) [165]. Because HDAC6 is involved in the aggresome formation and autophagic clearance of protein aggregates in response to increased misfolding (and impaired degradative capacity of the proteasome) [187], its induction in IPF–AECII was presumably caused by severe ER stress [18,20]. HDAC6 overexpression may represent an attempt of IPF–AECIIs to survive under conditions of irremediable ER stress but appear to be less able to counteract ER-stress-induced cell death. As described above, HDAC6 has also been widely reported as an eminent mediator of TGF-β-induced EMT in vitro, but AECIIs, as well as other epithelial cells, are not considered as cells giving rise to myofibroblasts in human IPF in vivo [40].

On the other hand, we could observe in our study that HDAC6 was also overexpressed in hyperplastic AEC cells without proSP-C expression (Figure 2) [165], which might suggest a role of HDAC6 in the differentiation of AECII to AECI or other AEC-like cells or to non-AEC epithelial cells. Interestingly, it has been reported very recently that human (but not murine) AECII transdifferentiate into metaplastic KRT5$^+$-expressing basal cells in response to fibrotic signalling in the lung mesenchyme in *h*AECII-derived organoids ex vivo and in *h*AECII xenotransplantation experiments with bleomycin-treated mice in vivo [301].

Although speculative, the upregulation of HDAC6 in AEC, as well as bronchiolar basal cells in IPF lungs versus normal lungs, could suggest an involvement of this HDAC enzyme in the reprogramming of hAECII towards metaplastic basal cells, which have been widely observed to colonise alveolar spaces in close proximity to AECII in IPF [52,118,302]. The crucial involvement of HDAC6 in Notch1 pathway activation and transformation of epithelial cells supports this speculation.

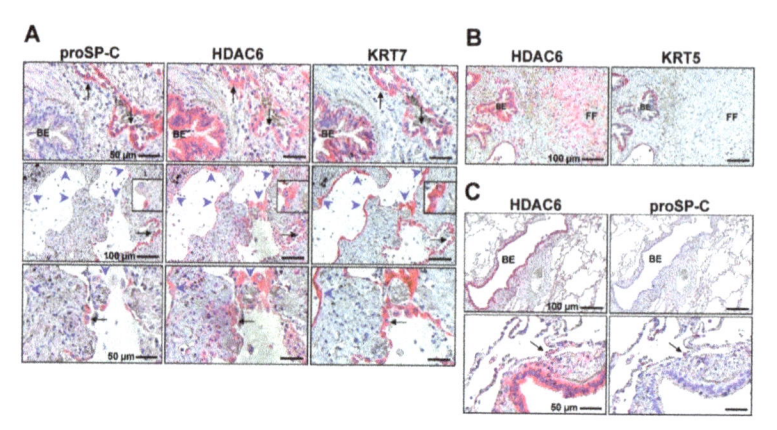

Figure 2. Expression and localisation of HDAC6 in IPF lungs and normal control lungs. (**A**) Representative immunohistochemistry (IHC) for proSP-C (AECII marker), HDAC6 and cytokeratin-7 (KRT7, marker for simple epithelia) in IPF lungs. Robust expression of HDAC6 was observed in AECII (proSP-C$^+$ KRT7$^+$, indicated by arrows) as well as hyperplastic AEC-like cells lining the alveoli (proSP-C$^-$ KRT7$^+$, indicated by blue arrowheads) and in bronchial epithelium (BE). (**B**) Robust expression of HDAC6 in fibroblast foci (FF) as well as KRT5$^+$ bronchiolar basal cells and ciliated bronchial cells. (**C**) Representative IHC for proSP-C and HDAC6 in normal control lungs. HDAC6 was expressed in ciliated bronchial epithelium but not in AECII or normal lungs. Faint HDAC6 immunostaining was observed in the interstitium of normal lungs. Taken with permission from the study by Korfei et al. (2015) [165] (supplement), with modifications.

2.3.2. HDAC6 Selective Inhibitors in Preclinical Models of Lung Fibrosis

In contrast to all other Class II HDACs, isoform-selective inhibitors have been developed for HDAC6 and not only evaluated in cancer but also lung fibrosis (Table 4) [174,190,191,235]. Similar to silencing of *HDAC6*, pharmacological inhibition of HDAC6 deacetylase acitivity by the small molecule inhibitor tubacin resulted in the abrogation of TGF-β-induced Notch1 signalling and EMT in A549 cells [190,191]. However, studies with tubacin were not undertaken in TGF-β-stimulated lung fibroblasts but with the other selective HDAC6-inhibitor tubastatin. In contrast to genetic knockdown of *HDAC6*, tubastatin was shown to lead to α-tubulin hyperacetylation (and thus successful HDAC6 inhibition) and to repress TGF-β-induced expression of type-I collagen (*COL1A1*) in lung fibroblasts by inducing AKT dephosphorylation at Ser43 through increasing the association of AKT with the specific phosphatase PHLPP (PH domain and leucine-rich repeat protein phosphatase), with consequent AKT inactivation [235]. In addition, the expression of downstream targets of the PI3K-AKT pathway, such as HIF-1α and VEGF, was repressed by tubastatin. In contrast, TGF-β activated SMAD2/3 signalling as well as p38MAPK and ERK pathways were not affected by tubastatin. Further results of this study indicated the significant amelioration of bleomycin-induced lung fibrosis in mice in vivo by tubastatin treatment [235].

Table 4. Class IIB isoform-selective inhibitors for treatment of pulmonary fibrosis.

Study	Lung Fibrosis Model	HDAC Inhibition	Effect/Involved Molecules
Campiani et al. (2021) [174]	Organoid cultures derived from IPF basal cells, Ex vivo human lung model of fibrosis	"Compound 6h" HDAC6	Basal cell proliferation ↓ Bronchosphere formation ↓ Tubulin acetylation ↑ TGF-β dependent ECM synthesis ↓
Shan et al. (2008) [190]	TGF-β-stimulated A549 cells	Tubacin HDAC6 HDAC6 siRNA	Tubulin-hyperacetylation, restoration of E-cadherin, SMAD3 phosphorylation ↓ PAI1 ↓ COL1A1 ↓ inhibition of EMT
Deskin et al. (2016) [191]	TGF-β-stimulated A549 cells	Tubacin HDAC6 HDAC6 siRNA	Abrogation of TGF-β induced Notch1 signalling (HEY1, HES1 ↓) Acetylation of HSP90 (Ac-K294) p38 pathway ↓
Saito et al. (2017) [235]	TGF-β-stimulated human normal lung fibroblasts, Bleomycin mouse model	Tubastatin A HDAC6	In vitro and in vivo: Tubulin hyperacetylation, inhibition of PI3K-AKT pathway, FMD ↓ ECM ↓ amelioration of lung fibrosis

Definition of abbreviations: IPF: idiopathic pulmonary fibrosis; EMT: epithelial–mesenchymal transition; ECM: extracellular matrix; FMD: fibroblast-to-myofibroblast differentiation; siRNA: small interfering RNA; ↑: upregulation; ↓: downregulation.

However, homozygous $Hdac6^{(-/-)}$ knockout mice were not protected against bleomycin-induced lung fibrosis despite pronounced hyperacetylation of α-tubulin. Similarly, TGF-β-induced collagen expression was not decreased in murine lung fibroblasts isolated from $Hdac6^{(-/-)}$ knockout mice compared to TGF-β-stimulated normal fibroblasts from wild-type mice. As mentioned above, RNAi-mediated knockout of HDAC6 in human lung fibroblasts did also not repress TGF-β-induced collagen expression. Together, these results suggested that tubastatin might have ameliorated bleomycin-induced lung fibrosis by targeting the PI3K-AKT pathway, likely through an HDAC6-independent mechanism, and that tubastatin might have significant off-target effects aside from HDAC6 [235]. On the other hand, besides its protein deacetylase activity, HDAC6 has also been reported to exhibit a significant ubiquitin-binding capability and sequester ubiquitylated protein aggregates into autophagosomes or aggresomes [187]. Thus, the authors of this very interesting study also suggested that, simply, the loss or inhibition of HDAC6's deacetylating function attenuated bleomycin-induced lung fibrosis by hyperacetylating target proteins, whereas in $Hdac6^{(-/-)}$ knockout mice, the additional loss of HDAC6 function to transport cytotoxic polyubiquitinated (misfolded) proteins into autophagosomes for their degradation, may aggravate bleomycin-induced lung fibrosis by causing defective autophagy [235].

Very recently, novel specific inhibitors for human HDAC6 enzyme have been developed as promising pharmaceutical tools for the treatment of IPF, with the aim of also investigating the role of HDAC6 in the abnormal bronchiolization process in IPF, as this enzyme isoform was found to be robustly overexpressed in bronchiolar basal cells of IPF lungs [174]. It could be shown that the newly developed, specific HDAC6 inhibitor "compound 6h" reduced basal cell proliferation and bronchosphere formation in 3D organoid cultures derived from airway basal cells of IPF patients. In addition, compound 6h significantly inhibited TGF-β dependent fibrogenesis in cultured human lung tissues ex vivo, as shown by diminished expression of ECM genes *ACTA2*, *COL1A1*, *COL3A1* and *FN*. The authors of this study concluded that HDAC6 confers the pronounced hyperproliferative and profibrotic effects to bronchiolar basal cells in IPF, thereby underscoring that inhibition of HDAC6's deacetylating function plays an important role in the treatment of IPF [174]. However, the effects of "compound 6h" on various non-canonical pathways activated by TGF-β were not evaluated in this study.

Taken together, HDAC6 deacetylase activity appears to mediate profibrotic responses and signalling through non-histone protein deacetylation, leading to altered cellular signalling, presumably involving HSP90 chaperone (a substrate of HDAC6)-mediated signalling and sustained AKT activation, which can be blocked by HDAC6 selective inhibitors. The selectivity of tubastatin to inhibit HDAC6 deacetylase activity should be re-checked.

3. Discussion of HDAC Inhibitors as Therapeutic Option for IPF

The summarised data provides evidence that abnormally increased HDAC activity in lung fibroblasts and bronchiolar basal cells versus a lack of HDAC activity in AECII is critical in the pathogenesis of lung fibrosis, which can be overcome by treatment with HDAC inhibitors. In particular, compelling evidence reveals a favourable therapeutic efficacy of pan-HDAC inhibitors in preclinical models of lung fibrosis (Table 1). Pan-HDAC inhibition through panobinostat inhibited FMD by reducing numerous ECM- and anti-apoptosis-related genes in IPF fibroblasts, while epigenetically repressed antifibrotic genes were restored by this drug. These beneficial effects were mediated largely through chromatin hyperacetylation and mechanisms involving non-histone protein acetylation and abrogation of p-STAT3 signalling [162,165,247,249]. In addition to the inactivation of Class I HDAC activity, panobinostat strongly inhibited HDAC6 activity (and also, therefore, with high probability, its profibrotic signalling) in IPF fibroblasts [249], which is in accordance with studies of its marvellous efficacy in various cancers [303]. Panobinostat also induced ER stress and proapoptotic signalling and thus led to the efficient inactivation of IPF fibroblasts [165]. Therefore, it is not surprising that a head-to-head comparison of the therapeutic effects of panobinostat versus the IPF drug pirfenidone has demonstrated the superior functionality of this pan-HDAC inhibitor over pirfenidone in acting against IPF-derived fibroblasts [249].

By employing an image-based screening assay with the use of α-SMA immunofluorescence intensity as the primary readout parameter of in vitro fibroblast activation (induced by TGF-β), Jones and coworkers (2019) tested and rank-ordered 99 modulators of epigenetic-regulating enzymes and identified the pan-HDAC inhibitor pracrinostat as the most effective small molecule in downregulating TGF-β-induced α-SMA expression [246]. Interestingly, panobinostat and SAHA were not included in this screening, but the first-discovered pan-HDAC inhibitor TSA (which is structurally related to SAHA) was evaluated and was 11th among the 99 compounds tested. Subsequent validation of pracrinostat revealed that it attenuated FMD through the derepression of the antifibrotic gene *PGC1A* and the suppression of various cytokine and ECM genes in TGF-β-stimulated IPF fibroblasts, which was, in part, attributed to the abrogation of HDAC7-mediated TGF-β signalling [246]. However, despite their beneficial effects on IPF fibroblasts, panobinostat and pracrinostat have yet not been evaluated in animal models of lung fibrosis in vivo. Additionally, two studies demonstrated the amelioration of pulmonary fibrosis and improved lung function in response to global HDAC inhibition by SAHA in bleomycin-treated C57Bl/6 mice in vivo [164,167]. The lung histopathology and health status of saline-treated control mice were not affected by SAHA [164]. SAHA was also shown to significantly attenuate paraquat-induced lung fibrosis in rats [252]. These findings indicate that hydroxamic-acid-based pan-HDAC inhibitors are well tolerated under conditions of lung fibrosis in vivo.

In IPF fibroblasts in vitro, SAHA suppressed genes associated with ECM and anti-apoptosis and upregulated proapoptotic genes through the modulation of chromatin acetylation and specific histone modifications associated with such genes and induced significant apoptosis in these cells [164,167]. In contrast, cell death was much less in normal control fibroblasts treated with SAHA [164]. This was similar to previously published studies showing that SAHA selectively induced malignant/tumour cells to undergo apoptosis but not normal cells [304]. This effect is important for the therapeutic efficacy of SAHA and tolerability in human patients. As mentioned in this article, panobinostat, pracrinostat and SAHA are FDA-approved drugs for cancer treatment but not the first-described pan-HDAC inhibitor TSA. Anyway, TSA was also shown in two studies to reduce the evolution of lung fibrosis in bleomycin-treated rodents [168,251]. In fibrotic fibroblasts, it derepressed *FAS* expression [163] and abrogated TGF-β-induced AKT phosphorylation with consequent suppression of *ACTA2* and *COL1A1* expression [250].

As outlined in Section 2.1., some Class I-specific HDAC inhibitors, in particular the FDA-approved drugs VPA and romidepsin, also indicated a significant therapeutic effect in preclinical models of lung fibrosis in vitro and in vivo (Table 2), suggesting that targeting Class I HDACs is effective enough to abolish lung fibrosis. In support of this notion, HDAC1, -2 and -3 contribute to fibroblast anti-apoptosis through p53 inactivation as well as through epigenetic repression of proapoptotic genes via chromatin remodelling [163]. Further, Class I HDACs contribute to profibrotic signalling through the epigenetic silencing of antifibrotic genes [162,247] and through their involvement in various fibrotic signalling pathways, including SMAD2/3 (HDAC1) [252], PI3K (HDAC3) [265], ERK (HDAC3) [265], and JAK2/p-STAT3 (HDAC1, -2, -3) [249,262–264]. Moreover, Class I HDAC inhibitors, including the anti-epileptic drug VPA, have been shown to enhance fibrinolytic capacity. Although not shown in the setting of lung fibrosis, VPA was demonstrated to upregulate the expression of tissue plasminogen activator (t-PA/*PLAT*) in the vasculature of mice and men while downregulating PAI-1 [305,306]. The stimulatory effect of VPA on t-PA expression was associated with increased acetylation at the *PLAT* promoter [307]. VPA also reduced fibrin deposition and thrombus formation in mice after mechanical vessel injury but was not associated with an increased risk of bleeding [305]. In human patients with coronary disease, VPA increased the capacity for endogenous t-PA release and decreased plasma PAI-1 antigen [308]. Considering these studies and the reported antifibrotic effects of VPA on lung fibrosis in vitro and in vivo (Table 2) and the fact that fibrinolytic activity is impaired in lung fibrosis, VPA could also exert beneficial therapeutic effects in patients with IPF. This also applies to romidepsin, as it demonstrated significant inhibition of fibrosis development in the mouse model of bleomycin-induced lung fibrosis and as it revealed anti-fibrotic effects in vitro and in vivo at low nanomolar concentrations [169].

Recently, a novel clinical-stage HDAC inhibitor, CG-745, specific for Class I HDACs and Class IIB HDAC6, revealed favourable therapeutic efficacy in bleomycin-treated mice as it significantly reduced inflammatory cell populations in BALF and lowered the collagen contents back to the levels of the control saline group. Interestingly, CG-745 also efficiently attenuated severe lung fibrosis in mice induced by polyhexamethylene guanidine (PHMG) [233].

However, in vitro and experimental studies for lung fibrosis/IPF described in this review were mainly restricted to the assessment of inflammation status and fibroblast/myofibroblast apoptosis, but not on the effects of HDAC inhibitors on AECII injury/AECII death and the aberrant bronchiolar re-epithelialization process. Although nearly all Class I and Class II HDAC enzymes appeared to be actually absent in differentiated proSP-C$^+$ IPF-AECII but abnormally upregulated in KRT5$^+$ bronchiolar basal cells [165], it can be speculated that hyperplastic dedifferentiated AEC-like cells without proSP-C expression, as recently described as transitional KRT8^{+high} progenitors in fibrotic lungs [301,309,310], might overexpress HDAC enzymes for their terminal differentiation into KRT5$^+$ basal cells. Interestingly, the administration of pan-HDAC inhibitors did not exert "deleterious" effects on fibrotic AECII in various rodent models of lung fibrosis but changed their abnormal phenotype. In the mouse model of bleomycin-induced lung fibrosis, Ota and coworkers (2015) showed that administration of the pan-HDAC inhibitor TSA from day 7 to 21 after bleomycin instillation restored *Sftpc* expression in FACS-isolated AECII in vivo [168]. Thus, although pan-HDAC inhibitors were shown to reduce lung fibrosis through the induction of significant myofibroblast apoptosis in bleomycin-treated mice, they appeared to reverse the aberrant hyperplastic (cytokine-releasing) phenotype of fibrotic AECII as well as to spare injured pro-apoptotic AECII from further apoptosis [164,168], thereby targeting two different AECII states in the fibrotic lung to promote proSP-C$^+$ AECII re-differentiation, proSP-C$^+$ AECII survival and proper re-epithelialization of the damaged alveolar epithelium as a therapeutic strategy. In renal fibrosis, it could be demonstrated in the murine model of unilateral ureteral obstruction that TSA led simultaneously to the inactivation of renal interstitial fibroblasts and the inhibition of renal tubular epithelial cell death [311]. However, the supposably beneficial effects of pan-HDAC inhibitors on AECII injury in experimental models of lung fibrosis as well as IPF *per se* are still underexplored.

Interestingly, a recent in vitro study showed that the weak pan-HDAC inhibitor 4-phenyl-butyrate (4-PBA) alleviated the aggregation and improved the secretion of IPF-associated mutant SP-A2 proteins in A549 cells through the upregulation of glucose-regulated protein (GRP)78 [255]. 4-PBA is an FDA-approved drug for the treatment of urea cycle disorders, and it is also well-known as a chemical chaperone exerting the proper folding of malfolded (mutant) proteins and the suppression of protein aggregation [224]. The study above suggests that the chaperone-like activity of 4-PBA may be (in part) mediated by its HDAC-inhibitor-function to upregulate genes involved in protein folding, but this remains to be elucidated. 4-PBA also attenuated bleomycin-induced lung fibrosis in rodents through the suppression of oxidative stress, NFκB activation and ER stress-mediated EMT induced by bleomycin [254,256] (Table 1).

However, the clinical use of pan-HDAC inhibitors in cancer patients has been, in part, associated with several challenges and side effects in some patients [312–314] that might be due to their broad activity across numerous HDAC isoforms and, thus, the concurrent inactivation of multiple HDAC family members, including their individual signalling. Significant side effects were also, in part, observed with romidepsin, suggesting that strong inhibition of more than one Class I isoform may be harmful to general cellular metabolism. On the other side, reports from clinical trials for NSCLC (non-small lung cancer) revealed that romidepsin and pan-HDAC inhibitors were well tolerated in patients [315]. Hence, the side effects are probably different depending on the genetic background as well as on the age of the patient. It might also be possible that lower doses of Class I/pan-HDAC inhibitors will be required in an IPF application compared to cancer.

The discussions about the side effects and improvement of therapeutic strategies have led to the development of HDAC isoform-selective inhibitors to overcome undesired effects [316]. Until now, most of the agents developed have selectivity for HDAC3, HDAC6 and HDAC8 and have been or are still currently evaluated in preclinical studies for cancer and lung fibrosis [171,189,234–238,258]. However, numerous HDACs have the very same targets. For example, HDACs 1, -2, -3 and -4 are well-known to be involved in the repression of $CIP1^{p21}$ expression, and the knockdown of each of these HDACs resulted in the derepression of $CIP1^{p21}$ expression. However, in each case, the magnitude of $CIP1^{p21}$ induction was markedly less than that induced by pan-HDAC inhibitors [198]. In agreement, some studies clearly indicated that the magnitude of growth inhibition and apoptosis induced upon selective HDAC3 inhibition in tumour cells was relatively modest compared to the effects induced by Class I or pan-HDAC inhibitors [317,318]. On the other hand, selective inhibition of HDAC3, HDAC6 or HDAC8 has recently been demonstrated to exert remarkable therapeutic effects in the bleomycin mouse model of lung fibrosis [171,235,258]. However, the integrity of isoform-selective inhibitors mentioned above is not yet evidently proven, and these still could have off-target effects on many cellular pathways. Further, the novel HDAC6 selective inhibitor "compound 6h" [174] remains to be evaluated in experimental fibrosis.

Taken together, it can be suggested that specific inhibition of single HDACs may yield some therapeutic benefit, whereas the use of pan-HDAC inhibitors is likely to yield a stronger therapeutic response. In conclusion, the published findings summarised in this review indicate that HDACs offer novel molecular targets for IPF therapy and that FDA-approved Class I and pan-HDAC inhibitors for cancer treatment may also be promising therapeutic agents for the treatment of IPF. The putative antifibrotic effects of HDAC-inhibitor treatment on IPF are illustrated in Figure 3.

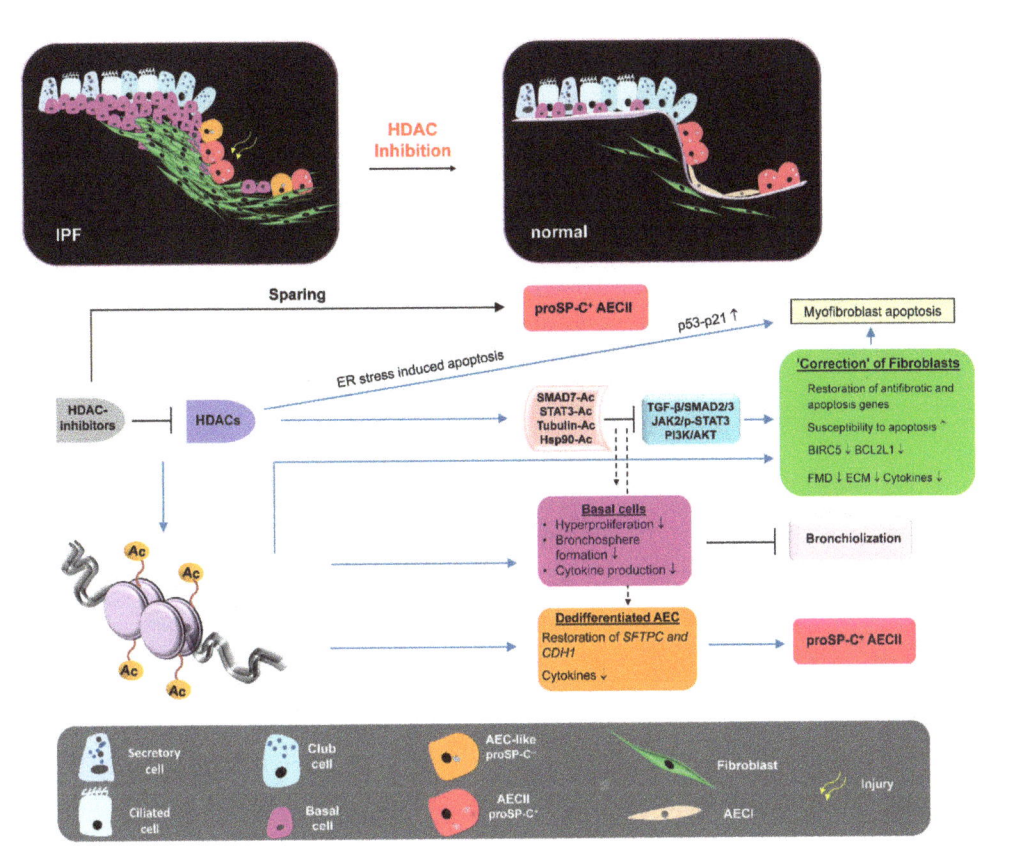

Figure 3. Summary of putative therapeutic effects of HDAC-inhibitor treatment on IPF. For details, see discussion. <u>Abbreviations</u>: IPF: idiopathic pulmonary fibrosis; ECM: extracellular matrix; FMD: fibroblast-to-myofibroblast differentiation; AECI/II: type-I/-II alveolar epithelial cell; Ac = acetylation; ↑: upregulation; ↓: downregulation.

4. Conclusions and Future Perspectives

Idiopathic pulmonary fibrosis is associated with a progressive loss of lung function and a poor prognosis. Loss of AECII, myofibroblast expansion and the ectopic appearance of basal cells in the alveoli are the hallmarks of IPF. The number of myofibroblast foci, as well as the extent of alveolar KRT5+ basal cells, directly correlate with mortality in IPF [175,319]. Approved antifibrotic drugs, nintedanib and pirfenidone, modify disease progression, but IPF remains incurable, and there is an urgent need for new therapies. The majority of the evidence generated to date indicates that the overexpression of Class I and Class II HDACs is associated with fibroblast proliferation and FMD, as well as accounts for the apoptosis-resistant, invasive phenotype of fibroblasts/myofibroblasts and bronchiolar basal cells in IPF. Consistent with such a role, preclinical studies have shown that various Class I and pan-HDAC inhibitors not only reduced profibrotic signalling and ECM production but also stimulated growth arrest and cell death through the p53-p21 pathway and/or ER stress-induced apoptosis in fibrotic fibroblasts/myofibroblasts [164,165,169,271], a prerequisite for resolution of organ fibrosis, while AECII in fibrotic lungs were apparently spared from HDAC-inhibitor-induced apoptosis. Despite the proven antifibrotic efficacy of FDA-approved HDAC inhibitors in preclinical models, none of them have been approved for fibrotic diseases yet but could be readily progressed into an IPF clinical trial.

We believe that pan-HDAC inhibitors can not only reverse the aberrant epigenetic response in (myo)fibroblasts and bronchiolar basal cells in IPF but also the activated senescent phenotype in the AECII of IPF lungs despite pro-apoptotic events and a lack of many HDACs in IPF–AECII. The mechanisms of HDAC inhibitors towards the injured alveolar epithelium (including the aberrant epithelial repair mechanisms) in IPF have not yet been addressed and should be elucidated in future studies.

Author Contributions: M.K. wrote and revised the manuscript. P.M. helped with the revision of the article and produced figures/artwork. A.G. revised, edited and corrected the manuscript. All authors have read and agreed to the published version of the manuscript.

Funding: This work has been supported by grants of the German Ministry of Science and Education ["German Center for Lung Research (DZL)"], and by a grant funded by the European Joint Programme on Rare Diseases (EJP RD), administrated by the German Research Council (DFG, GU 405/16-1), with the title: "Raising diagnostic accuracy and therapeutic perspectives in interstitial lung diseases (RARE-ILD)".

Institutional Review Board Statement: All data are extracted and summarized from published studies, please refer to the original publications.

Informed Consent Statement: Informed consent was obtained from all subjects involved in the study.

Data Availability Statement: Not applicable.

Conflicts of Interest: The authors declare no conflict of interest.

References

1. Raghu, G.; Collard, H.R.; Egan, J.J.; Martinez, F.J.; Behr, J.; Brown, K.K.; Colby, T.V.; Cordier, J.F.; Flaherty, K.R.; Lasky, J.A.; et al. An official ATS/ERS/JRS/ALAT statement: Idiopathic pulmonary fibrosis: Evidence-based guidelines for diagnosis and management. *Am. J. Respir. Crit. Care Med.* **2011**, *183*, 788–824. [PubMed]
2. Raghu, G.; Weycker, D.; Edelsberg, J.; Bradford, W.Z.; Oster, G. Incidence and prevalence of idiopathic pulmonary fibrosis. *Am. J. Respir. Crit. Care Med.* **2006**, *174*, 810–816. [CrossRef] [PubMed]
3. Noble, P.W.; Albera, C.; Bradford, W.Z.; Costabel, U.; Glassberg, M.K.; Kardatzke, D.; King, T.E., Jr.; Lancaster, L.; Sahn, S.A.; Szwarcberg, J.; et al. Pirfenidone in patients with idiopathic pulmonary fibrosis (CAPACITY): Two randomised trials. *Lancet* **2011**, *377*, 1760–1769. [CrossRef]
4. Richeldi, L.; du Bois, R.M.; Raghu, G.; Azuma, A.; Brown, K.K.; Costabel, U.; Cottin, V.; Flaherty, K.R.; Hansell, D.M.; Inoue, Y.; et al. Efficacy and safety of nintedanib in idiopathic pulmonary fibrosis. *N. Engl. J. Med.* **2014**, *370*, 2071–2082. [CrossRef]
5. Cerri, S.; Monari, M.; Guerrieri, A.; Donatelli, P.; Bassi, I.; Garuti, M.; Luppi, F.; Betti, S.; Bandelli, G.; Carpano, M.; et al. Real-life comparison of pirfenidone and nintedanib in patients with idiopathic pulmonary fibrosis: A 24-month assessment. *Respir. Med.* **2019**, *159*, 105803. [CrossRef]
6. Richeldi, L.; Collard, H.R.; Jones, M.G. Idiopathic pulmonary fibrosis. *Lancet* **2017**, *389*, 1941–1952.
7. Selman, M.; Pardo, A. Revealing the pathogenic and aging-related mechanisms of the enigmatic idiopathic pulmonary fibrosis. an integral model. *Am. J. Respir. Crit. Care Med.* **2014**, *189*, 1161–1172. [CrossRef]
8. Selman, M.; Pardo, A. The leading role of epithelial cells in the pathogenesis of idiopathic pulmonary fibrosis. *Cell Signal.* **2020**, *66*, 109482.
9. Hinz, B.; Phan, S.H.; Thannickal, V.J.; Prunotto, M.; Desmouliere, A.; Varga, J.; De Wever, O.; Mareel, M.; Gabbiani, G. Recent developments in myofibroblast biology: Paradigms for connective tissue remodeling. *Am. J. Pathol.* **2012**, *180*, 1340–1355. [CrossRef]
10. Chilosi, M.; Poletti, V.; Murer, B.; Lestani, M.; Cancellieri, A.; Montagna, L.; Piccoli, P.; Cangi, G.; Semenzato, G.; Doglioni, C. Abnormal re-epithelialization and lung remodeling in idiopathic pulmonary fibrosis: The role of deltaN-p63. *Lab. Investig.* **2002**, *82*, 1335–1345. [CrossRef]
11. Plantier, L.; Crestani, B.; Wert, S.E.; Dehoux, M.; Zweytick, B.; Guenther, A.; Whitsett, J.A. Ectopic respiratory epithelial cell differentiation in bronchiolised distal airspaces in idiopathic pulmonary fibrosis. *Thorax* **2011**, *66*, 651–657. [CrossRef]
12. Zuo, W.L.; Rostami, M.R.; LeBlanc, M.; Kaner, R.J.; O'Beirne, S.L.; Mezey, J.G.; Leopold, P.L.; Quast, K.; Visvanathan, S.; Fine, J.S.; et al. Dysregulation of club cell biology in idiopathic pulmonary fibrosis. *PLoS ONE* **2020**, *15*, e0237529. [CrossRef]
13. Chilosi, M.; Zamo, A.; Doglioni, C.; Reghellin, D.; Lestani, M.; Montagna, L.; Pedron, S.; Ennas, M.G.; Cancellieri, A.; Murer, B.; et al. Migratory marker expression in fibroblast foci of idiopathic pulmonary fibrosis. *Respir. Res.* **2006**, *7*, 95. [CrossRef]
14. Myers, J.L.; Katzenstein, A.L. Epithelial necrosis and alveolar collapse in the pathogenesis of usual interstitial pneumonia. *Chest* **1988**, *94*, 1309–1311.
15. Uhal, B.D.; Joshi, I.; Hughes, W.F.; Ramos, C.; Pardo, A.; Selman, M. Alveolar epithelial cell death adjacent to underlying myofibroblasts in advanced fibrotic human lung. *Am. J. Physiol.* **1998**, *275*, L1192–L1199.

16. Barbas-Filho, J.V.; Ferreira, M.A.; Sesso, A.; Kairalla, R.A.; Carvalho, C.R.; Capelozzi, V.L. Evidence of type II pneumocyte apoptosis in the pathogenesis of idiopathic pulmonary fibrosis (IFP)/usual interstitial pneumonia (UIP). *J. Clin. Pathol.* **2001**, *54*, 132–138. [CrossRef]
17. Kuwano, K.; Kunitake, R.; Kawasaki, M.; Nomoto, Y.; Hagimoto, N.; Nakanishi, Y.; Hara, N. P21Waf1/Cip1/Sdi1 and p53 expression in association with DNA strand breaks in idiopathic pulmonary fibrosis. *Am. J. Respir. Crit. Care Med.* **1996**, *154 (2 Pt 1)*, 477–483. [CrossRef]
18. Korfei, M.; Ruppert, C.; Mahavadi, P.; Henneke, I.; Markart, P.; Koch, M.; Lang, G.; Fink, L.; Bohle, R.M.; Seeger, W.; et al. Epithelial endoplasmic reticulum stress and apoptosis in sporadic idiopathic pulmonary fibrosis. *Am. J. Respir. Crit. Care Med.* **2008**, *178*, 838–846. [CrossRef]
19. Lawson, W.E.; Crossno, P.F.; Polosukhin, V.V.; Roldan, J.; Cheng, D.S.; Lane, K.B.; Blackwell, T.R.; Xu, C.; Markin, C.; Ware, L.B.; et al. Endoplasmic reticulum stress in alveolar epithelial cells is prominent in IPF: Association with altered surfactant protein processing and herpesvirus infection. *Am. J. Physiol. Lung Cell Mol. Physiol.* **2008**, *294*, L1119–L1126. [CrossRef]
20. Cha, S.I.; Ryerson, C.J.; Lee, J.S.; Kukreja, J.; Barry, S.S.; Jones, K.D.; Elicker, B.M.; Kim, D.S.; Papa, F.R.; Collard, H.R.; et al. Cleaved cytokeratin-18 is a mechanistically informative biomarker in idiopathic pulmonary fibrosis. *Respir. Res.* **2012**, *13*, 105. [CrossRef]
21. Klymenko, O.; Huehn, M.; Wilhelm, J.; Wasnick, R.; Shalashova, I.; Ruppert, C.; Henneke, I.; Hezel, S.; Guenther, K.; Mahavadi, P.; et al. Regulation and role of the ER stress transcription factor CHOP in alveolar epithelial type-II cells. *J. Mol. Med.* **2019**, *97*, 973–990. [PubMed]
22. Thomas, A.Q.; Lane, K.; Phillips, J., 3rd; Prince, M.; Markin, C.; Speer, M.; Schwartz, D.A.; Gaddipati, R.; Marney, A.; Johnson, J.; et al. Heterozygosity for a surfactant protein C gene mutation associated with usual interstitial pneumonitis and cellular nonspecific interstitial pneumonitis in one kindred. *Am. J. Respir. Crit. Care Med.* **2002**, *165*, 1322–1328. [PubMed]
23. Mulugeta, S.; Nguyen, V.; Russo, S.J.; Muniswamy, M.; Beers, M.F. A surfactant protein C precursor protein BRICHOS domain mutation causes endoplasmic reticulum stress, proteasome dysfunction, and caspase 3 activation. *Am. J. Respir. Cell Mol. Biol.* **2005**, *32*, 521–530. [PubMed]
24. Wang, Y.; Kuan, P.J.; Xing, C.; Cronkhite, J.T.; Torres, F.; Rosenblatt, R.L.; DiMaio, J.M.; Kinch, L.N.; Grishin, N.V.; Garcia, C.K. Genetic defects in surfactant protein A2 are associated with pulmonary fibrosis and lung cancer. *Am. J. Hum. Genet.* **2009**, *84*, 52–59.
25. Maitra, M.; Wang, Y.; Gerard, R.D.; Mendelson, C.R.; Garcia, C.K. Surfactant protein A2 mutations associated with pulmonary fibrosis lead to protein instability and endoplasmic reticulum stress. *J. Biol. Chem.* **2010**, *285*, 22103–22113. [CrossRef]
26. Katzen, J.; Wagner, B.D.; Venosa, A.; Kopp, M.; Tomer, Y.; Russo, S.J.; Headen, A.C.; Basil, M.C.; Stark, J.M.; Mulugeta, S.; et al. An SFTPC BRICHOS mutant links epithelial ER stress and spontaneous lung fibrosis. *JCI Insight* **2019**, *4*, e126125. [CrossRef]
27. Armanios, M.Y.; Chen, J.J.; Cogan, J.D.; Alder, J.K.; Ingersoll, R.G.; Markin, C.; Lawson, W.E.; Xie, M.; Vulto, I.; Phillips, J.A., 3rd; et al. Telomerase mutations in families with idiopathic pulmonary fibrosis. *N. Engl. J. Med.* **2007**, *356*, 1317–1326.
28. Tsakiri, K.D.; Cronkhite, J.T.; Kuan, P.J.; Xing, C.; Raghu, G.; Weissler, J.C.; Rosenblatt, R.L.; Shay, J.W.; Garcia, C.K. Adult-onset pulmonary fibrosis caused by mutations in telomerase. *Proc. Natl. Acad. Sci. USA* **2007**, *104*, 7552–7557. [CrossRef]
29. Kropski, J.A.; Mitchell, D.B.; Markin, C.; Polosukhin, V.V.; Choi, L.; Johnson, J.E.; Lawson, W.E.; Phillips, J.A., 3rd; Cogan, J.D.; Blackwell, T.S.; et al. A novel dyskerin (DKC1) mutation is associated with familial interstitial pneumonia. *Chest* **2014**, *146*, e1–e7.
30. Fukuhara, A.; Tanino, Y.; Ishii, T.; Inokoshi, Y.; Saito, K.; Fukuhara, N.; Sato, S.; Saito, J.; Ishida, T.; Yamaguchi, H.; et al. Pulmonary fibrosis in dyskeratosis congenita with TINF2 gene mutation. *Eur. Respir. J.* **2013**, *42*, 1757–1759.
31. Stuart, B.D.; Choi, J.; Zaidi, S.; Xing, C.; Holohan, B.; Chen, R.; Choi, M.; Dharwadkar, P.; Torres, F.; Girod, C.E.; et al. Exome sequencing links mutations in PARN and RTEL1 with familial pulmonary fibrosis and telomere shortening. *Nat. Genet.* **2015**, *47*, 512–517. [CrossRef]
32. Naikawadi, R.P.; Disayabutr, S.; Mallavia, B.; Donne, M.L.; Green, G.; La, J.L.; Rock, J.R.; Looney, M.R.; Wolters, P.J. Telomere dysfunction in alveolar epithelial cells causes lung remodeling and fibrosis. *JCI Insight* **2016**, *1*, e86704. [CrossRef]
33. Kropski, J.A.; Lawson, W.E.; Young, L.R.; Blackwell, T.S. Genetic studies provide clues on the pathogenesis of idiopathic pulmonary fibrosis. *Dis. Model. Mech.* **2013**, *6*, 9–17. [CrossRef]
34. Courtwright, A.M.; El-Chemaly, S. Telomeres in Interstitial Lung Disease: The Short and the Long of It. *Ann. Am. Thorac. Soc.* **2019**, *16*, 175–181. [CrossRef]
35. Seibold, M.A.; Wise, A.L.; Speer, M.C.; Steele, M.P.; Brown, K.K.; Loyd, J.E.; Fingerlin, T.E.; Zhang, W.; Gudmundsson, G.; Groshong, S.D.; et al. A common MUC5B promoter polymorphism and pulmonary fibrosis. *N. Engl. J. Med.* **2011**, *364*, 1503–1512. [CrossRef]
36. Noth, I.; Zhang, Y.; Ma, S.F.; Flores, C.; Barber, M.; Huang, Y.; Broderick, S.M.; Wade, M.S.; Hysi, P.; Scuirba, J.; et al. Genetic variants associated with idiopathic pulmonary fibrosis susceptibility and mortality: A genome-wide association study. *Lancet Respir. Med.* **2013**, *1*, 309–317. [CrossRef]
37. Evans, C.M.; Fingerlin, T.E.; Schwarz, M.I.; Lynch, D.; Kurche, J.; Warg, L.; Yang, I.V.; Schwartz, D.A. Idiopathic Pulmonary Fibrosis: A Genetic Disease That Involves Mucociliary Dysfunction of the Peripheral Airways. *Physiol. Rev.* **2016**, *96*, 1567–1591. [CrossRef]

38. Hancock, L.A.; Hennessy, C.E.; Solomon, G.M.; Dobrinskikh, E.; Estrella, A.; Hara, N.; Hill, D.B.; Kissner, W.J.; Markovetz, M.R.; Grove Villalon, D.E.; et al. Muc5b overexpression causes mucociliary dysfunction and enhances lung fibrosis in mice. *Nat. Commun.* **2018**, *9*, 5363. [CrossRef]
39. Parimon, T.; Yao, C.; Stripp, B.R.; Noble, P.W.; Chen, P. Alveolar Epithelial Type II Cells as Drivers of Lung Fibrosis in Idiopathic Pulmonary Fibrosis. *Int. J. Mol. Sci.* **2020**, *21*, 2269.
40. Rock, J.R.; Barkauskas, C.E.; Cronce, M.J.; Xue, Y.; Harris, J.R.; Liang, J.; Noble, P.W.; Hogan, B.L. Multiple stromal populations contribute to pulmonary fibrosis without evidence for epithelial to mesenchymal transition. *Proc. Natl. Acad. Sci. USA* **2011**, *108*, E1475–E1483.
41. Bouros, E.; Filidou, E.; Arvanitidis, K.; Mikroulis, D.; Steiropoulos, P.; Bamias, G.; Bouros, D.; Kolios, G. Lung fibrosis-associated soluble mediators and bronchoalveolar lavage from idiopathic pulmonary fibrosis patients promote the expression of fibrogenic factors in subepithelial lung myofibroblasts. *Pulm. Pharmacol. Ther.* **2017**, *46*, 78–87.
42. Yang, J.; Velikoff, M.; Canalis, E.; Horowitz, J.C.; Kim, K.K. Activated alveolar epithelial cells initiate fibrosis through autocrine and paracrine secretion of connective tissue growth factor. *Am. J. Physiol. Lung Cell. Mol. Physiol.* **2014**, *306*, L786–L796.
43. Osterholzer, J.J.; Christensen, P.J.; Lama, V.; Horowitz, J.C.; Hattori, N.; Subbotina, N.; Cunningham, A.; Lin, Y.; Murdock, B.J.; Morey, R.E.; et al. PAI-1 promotes the accumulation of exudate macrophages and worsens pulmonary fibrosis following type II alveolar epithelial cell injury. *J. Pathol.* **2012**, *228*, 170–180.
44. Kim, K.K.; Dotson, M.R.; Agarwal, M.; Yang, J.; Bradley, P.B.; Subbotina, N.; Osterholzer, J.J.; Sisson, T.H. Efferocytosis of apoptotic alveolar epithelial cells is sufficient to initiate lung fibrosis. *Cell Death Dis.* **2018**, *9*, 1056.
45. Camelo, A.; Dunmore, R.; Sleeman, M.A.; Clarke, D.L. The epithelium in idiopathic pulmonary fibrosis: Breaking the barrier. *Front. Pharmacol.* **2014**, *4*, 173.
46. Waghray, M.; Cui, Z.; Horowitz, J.C.; Subramanian, I.M.; Martinez, F.J.; Toews, G.B.; Thannickal, V.J. Hydrogen peroxide is a diffusible paracrine signal for the induction of epithelial cell death by activated myofibroblasts. *FASEB J.* **2005**, *19*, 854–856.
47. Hecker, L.; Vittal, R.; Jones, T.; Jagirdar, R.; Luckhardt, T.R.; Horowitz, J.C.; Pennathur, S.; Martinez, F.J.; Thannickal, V.J. NADPH oxidase-4 mediates myofibroblast activation and fibrogenic responses to lung injury. *Nat. Med.* **2009**, *15*, 1077–1081.
48. Amara, N.; Goven, D.; Prost, F.; Muloway, R.; Crestani, B.; Boczkowski, J. NOX4/NADPH oxidase expression is increased in pulmonary fibroblasts from patients with idiopathic pulmonary fibrosis and mediates TGFbeta1-induced fibroblast differentiation into myofibroblasts. *Thorax* **2010**, *65*, 733–738.
49. Sisson, T.H.; Maher, T.M.; Ajayi, I.O.; King, J.E.; Higgins, P.D.; Booth, A.J.; Sagana, R.L.; Huang, S.K.; White, E.S.; Moore, B.B.; et al. Increased survivin expression contributes to apoptosis-resistance in IPF fibroblasts. *Adv. Biosci. Biotechnol.* **2012**, *3*, 657–664.
50. Predescu, S.A.; Zhang, J.; Bardita, C.; Patel, M.; Godbole, V.; Predescu, D.N. Mouse Lung Fibroblast Resistance to Fas-Mediated Apoptosis Is Dependent on the Baculoviral Inhibitor of Apoptosis Protein 4 and the Cellular FLICE-Inhibitory Protein. *Front. Physiol.* **2017**, *8*, 128.
51. Golan-Gerstl, R.; Wallach-Dayan, S.B.; Zisman, P.; Cardoso, W.V.; Goldstein, R.H.; Breuer, R. Cellular FLICE-like inhibitory protein deviates myofibroblast fas-induced apoptosis toward proliferation during lung fibrosis. *Am. J. Respir. Cell Mol. Biol.* **2012**, *47*, 271–279. [CrossRef] [PubMed]
52. Conte, E.; Gili, E.; Fruciano, M.; Korfei, M.; Fagone, E.; Iemmolo, M.; Lo Furno, D.; Giuffrida, R.; Crimi, N.; Guenther, A.; et al. PI3K p110gamma overexpression in idiopathic pulmonary fibrosis lung tissue and fibroblast cells: In vitro effects of its inhibition. *Lab. Investig.* **2013**, *93*, 566–576. [CrossRef] [PubMed]
53. Chang, W.; Wei, K.; Jacobs, S.S.; Upadhyay, D.; Weill, D.; Rosen, G.D. SPARC suppresses apoptosis of idiopathic pulmonary fibrosis fibroblasts through constitutive activation of beta-catenin. *J. Biol. Chem.* **2010**, *285*, 8196–8206. [PubMed]
54. Ajayi, I.O.; Sisson, T.H.; Higgins, P.D.; Booth, A.J.; Sagana, R.L.; Huang, S.K.; White, E.S.; King, J.E.; Moore, B.B.; Horowitz, J.C. X-linked inhibitor of apoptosis regulates lung fibroblast resistance to Fas-mediated apoptosis. *Am. J. Respir. Cell Mol. Biol.* **2013**, *49*, 86–95. [CrossRef]
55. Santibanez, J.F.; Quintanilla, M.; Bernabeu, C. TGF-beta/TGF-beta receptor system and its role in physiological and pathological conditions. *Clin. Sci.* **2011**, *121*, 233–251. [CrossRef]
56. Daniels, C.E.; Wilkes, M.C.; Edens, M.; Kottom, T.J.; Murphy, S.J.; Limper, A.H.; Leof, E.B. Imatinib mesylate inhibits the profibrogenic activity of TGF-beta and prevents bleomycin-mediated lung fibrosis. *J. Clin. Investig.* **2004**, *114*, 1308–1316. [CrossRef]
57. Zhang, Y.; Dees, C.; Beyer, C.; Lin, N.Y.; Distler, A.; Zerr, P.; Palumbo, K.; Susok, L.; Kreuter, A.; Distler, O.; et al. Inhibition of casein kinase II reduces TGFbeta induced fibroblast activation and ameliorates experimental fibrosis. *Ann. Rheum. Dis.* **2015**, *74*, 936–943. [CrossRef]
58. Milara, J.; Ballester, B.; Morell, A.; Ortiz, J.L.; Escriva, J.; Fernandez, E.; Perez-Vizcaino, F.; Cogolludo, A.; Pastor, E.; Artigues, E.; et al. JAK2 mediates lung fibrosis, pulmonary vascular remodelling and hypertension in idiopathic pulmonary fibrosis: An experimental study. *Thorax* **2018**, *73*, 519–529.
59. Wang, J.; Hu, K.; Cai, X.; Yang, B.; He, Q.; Wang, J.; Weng, Q. Targeting PI3K/AKT signaling for treatment of idiopathic pulmonary fibrosis. *Acta Pharm. Sin. B* **2022**, *12*, 18–32. [CrossRef]
60. Hu, Y.; Peng, J.; Feng, D.; Chu, L.; Li, X.; Jin, Z.; Lin, Z.; Zeng, Q. Role of extracellular signal-regulated kinase, p38 kinase, and activator protein-1 in transforming growth factor-beta1-induced alpha smooth muscle actin expression in human fetal lung fibroblasts in vitro. *Lung* **2006**, *184*, 33–42.

61. Xia, H.; Khalil, W.; Kahm, J.; Jessurun, J.; Kleidon, J.; Henke, C.A. Pathologic caveolin-1 regulation of PTEN in idiopathic pulmonary fibrosis. *Am. J. Pathol.* **2010**, *176*, 2626–2637. [CrossRef]
62. Conte, E.; Fruciano, M.; Fagone, E.; Gili, E.; Caraci, F.; Iemmolo, M.; Crimi, N.; Vancheri, C. Inhibition of PI3K prevents the proliferation and differentiation of human lung fibroblasts into myofibroblasts: The role of class I P110 isoforms. *PLoS ONE* **2011**, *6*, e24663.
63. Zhang, X.L.; Xing, R.G.; Chen, L.; Liu, C.R.; Miao, Z.G. PI3K/Akt signaling is involved in the pathogenesis of bleomycin-induced pulmonary fibrosis via regulation of epithelial-mesenchymal transition. *Mol. Med. Rep.* **2016**, *14*, 5699–5706. [CrossRef]
64. Wei, X.; Han, J.; Chen, Z.Z.; Qi, B.W.; Wang, G.C.; Ma, Y.H.; Zheng, H.; Luo, Y.F.; Wei, Y.Q.; Chen, L.J. A phosphoinositide 3-kinase-gamma inhibitor, AS605240 prevents bleomycin-induced pulmonary fibrosis in rats. *Biochem. Biophys. Res. Commun.* **2010**, *397*, 311–317. [CrossRef]
65. Guerreiro, A.S.; Fattet, S.; Kulesza, D.W.; Atamer, A.; Elsing, A.N.; Shalaby, T.; Jackson, S.P.; Schoenwaelder, S.M.; Grotzer, M.A.; Delattre, O.; et al. A sensitized RNA interference screen identifies a novel role for the PI3K p110gamma isoform in medulloblastoma cell proliferation and chemoresistance. *Mol. Cancer Res.* **2011**, *9*, 925–935. [CrossRef]
66. Lu, Y.; Azad, N.; Wang, L.; Iyer, A.K.; Castranova, V.; Jiang, B.H.; Rojanasakul, Y. Phosphatidylinositol-3-kinase/Akt regulates bleomycin-induced fibroblast proliferation and collagen production. *Am. J. Respir. Cell Mol. Biol.* **2010**, *42*, 432–441. [CrossRef]
67. Spassov, S.G.; Donus, R.; Ihle, P.M.; Engelstaedter, H.; Hoetzel, A.; Faller, S. Hydrogen Sulfide Prevents Formation of Reactive Oxygen Species through PI3K/Akt Signaling and Limits Ventilator-Induced Lung Injury. *Oxid. Med. Cell. Longev.* **2017**, *2017*, 3715037. [CrossRef]
68. O'Donoghue, R.J.; Knight, D.A.; Richards, C.D.; Prele, C.M.; Lau, H.L.; Jarnicki, A.G.; Jones, J.; Bozinovski, S.; Vlahos, R.; Thiem, S.; et al. Genetic partitioning of interleukin-6 signalling in mice dissociates Stat3 from Smad3-mediated lung fibrosis. *EMBO Mol. Med.* **2012**, *4*, 939–951. [CrossRef]
69. Pedroza, M.; Le, T.T.; Lewis, K.; Karmouty-Quintana, H.; To, S.; George, A.T.; Blackburn, M.R.; Tweardy, D.J.; Agarwal, S.K. STAT-3 contributes to pulmonary fibrosis through epithelial injury and fibroblast-myofibroblast differentiation. *FASEB J.* **2016**, *30*, 129–140. [CrossRef]
70. Ruan, H.; Luan, J.; Gao, S.; Li, S.; Jiang, Q.; Liu, R.; Liang, Q.; Zhang, R.; Zhang, F.; Li, X.; et al. Fedratinib Attenuates Bleomycin-Induced Pulmonary Fibrosis via the JAK2/STAT3 and TGF-beta1 Signaling Pathway. *Molecules* **2021**, *26*, 4491. [CrossRef]
71. Chuang, Y.F.; Huang, S.W.; Hsu, Y.F.; Yu, M.C.; Ou, G.; Huang, W.J.; Hsu, M.J. WMJ-8-B, a novel hydroxamate derivative, induces MDA-MB-231 breast cancer cell death via the SHP-1-STAT3-survivin cascade. *Br. J. Pharmacol.* **2017**, *174*, 2941–2961. [CrossRef]
72. Prele, C.M.; Yao, E.; O'Donoghue, R.J.; Mutsaers, S.E.; Knight, D.A. STAT3: A central mediator of pulmonary fibrosis? *Proc. Am. Thorac. Soc.* **2012**, *9*, 177–182. [CrossRef]
73. Milara, J.; Hernandez, G.; Ballester, B.; Morell, A.; Roger, I.; Montero, P.; Escriva, J.; Lloris, J.M.; Molina-Molina, M.; Morcillo, E.; et al. The JAK2 pathway is activated in idiopathic pulmonary fibrosis. *Respir. Res.* **2018**, *19*, 24. [CrossRef]
74. Chambers, R.C. Procoagulant signalling mechanisms in lung inflammation and fibrosis: Novel opportunities for pharmacological intervention? *Br. J. Pharmacol.* **2008**, *153*, S367–S378. [CrossRef]
75. Howell, D.C.; Laurent, G.J.; Chambers, R.C. Role of thrombin and its major cellular receptor, protease-activated receptor-1, in pulmonary fibrosis. *Biochem. Soc. Trans.* **2002**, *30*, 211–216. [CrossRef]
76. Scotton, C.J.; Krupiczojc, M.A.; Konigshoff, M.; Mercer, P.F.; Lee, Y.C.; Kaminski, N.; Morser, J.; Post, J.M.; Maher, T.M.; Nicholson, A.G.; et al. Increased local expression of coagulation factor X contributes to the fibrotic response in human and murine lung injury. *J. Clin. Investig.* **2009**, *119*, 2550–2563. [CrossRef]
77. Bai, K.J.; Chen, B.C.; Pai, H.C.; Weng, C.M.; Yu, C.C.; Hsu, M.J.; Yu, M.C.; Ma, H.P.; Wu, C.H.; Hong, C.Y.; et al. Thrombin-induced CCN2 expression in human lung fibroblasts requires the c-Src/JAK2/STAT3 pathway. *J. Leukoc. Biol.* **2013**, *93*, 101–112. [CrossRef]
78. Atanelishvili, I.; Liang, J.; Akter, T.; Spyropoulos, D.D.; Silver, R.M.; Bogatkevich, G.S. Thrombin increases lung fibroblast survival while promoting alveolar epithelial cell apoptosis via the endoplasmic reticulum stress marker, CCAAT enhancer-binding homologous protein. *Am. J. Respir. Cell Mol. Biol.* **2014**, *50*, 893–902. [CrossRef]
79. Li, H.; Zhao, X.; Shan, H.; Liang, H. MicroRNAs in idiopathic pulmonary fibrosis: Involvement in pathogenesis and potential use in diagnosis and therapeutics. *Acta Pharm. Sin. B* **2016**, *6*, 531–539. [CrossRef]
80. Yang, G.; Yang, L.; Wang, W.; Wang, J.; Wang, J.; Xu, Z. Discovery and validation of extracellular/circulating microRNAs during idiopathic pulmonary fibrosis disease progression. *Gene* **2015**, *562*, 138–144. [CrossRef]
81. Yang, S.; Banerjee, S.; de Freitas, A.; Sanders, Y.Y.; Ding, Q.; Matalon, S.; Thannickal, V.J.; Abraham, E.; Liu, G. Participation of miR-200 in pulmonary fibrosis. *Am. J. Pathol.* **2012**, *180*, 484–493. [CrossRef] [PubMed]
82. Liu, G.; Friggeri, A.; Yang, Y.; Milosevic, J.; Ding, Q.; Thannickal, V.J.; Kaminski, N.; Abraham, E. miR-21 mediates fibrogenic activation of pulmonary fibroblasts and lung fibrosis. *J. Exp. Med.* **2010**, *207*, 1589–1597. [CrossRef]
83. Liu, L.; Qian, H. Up-regulation of miR-21 promotes cell proliferation and collagen synthesis in pulmonary fibroblasts. *Xi Bao Yu Fen Zi Mian Yi Xue Za Zhi = Chin. J. Cell. Mol. Immunol.* **2015**, *31*, 918–922.
84. Lino Cardenas, C.L.; Henaoui, I.S.; Courcot, E.; Roderburg, C.; Cauffiez, C.; Aubert, S.; Copin, M.C.; Wallaert, B.; Glowacki, F.; Dewaeles, E.; et al. miR-199a-5p is upregulated during fibrogenic response to tissue injury and mediates TGFbeta-induced lung fibroblast activation by targeting caveolin-1. *PLoS Genet.* **2013**, *9*, e1003291. [CrossRef]

85. Liang, H.; Xu, C.; Pan, Z.; Zhang, Y.; Xu, Z.; Chen, Y.; Li, T.; Li, X.; Liu, Y.; Huangfu, L.; et al. The antifibrotic effects and mechanisms of microRNA-26a action in idiopathic pulmonary fibrosis. *Mol. Ther.* **2014**, *22*, 1122–1133. [CrossRef] [PubMed]
86. Fierro-Fernandez, M.; Busnadiego, O.; Sandoval, P.; Espinosa-Diez, C.; Blanco-Ruiz, E.; Rodriguez, M.; Pian, H.; Ramos, R.; Lopez-Cabrera, M.; Garcia-Bermejo, M.L.; et al. miR-9-5p suppresses pro-fibrogenic transformation of fibroblasts and prevents organ fibrosis by targeting NOX4 and TGFBR2. *EMBO Rep.* **2015**, *16*, 1358–1377. [CrossRef] [PubMed]
87. Herrera, J.; Beisang, D.J.; Peterson, M.; Forster, C.; Gilbertsen, A.; Benyumov, A.; Smith, K.; Korenczuk, C.E.; Barocas, V.H.; Guenther, K.; et al. Dicer1 Deficiency in the Idiopathic Pulmonary Fibrosis Fibroblastic Focus Promotes Fibrosis by Suppressing MicroRNA Biogenesis. *Am. J. Respir. Crit. Care Med.* **2018**, *198*, 486–496. [CrossRef]
88. Pandit, K.V.; Corcoran, D.; Yousef, H.; Yarlagadda, M.; Tzouvelekis, A.; Gibson, K.F.; Konishi, K.; Yousem, S.A.; Singh, M.; Handley, D.; et al. Inhibition and role of let-7d in idiopathic pulmonary fibrosis. *Am. J. Respir. Crit. Care Med.* **2010**, *182*, 220–229. [CrossRef]
89. Moimas, S.; Salton, F.; Kosmider, B.; Ring, N.; Volpe, M.C.; Bahmed, K.; Braga, L.; Rehman, M.; Vodret, S.; Graziani, M.L.; et al. miR-200 family members reduce senescence and restore idiopathic pulmonary fibrosis type II alveolar epithelial cell transdifferentiation. *ERJ Open Res.* **2019**, *5*, 00138–02019. [CrossRef]
90. Ge, L.; Habiel, D.M.; Hansbro, P.M.; Kim, R.Y.; Gharib, S.A.; Edelman, J.D.; Konigshoff, M.; Parimon, T.; Brauer, R.; Huang, Y.; et al. miR-323a-3p regulates lung fibrosis by targeting multiple profibrotic pathways. *JCI Insight* **2016**, *1*, e90301. [CrossRef]
91. Hayton, C.; Chaudhuri, N. Managing Idiopathic Pulmonary Fibrosis: Which Drug for Which Patient? *Drugs Aging* **2017**, *34*, 647–653. [CrossRef] [PubMed]
92. Krauss, E.; Tello, S.; Wilhelm, J.; Schmidt, J.; Stoehr, M.; Seeger, W.; Dartsch, R.C.; Crestani, B.; Guenther, A. Assessing the Effectiveness of Pirfenidone in Idiopathic Pulmonary Fibrosis: Long-Term, Real-World Data from European IPF Registry (eurIPFreg). *J. Clin. Med.* **2020**, *9*, 3763. [CrossRef] [PubMed]
93. Wollin, L.; Wex, E.; Pautsch, A.; Schnapp, G.; Hostettler, K.E.; Stowasser, S.; Kolb, M. Mode of action of nintedanib in the treatment of idiopathic pulmonary fibrosis. *Eur. Respir. J.* **2015**, *45*, 1434–1445. [CrossRef] [PubMed]
94. Iyer, S.N.; Gurujeyalakshmi, G.; Giri, S.N. Effects of pirfenidone on transforming growth factor-beta gene expression at the transcriptional level in bleomycin hamster model of lung fibrosis. *J. Pharmacol. Exp. Ther.* **1999**, *291*, 367–373. [PubMed]
95. Oku, H.; Shimizu, T.; Kawabata, T.; Nagira, M.; Hikita, I.; Ueyama, A.; Matsushima, S.; Torii, M.; Arimura, A. Antifibrotic action of pirfenidone and prednisolone: Different effects on pulmonary cytokines and growth factors in bleomycin-induced murine pulmonary fibrosis. *Eur. J. Pharmacol.* **2008**, *590*, 400–408. [CrossRef]
96. Gurujeyalakshmi, G.; Hollinger, M.A.; Giri, S.N. Pirfenidone inhibits PDGF isoforms in bleomycin hamster model of lung fibrosis at the translational level. *Am. J. Physiol.* **1999**, *276*, L311–L318. [CrossRef]
97. Grattendick, K.J.; Nakashima, J.M.; Feng, L.; Giri, S.N.; Margolin, S.B. Effects of three anti-TNF-alpha drugs: Etanercept, infliximab and pirfenidone on release of TNF-alpha in medium and TNF-alpha associated with the cell in vitro. *Int. Immunopharmacol.* **2008**, *8*, 679–687. [CrossRef]
98. Conte, E.; Gili, E.; Fagone, E.; Fruciano, M.; Iemmolo, M.; Vancheri, C. Effect of pirfenidone on proliferation, TGF-beta-induced myofibroblast differentiation and fibrogenic activity of primary human lung fibroblasts. *Eur. J. Pharm. Sci.* **2014**, *58*, 13–19. [CrossRef]
99. Lehmann, M.; Buhl, L.; Alsafadi, H.N.; Klee, S.; Hermann, S.; Mutze, K.; Ota, C.; Lindner, M.; Behr, J.; Hilgendorff, A.; et al. Differential effects of Nintedanib and Pirfenidone on lung alveolar epithelial cell function in ex vivo murine and human lung tissue cultures of pulmonary fibrosis. *Respir. Res.* **2018**, *19*, 175. [CrossRef]
100. Liu, Y.; Lu, F.; Kang, L.; Wang, Z.; Wang, Y. Pirfenidone attenuates bleomycin-induced pulmonary fibrosis in mice by regulating Nrf2/Bach1 equilibrium. *BMC Pulm. Med.* **2017**, *17*, 63. [CrossRef]
101. Pourgholamhossein, F.; Rasooli, R.; Pournamdari, M.; Pourgholi, L.; Samareh-Fekri, M.; Ghazi-Khansari, M.; Iranpour, M.; Poursalehi, H.R.; Heidari, M.R.; Mandegary, A. Pirfenidone protects against paraquat-induced lung injury and fibrosis in mice by modulation of inflammation, oxidative stress, and gene expression. *Food Chem. Toxicol.* **2018**, *112*, 39–46. [CrossRef]
102. King, T.E., Jr.; Bradford, W.Z.; Castro-Bernardini, S.; Fagan, E.A.; Glaspole, I.; Glassberg, M.K.; Gorina, E.; Hopkins, P.M.; Kardatzke, D.; Lancaster, L.; et al. A phase 3 trial of pirfenidone in patients with idiopathic pulmonary fibrosis. *N. Engl. J. Med.* **2014**, *370*, 2083–2092. [CrossRef]
103. Crestani, B.; Huggins, J.T.; Kaye, M.; Costabel, U.; Glaspole, I.; Ogura, T.; Song, J.W.; Stansen, W.; Quaresma, M.; Stowasser, S.; et al. Long-term safety and tolerability of nintedanib in patients with idiopathic pulmonary fibrosis: Results from the open-label extension study, INPULSIS-ON. *Lancet Respir. Med.* **2019**, *7*, 60–68. [CrossRef]
104. Vancheri, C.; Kreuter, M.; Richeldi, L.; Ryerson, C.J.; Valeyre, D.; Grutters, J.C.; Wiebe, S.; Stansen, W.; Quaresma, M.; Stowasser, S.; et al. Nintedanib with Add-on Pirfenidone in Idiopathic Pulmonary Fibrosis. Results of the INJOURNEY Trial. *Am. J. Respir. Crit. Care Med.* **2018**, *197*, 356–363. [CrossRef]
105. Koli, K.; Myllarniemi, M.; Keski-Oja, J.; Kinnula, V.L. Transforming growth factor-beta activation in the lung: Focus on fibrosis and reactive oxygen species. *Antioxid. Redox Signal.* **2008**, *10*, 333–342. [CrossRef]
106. Saini, G.; Porte, J.; Weinreb, P.H.; Violette, S.M.; Wallace, W.A.; McKeever, T.M.; Jenkins, G. αvβ6 integrin may be a potential prognostic biomarker in interstitial lung disease. *Eur. Respir. J.* **2015**, *46*, 486–494. [CrossRef]
107. Zhang, J.; Wang, T.; Saigal, A.; Johnson, J.; Morrison, J.; Tabrizifard, S.; Hollingsworth, S.A.; Eddins, M.J.; Mao, W.; O'Neill, K.; et al. Discovery of a new class of integrin antibodies for fibrosis. *Sci. Rep.* **2021**, *11*, 2118. [CrossRef]

108. John, A.E.; Graves, R.H.; Pun, K.T.; Vitulli, G.; Forty, E.J.; Mercer, P.F.; Morrell, J.L.; Barrett, J.W.; Rogers, R.F.; Hafeji, M.; et al. Translational pharmacology of an inhaled small molecule alphavbeta6 integrin inhibitor for idiopathic pulmonary fibrosis. *Nat. Commun.* 2020, *11*, 4659. [CrossRef]
109. Mullally, A.; Hood, J.; Harrison, C.; Mesa, R. Fedratinib in myelofibrosis. *Blood Adv.* 2020, *4*, 1792–1800.
110. D'Alessandro, M.; Perillo, F.; Metella Refini, R.; Bergantini, L.; Bellisai, F.; Selvi, E.; Cameli, P.; Manganelli, S.; Conticini, E.; Cantarini, L.; et al. Efficacy of baricitinib in treating rheumatoid arthritis: Modulatory effects on fibrotic and inflammatory biomarkers in a real-life setting. *Int. Immunopharmacol.* 2020, *86*, 106748. [CrossRef]
111. Strand, V.; van Vollenhoven, R.F.; Lee, E.B.; Fleischmann, R.; Zwillich, S.H.; Gruben, D.; Koncz, T.; Wilkinson, B.; Wallenstein, G. Tofacitinib or adalimumab versus placebo: Patient-reported outcomes from a phase 3 study of active rheumatoid arthritis. *Rheumatology* 2016, *55*, 1031–1041. [CrossRef]
112. O'Shea, J.J.; Schwartz, D.M.; Villarino, A.V.; Gadina, M.; McInnes, I.B.; Laurence, A. The JAK-STAT pathway: Impact on human disease and therapeutic intervention. *Annu. Rev. Med.* 2015, *66*, 311–328. [CrossRef]
113. Zhang, Y.; Liang, R.; Chen, C.W.; Mallano, T.; Dees, C.; Distler, A.; Reich, A.; Bergmann, C.; Ramming, A.; Gelse, K.; et al. JAK1-dependent transphosphorylation of JAK2 limits the antifibrotic effects of selective JAK2 inhibitors on long-term treatment. *Ann. Rheum. Dis.* 2017, *76*, 1467–1475. [CrossRef]
114. Emery, P.; Keystone, E.; Tony, H.P.; Cantagrel, A.; van Vollenhoven, R.; Sanchez, A.; Alecock, E.; Lee, J.; Kremer, J. IL-6 receptor inhibition with tocilizumab improves treatment outcomes in patients with rheumatoid arthritis refractory to anti-tumour necrosis factor biologicals: Results from a 24-week multicentre randomised placebo-controlled trial. *Ann. Rheum. Dis.* 2008, *67*, 1516–1523. [CrossRef]
115. Abidi, E.; El Nekidy, W.S.; Alefishat, E.; Rahman, N.; Petroianu, G.A.; El-Lababidi, R.; Mallat, J. Tocilizumab and COVID-19: Timing of Administration and Efficacy. *Front. Pharmacol.* 2022, *13*, 825749. [CrossRef]
116. Coltro, G.; Vannucchi, A.M. The safety of JAK kinase inhibitors for the treatment of myelofibrosis. *Expert Opin. Drug Saf.* 2021, *20*, 139–154. [CrossRef]
117. Merkt, W.; Bueno, M.; Mora, A.L.; Lagares, D. Senotherapeutics: Targeting senescence in idiopathic pulmonary fibrosis. *Semin. Cell Dev. Biol.* 2020, *101*, 104–110. [CrossRef]
118. Lehmann, M.; Korfei, M.; Mutze, K.; Klee, S.; Skronska-Wasek, W.; Alsafadi, H.N.; Ota, C.; Costa, R.; Schiller, H.B.; Lindner, M.; et al. Senolytic drugs target alveolar epithelial cell function and attenuate experimental lung fibrosis ex vivo. *Eur. Respir. J.* 2017, *50*, 1602367. [CrossRef]
119. Xu, Y.; Mizuno, T.; Sridharan, A.; Du, Y.; Guo, M.; Tang, J.; Wikenheiser-Brokamp, K.A.; Perl, A.T.; Funari, V.A.; Gokey, J.J.; et al. Single-cell RNA sequencing identifies diverse roles of epithelial cells in idiopathic pulmonary fibrosis. *JCI Insight* 2016, *1*, e90558. [CrossRef] [PubMed]
120. Yao, C.; Guan, X.; Carraro, G.; Parimon, T.; Liu, X.; Huang, G.; Mulay, A.; Soukiasian, H.J.; David, G.; Weigt, S.S.; et al. Senescence of Alveolar Type 2 Cells Drives Progressive Pulmonary Fibrosis. *Am. J. Respir. Crit. Care Med.* 2021, *203*, 707–717. [CrossRef] [PubMed]
121. Schafer, M.J.; White, T.A.; Iijima, K.; Haak, A.J.; Ligresti, G.; Atkinson, E.J.; Oberg, A.L.; Birch, J.; Salmonowicz, H.; Zhu, Y.; et al. Cellular senescence mediates fibrotic pulmonary disease. *Nat. Commun.* 2017, *8*, 14532. [CrossRef]
122. Luo, S.; Kan, J.; Zhang, J.; Ye, P.; Wang, D.; Jiang, X.; Li, M.; Zhu, L.; Gu, Y. Bioactive Compounds from Coptidis Rhizoma Alleviate Pulmonary Arterial Hypertension by Inhibiting Pulmonary Artery Smooth Muscle Cells' Proliferation and Migration. *J. Cardiovasc. Pharmacol.* 2021, *78*, 253–262. [CrossRef] [PubMed]
123. Carnesecchi, S.; Deffert, C.; Donati, Y.; Basset, O.; Hinz, B.; Preynat-Seauve, O.; Guichard, C.; Arbiser, J.L.; Banfi, B.; Pache, J.C.; et al. A key role for NOX4 in epithelial cell death during development of lung fibrosis. *Antioxid. Redox Signal.* 2011, *15*, 607–619. [CrossRef]
124. Hohmann, M.S.; Habiel, D.M.; Coelho, A.L.; Verri, W.A., Jr.; Hogaboam, C.M. Quercetin Enhances Ligand-induced Apoptosis in Senescent Idiopathic Pulmonary Fibrosis Fibroblasts and Reduces Lung Fibrosis In Vivo. *Am. J. Respir. Cell Mol. Biol.* 2019, *60*, 28–40. [CrossRef]
125. Justice, J.N.; Nambiar, A.M.; Tchkonia, T.; LeBrasseur, N.K.; Pascual, R.; Hashmi, S.K.; Prata, L.; Masternak, M.M.; Kritchevsky, S.B.; Musi, N.; et al. Senolytics in idiopathic pulmonary fibrosis: Results from a first-in-human, open-label, pilot study. *EBioMedicine* 2019, *40*, 554–563. [CrossRef]
126. Van Deursen, J.M. Senolytic therapies for healthy longevity. *Science* 2019, *364*, 636–637. [CrossRef]
127. Ozgur Yurttas, N.; Eskazan, A.E. Dasatinib-induced pulmonary arterial hypertension. *Br. J. Clin. Pharmacol.* 2018, *84*, 835–845. [CrossRef]
128. Shea, B.S.; Tager, A.M. Role of the lysophospholipid mediators lysophosphatidic acid and sphingosine 1-phosphate in lung fibrosis. *Proc. Am. Thorac. Soc.* 2012, *9*, 102–110. [CrossRef]
129. Ninou, I.; Kaffe, E.; Muller, S.; Budd, D.C.; Stevenson, C.S.; Ullmer, C.; Aidinis, V. Pharmacologic targeting of the ATX/LPA axis attenuates bleomycin-induced pulmonary fibrosis. *Pulm. Pharmacol. Ther.* 2018, *52*, 32–40. [CrossRef]
130. Tager, A.M.; LaCamera, P.; Shea, B.S.; Campanella, G.S.; Selman, M.; Zhao, Z.; Polosukhin, V.; Wain, J.; Karimi-Shah, B.A.; Kim, N.D.; et al. The lysophosphatidic acid receptor LPA1 links pulmonary fibrosis to lung injury by mediating fibroblast recruitment and vascular leak. *Nat. Med.* 2008, *14*, 45–54. [CrossRef]

131. Gill, M.W.; Sivaraman, L.; Cheng, P.T.W.; Murphy, B.J.; Chadwick, K.; Lehman-McKeeman, L.; Graziano, M.; Bristol-Myers Squibb. BMS-986278, an LPA_1 receptor antagonist for idiopathic pulmonary fibrosis: Preclinical assessments of potential hepatobiliary toxicity [abstract]. *Am. J. Respir. Crit. Care Med.* **2019**, *199*, 8755.
132. Corte, T.J.; Lancaster, L.; Swigris, J.J.; Maher, T.M.; Goldin, J.G.; Palmer, S.M.; Suda, T.; Ogura, T.; Minnich, A.; Zhan, X.; et al. Phase 2 trial design of BMS-986278, a lysophosphatidic acid receptor 1 (LPA1) antagonist, in patients with idiopathic pulmonary fibrosis (IPF) or progressive fibrotic interstitial lung disease (PF-ILD). *BMJ Open Respir. Res.* **2021**, *8*, e001026. [CrossRef] [PubMed]
133. Richeldi, L.; Fernandez Perez, E.R.; Costabel, U.; Albera, C.; Lederer, D.J.; Flaherty, K.R.; Ettinger, N.; Perez, R.; Scholand, M.B.; Goldin, J.; et al. Pamrevlumab, an anti-connective tissue growth factor therapy, for idiopathic pulmonary fibrosis (PRAISE): A phase 2, randomised, double-blind, placebo-controlled trial. *Lancet Respir. Med.* **2020**, *8*, 25–33. [CrossRef]
134. Pilling, D.; Galvis-Carvajal, E.; Karhadkar, T.R.; Cox, N.; Gomer, R.H. Monocyte differentiation and macrophage priming are regulated differentially by pentraxins and their ligands. *BMC Immunol.* **2017**, *18*, 30. [CrossRef]
135. Murray, L.A.; Chen, Q.; Kramer, M.S.; Hesson, D.P.; Argentieri, R.L.; Peng, X.; Gulati, M.; Homer, R.J.; Russell, T.; van Rooijen, N.; et al. TGF-beta driven lung fibrosis is macrophage dependent and blocked by Serum amyloid P. *Int. J. Biochem. Cell Biol.* **2011**, *43*, 154–162. [CrossRef]
136. Korfei, M.; von der Beck, D.; Henneke, I.; Markart, P.; Ruppert, C.; Mahavadi, P.; Ghanim, B.; Klepetko, W.; Fink, L.; Meiners, S.; et al. Comparative proteome analysis of lung tissue from patients with idiopathic pulmonary fibrosis (IPF), non-specific interstitial pneumonia (NSIP) and organ donors. *J. Proteom.* **2013**, *85*, 109–128. [CrossRef]
137. Raghu, G.; van den Blink, B.; Hamblin, M.J.; Brown, A.W.; Golden, J.A.; Ho, L.A.; Wijsenbeek, M.S.; Vasakova, M.; Pesci, A.; Antin-Ozerkis, D.E.; et al. Effect of Recombinant Human Pentraxin 2 vs Placebo on Change in Forced Vital Capacity in Patients with Idiopathic Pulmonary Fibrosis: A Randomized Clinical Trial. *JAMA* **2018**, *319*, 2299–2307. [CrossRef]
138. Jia, W.; Wang, Z.; Gao, C.; Wu, J.; Wu, Q. Trajectory modeling of endothelial-to-mesenchymal transition reveals galectin-3 as a mediator in pulmonary fibrosis. *Cell Death Dis.* **2021**, *12*, 327. [CrossRef]
139. Mackinnon, A.C.; Gibbons, M.A.; Farnworth, S.L.; Leffler, H.; Nilsson, U.J.; Delaine, T.; Simpson, A.J.; Forbes, S.J.; Hirani, N.; Gauldie, J.; et al. Regulation of transforming growth factor-beta1-driven lung fibrosis by galectin-3. *Am. J. Respir. Crit. Care Med.* **2012**, *185*, 537–546. [CrossRef]
140. Hirani, N.; MacKinnon, A.C.; Nicol, L.; Ford, P.; Schambye, H.; Pedersen, A.; Nilsson, U.J.; Leffler, H.; Sethi, T.; Tantawi, S.; et al. Target inhibition of galectin-3 by inhaled TD139 in patients with idiopathic pulmonary fibrosis. *Eur. Respir. J.* **2021**, *57*, 2002559. [CrossRef]
141. Noth, I.; Anstrom, K.J.; Calvert, S.B.; de Andrade, J.; Flaherty, K.R.; Glazer, C.; Kaner, R.J.; Olman, M.A.; Idiopathic Pulmonary Fibrosis Clinical Research Network. A placebo-controlled randomized trial of warfarin in idiopathic pulmonary fibrosis. *Am. J. Respir. Crit. Care Med.* **2012**, *186*, 88–95. [CrossRef] [PubMed]
142. Idiopathic Pulmonary Fibrosis Clinical Research Network; Raghu, G.; Anstrom, K.J.; King, T.E., Jr.; Lasky, J.A.; Martinez, F.J. Prednisone, azathioprine, and N-acetylcysteine for pulmonary fibrosis. *N. Engl. J. Med.* **2012**, *366*, 1968–1977.
143. Behr, J.; Bendstrup, E.; Crestani, B.; Gunther, A.; Olschewski, H.; Skold, C.M.; Wells, A.; Wuyts, W.; Koschel, D.; Kreuter, M.; et al. Safety and tolerability of acetylcysteine and pirfenidone combination therapy in idiopathic pulmonary fibrosis: A randomised, double-blind, placebo-controlled, phase 2 trial. *Lancet Respir. Med.* **2016**, *4*, 445–453. [CrossRef]
144. King, T.E., Jr.; Brown, K.K.; Raghu, G.; du Bois, R.M.; Lynch, D.A.; Martinez, F.; Valeyre, D.; Leconte, I.; Morganti, A.; Roux, S.; et al. BUILD-3: A randomized, controlled trial of bosentan in idiopathic pulmonary fibrosis. *Am. J. Respir. Crit. Care Med.* **2011**, *184*, 92–99. [CrossRef]
145. Raghu, G.; Behr, J.; Brown, K.K.; Egan, J.J.; Kawut, S.M.; Flaherty, K.R.; Martinez, F.J.; Nathan, S.D.; Wells, A.U.; Collard, H.R.; et al. Treatment of idiopathic pulmonary fibrosis with ambrisentan: A parallel, randomized trial. *Ann. Intern Med.* **2013**, *158*, 641–649. [CrossRef]
146. Kolb, M.; Raghu, G.; Wells, A.U.; Behr, J.; Richeldi, L.; Schinzel, B.; Quaresma, M.; Stowasser, S.; Martinez, F.J.; INSTAGE Investigators. Nintedanib plus Sildenafil in Patients with Idiopathic Pulmonary Fibrosis. *N. Engl. J. Med.* **2018**, *379*, 1722–1731. [CrossRef]
147. Daniels, C.E.; Lasky, J.A.; Limper, A.H.; Mieras, K.; Gabor, E.; Schroeder, D.R.; Imatinib-IPF Study Investigators. Imatinib treatment for idiopathic pulmonary fibrosis: Randomized placebo-controlled trial results. *Am. J. Respir. Crit. Care Med.* **2010**, *181*, 604–610. [CrossRef]
148. Collard, H.R.; Ryu, J.H.; Douglas, W.W.; Schwarz, M.I.; Curran-Everett, D.; King, T.E., Jr.; Brown, K.K. Combined corticosteroid and cyclophosphamide therapy does not alter survival in idiopathic pulmonary fibrosis. *Chest* **2004**, *125*, 2169–2174. [CrossRef]
149. King, T.E., Jr.; Albera, C.; Bradford, W.Z.; Costabel, U.; Hormel, P.; Lancaster, L.; Noble, P.W.; Sahn, S.A.; Szwarcberg, J.; Thomeer, M.; et al. Effect of interferon gamma-1b on survival in patients with idiopathic pulmonary fibrosis (INSPIRE): A multicentre, randomised, placebo-controlled trial. *Lancet* **2009**, *374*, 222–228. [CrossRef]
150. Raghu, G.; Brown, K.K.; Collard, H.R.; Cottin, V.; Gibson, K.F.; Kaner, R.J.; Lederer, D.J.; Martinez, F.J.; Noble, P.W.; Song, J.W.; et al. Efficacy of simtuzumab versus placebo in patients with idiopathic pulmonary fibrosis: A randomised, double-blind, controlled, phase 2 trial. *Lancet Respir. Med.* **2017**, *5*, 22–32. [CrossRef]
151. Wheaton, A.K.; Velikoff, M.; Agarwal, M.; Loo, T.T.; Horowitz, J.C.; Sisson, T.H.; Kim, K.K. The vitronectin RGD motif regulates TGF-beta-induced alveolar epithelial cell apoptosis. *Am. J. Physiol. Lung Cell. Mol. Physiol.* **2016**, *310*, L1206–L1217. [CrossRef]

152. Distler, J.H.W.; Gyorfi, A.H.; Ramanujam, M.; Whitfield, M.L.; Konigshoff, M.; Lafyatis, R. Shared and distinct mechanisms of fibrosis. *Nat. Rev. Rheumatol.* **2019**, *15*, 705–730. [CrossRef]
153. Li, Y.; Jiang, D.; Liang, J.; Meltzer, E.B.; Gray, A.; Miura, R.; Wogensen, L.; Yamaguchi, Y.; Noble, P.W. Severe lung fibrosis requires an invasive fibroblast phenotype regulated by hyaluronan and CD44. *J. Exp. Med.* **2011**, *208*, 1459–1471. [CrossRef]
154. White, E.S.; Thannickal, V.J.; Carskadon, S.L.; Dickie, E.G.; Livant, D.L.; Markwart, S.; Toews, G.B.; Arenberg, D.A. Integrin alpha4beta1 regulates migration across basement membranes by lung fibroblasts: A role for phosphatase and tensin homologue deleted on chromosome 10. *Am. J. Respir. Crit. Care Med.* **2003**, *168*, 436–442. [CrossRef]
155. Wolters, P.J.; Collard, H.R.; Jones, K.D. Pathogenesis of idiopathic pulmonary fibrosis. *Annu. Rev. Pathol.* **2014**, *9*, 157–179. [CrossRef]
156. Vancheri, C. Idiopathic pulmonary fibrosis and cancer: Do they really look similar? *BMC Med.* **2015**, *13*, 220. [CrossRef]
157. Qi, Y.; Huang, Y.; Pang, L.; Gu, W.; Wang, N.; Hu, J.; Cui, X.; Zhang, J.; Zhao, J.; Liu, C.; et al. Prognostic value of the MicroRNA-29 family in multiple human cancers: A meta-analysis and systematic review. *Clin. Exp. Pharmacol. Physiol.* **2017**, *44*, 441–454. [CrossRef]
158. Babaei, G.; Raei, N.; Toofani Milani, A.; Gholizadeh-Ghaleh Aziz, S.; Pourjabbar, N.; Geravand, F. The emerging role of miR-200 family in metastasis: Focus on EMT, CSCs, angiogenesis, and anoikis. *Mol. Biol. Rep.* **2021**, *48*, 6935–6947. [CrossRef]
159. De Santis, C.; Gotte, M. The Role of microRNA Let-7d in Female Malignancies and Diseases of the Female Reproductive Tract. *Int. J. Mol. Sci.* **2021**, *22*, 7359. [CrossRef]
160. Lettieri, S.; Oggionni, T.; Lancia, A.; Bortolotto, C.; Stella, G.M. Immune Stroma in Lung Cancer and Idiopathic Pulmonary Fibrosis: A Common Biologic Landscape? *Int. J. Mol. Sci.* **2021**, *22*, 2882. [CrossRef]
161. Singh, A.; Singh, A.K.; Giri, R.; Kumar, D.; Sharma, R.; Valis, M.; Kuca, K.; Garg, N. The role of microRNA-21 in the onset and progression of cancer. *Future Med. Chem.* **2021**, *13*, 1885–1906. [CrossRef] [PubMed]
162. Coward, W.R.; Watts, K.; Feghali-Bostwick, C.A.; Knox, A.; Pang, L. Defective histone acetylation is responsible for the diminished expression of cyclooxygenase 2 in idiopathic pulmonary fibrosis. *Mol. Cell. Biol.* **2009**, *29*, 4325–4339. [CrossRef] [PubMed]
163. Huang, S.K.; Scruggs, A.M.; Donaghy, J.; Horowitz, J.C.; Zaslona, Z.; Przybranowski, S.; White, E.S.; Peters-Golden, M. Histone modifications are responsible for decreased Fas expression and apoptosis resistance in fibrotic lung fibroblasts. *Cell Death Dis.* **2013**, *4*, e621. [CrossRef] [PubMed]
164. Sanders, Y.Y.; Hagood, J.S.; Liu, H.; Zhang, W.; Ambalavanan, N.; Thannickal, V.J. Histone deacetylase inhibition promotes fibroblast apoptosis and ameliorates pulmonary fibrosis in mice. *Eur. Respir. J.* **2014**, *43*, 1448–1458. [CrossRef]
165. Korfei, M.; Skwarna, S.; Henneke, I.; MacKenzie, B.; Klymenko, O.; Saito, S.; Ruppert, C.; von der Beck, D.; Mahavadi, P.; Klepetko, W.; et al. Aberrant expression and activity of histone deacetylases in sporadic idiopathic pulmonary fibrosis. *Thorax* **2015**, *70*, 1022–1032. [CrossRef]
166. Parbin, S.; Kar, S.; Shilpi, A.; Sengupta, D.; Deb, M.; Rath, S.K.; Patra, S.K. Histone deacetylases: A saga of perturbed acetylation homeostasis in cancer. *J. Histochem. Cytochem.* **2014**, *62*, 11–33. [CrossRef]
167. Zhang, X.; Liu, H.; Hock, T.; Thannickal, V.J.; Sanders, Y.Y. Histone deacetylase inhibition downregulates collagen 3A1 in fibrotic lung fibroblasts. *Int. J. Mol. Sci.* **2013**, *14*, 19605–19617. [CrossRef]
168. Ota, C.; Yamada, M.; Fujino, N.; Motohashi, H.; Tando, Y.; Takei, Y.; Suzuki, T.; Takahashi, T.; Kamata, S.; Makiguchi, T.; et al. Histone deacetylase inhibitor restores surfactant protein-C expression in alveolar-epithelial type II cells and attenuates bleomycin-induced pulmonary fibrosis in vivo. *Exp. Lung Res.* **2015**, *41*, 422–434. [CrossRef]
169. Conforti, F.; Davies, E.R.; Calderwood, C.J.; Thatcher, T.H.; Jones, M.G.; Smart, D.E.; Mahajan, S.; Alzetani, A.; Havelock, T.; Maher, T.M.; et al. The histone deacetylase inhibitor, romidepsin, as a potential treatment for pulmonary fibrosis. *Oncotarget* **2017**, *8*, 48737–48754. [CrossRef]
170. Chen, L.; Alam, J.; Pac-Soo, A.; Chen, Q.; Shang, Y.; Zhao, H.; Yao, S.; Ma, D. Pretreatment with valproic acid alleviates pulmonary fibrosis through epithelial-mesenchymal transition inhibition in vitro and in vivo. *Lab. Investig.* **2021**, *101*, 1166–1175. [CrossRef]
171. Saito, S.; Zhuang, Y.; Suzuki, T.; Ota, Y.; Bateman, M.E.; Alkhatib, A.L.; Morris, G.F.; Lasky, J.A. HDAC8 inhibition ameliorates pulmonary fibrosis. *Am. J. Physiol. Lung Cell Mol. Physiol.* **2019**, *316*, L175–L186. [CrossRef]
172. Xu, W.S.; Parmigiani, R.B.; Marks, P.A. Histone deacetylase inhibitors: Molecular mechanisms of action. *Oncogene* **2007**, *26*, 5541–5552. [CrossRef]
173. Qiu, L.; Burgess, A.; Fairlie, D.P.; Leonard, H.; Parsons, P.G.; Gabrielli, B.G. Histone deacetylase inhibitors trigger a G2 checkpoint in normal cells that is defective in tumor cells. *Mol. Biol. Cell* **2000**, *11*, 2069–2083. [CrossRef]
174. Campiani, G.; Cavella, C.; Osko, J.D.; Brindisi, M.; Relitti, N.; Brogi, S.; Saraswati, A.P.; Federico, S.; Chemi, G.; Maramai, S.; et al. Harnessing the Role of HDAC6 in Idiopathic Pulmonary Fibrosis: Design, Synthesis, Structural Analysis, and Biological Evaluation of Potent Inhibitors. *J. Med. Chem.* **2021**, *64*, 9960–9988. [CrossRef]
175. Prasse, A.; Binder, H.; Schupp, J.C.; Kayser, G.; Bargagli, E.; Jaeger, B.; Hess, M.; Rittinghausen, S.; Vuga, L.; Lynn, H.; et al. BAL Cell Gene Expression Is Indicative of Outcome and Airway Basal Cell Involvement in Idiopathic Pulmonary Fibrosis. *Am. J. Respir. Crit. Care Med.* **2019**, *199*, 622–630. [CrossRef]
176. Yang, X.J.; Seto, E. The Rpd3/Hda1 family of lysine deacetylases: From bacteria and yeast to mice and men. *Nat. Rev. Mol. Cell Biol.* **2008**, *9*, 206–218. [CrossRef]
177. Haberland, M.; Montgomery, R.L.; Olson, E.N. The many roles of histone deacetylases in development and physiology: Implications for disease and therapy. *Nat. Rev. Genet.* **2009**, *10*, 32–42. [CrossRef]

178. Eberharter, A.; Becker, P.B. Histone acetylation: A switch between repressive and permissive chromatin. Second in review series on chromatin dynamics. *EMBO Rep.* **2002**, *3*, 224–229. [CrossRef]
179. Kanno, T.; Kanno, Y.; Siegel, R.M.; Jang, M.K.; Lenardo, M.J.; Ozato, K. Selective recognition of acetylated histones by bromodomain proteins visualized in living cells. *Mol. Cell* **2004**, *13*, 33–43. [CrossRef]
180. Spange, S.; Wagner, T.; Heinzel, T.; Kramer, O.H. Acetylation of non-histone proteins modulates cellular signalling at multiple levels. *Int. J. Biochem. Cell Biol.* **2009**, *41*, 185–198. [CrossRef]
181. Buchwald, M.; Kramer, O.H.; Heinzel, T. HDACi—Targets beyond chromatin. *Cancer Lett.* **2009**, *280*, 160–167. [CrossRef]
182. Kramer, O.H. HDAC2: A critical factor in health and disease. *Trends Pharm. Sci* **2009**, *30*, 647–655. [CrossRef]
183. Fritsche, P.; Seidler, B.; Schuler, S.; Schnieke, A.; Gottlicher, M.; Schmid, R.M.; Saur, D.; Schneider, G. HDAC2 mediates therapeutic resistance of pancreatic cancer cells via the BH3-only protein NOXA. *Gut* **2009**, *58*, 1399–1409. [CrossRef]
184. Parmigiani, R.B.; Xu, W.S.; Venta-Perez, G.; Erdjument-Bromage, H.; Yaneva, M.; Tempst, P.; Marks, P.A. HDAC6 is a specific deacetylase of peroxiredoxins and is involved in redox regulation. *Proc. Natl. Acad. Sci. USA* **2008**, *105*, 9633–9638. [CrossRef]
185. Li, Y.; Shin, D.; Kwon, S.H. Histone deacetylase 6 plays a role as a distinct regulator of diverse cellular processes. *FEBS J.* **2013**, *280*, 775–793. [CrossRef]
186. Liu, P.; Xiao, J.; Wang, Y.; Song, X.; Huang, L.; Ren, Z.; Kitazato, K. Posttranslational modification and beyond: Interplay between histone deacetylase 6 and heat-shock protein 90. *Mol. Med.* **2021**, *27*, 110. [CrossRef]
187. Lee, J.Y.; Koga, H.; Kawaguchi, Y.; Tang, W.; Wong, E.; Gao, Y.S.; Pandey, U.B.; Kaushik, S.; Tresse, E.; Lu, J.; et al. HDAC6 controls autophagosome maturation essential for ubiquitin-selective quality-control autophagy. *EMBO J.* **2010**, *29*, 969–980. [CrossRef]
188. Trepel, J.; Mollapour, M.; Giaccone, G.; Neckers, L. Targeting the dynamic HSP90 complex in cancer. *Nat. Rev. Cancer* **2010**, *10*, 537–549. [CrossRef]
189. Lee, S.W.; Yeon, S.K.; Kim, G.W.; Lee, D.H.; Jeon, Y.H.; Yoo, J.; Kim, S.Y.; Kwon, S.H. HDAC6-Selective Inhibitor Overcomes Bortezomib Resistance in Multiple Myeloma. *Int. J. Mol. Sci.* **2021**, *22*, 1341. [CrossRef]
190. Shan, B.; Yao, T.P.; Nguyen, H.T.; Zhuo, Y.; Levy, D.R.; Klingsberg, R.C.; Tao, H.; Palmer, M.L.; Holder, K.N.; Lasky, J.A. Requirement of HDAC6 for transforming growth factor-beta1-induced epithelial-mesenchymal transition. *J. Biol. Chem.* **2008**, *283*, 21065–21073. [CrossRef]
191. Deskin, B.; Lasky, J.; Zhuang, Y.; Shan, B. Requirement of HDAC6 for activation of Notch1 by TGF-beta1. *Sci. Rep.* **2016**, *6*, 31086. [CrossRef] [PubMed]
192. Losson, H.; Schnekenburger, M.; Dicato, M.; Diederich, M. HDAC6-an Emerging Target Against Chronic Myeloid Leukemia? *Cancers* **2020**, *12*, 318. [CrossRef] [PubMed]
193. Lafon-Hughes, L.; Di Tomaso, M.V.; Mendez-Acuna, L.; Martinez-Lopez, W. Chromatin-remodelling mechanisms in cancer. *Mutat. Res.* **2008**, *658*, 191–214. [CrossRef] [PubMed]
194. Zhang, H.; Shang, Y.P.; Chen, H.Y.; Li, J. Histone deacetylases function as novel potential therapeutic targets for cancer. *Hepatol. Res.* **2017**, *47*, 149–159. [CrossRef]
195. Harms, K.L.; Chen, X. Histone deacetylase 2 modulates p53 transcriptional activities through regulation of p53-DNA binding activity. *Cancer Res.* **2007**, *67*, 3145–3152. [CrossRef]
196. Jung, K.H.; Noh, J.H.; Kim, J.K.; Eun, J.W.; Bae, H.J.; Xie, H.J.; Chang, Y.G.; Kim, M.G.; Park, H.; Lee, J.Y.; et al. HDAC2 overexpression confers oncogenic potential to human lung cancer cells by deregulating expression of apoptosis and cell cycle proteins. *J. Cell. Biochem.* **2012**, *113*, 2167–2177. [CrossRef]
197. Von Burstin, J.; Eser, S.; Paul, M.C.; Seidler, B.; Brandl, M.; Messer, M.; von Werder, A.; Schmidt, A.; Mages, J.; Pagel, P.; et al. E-cadherin regulates metastasis of pancreatic cancer in vivo and is suppressed by a SNAIL/HDAC1/HDAC2 repressor complex. *Gastroenterology* **2009**, *137*, 361–371.e5. [CrossRef]
198. Mariadason, J.M. Dissecting HDAC3-mediated tumor progression. *Cancer Biol. Ther.* **2008**, *7*, 1581–1583. [CrossRef]
199. Zhang, L.; Cao, W. Histone deacetylase 3 (HDAC3) as an important epigenetic regulator of kidney diseases. *J. Mol. Med.* **2022**, *100*, 43–51. [CrossRef]
200. Wilson, A.J.; Byun, D.S.; Nasser, S.; Murray, L.B.; Ayyanar, K.; Arango, D.; Figueroa, M.; Melnick, A.; Kao, G.D.; Augenlicht, L.H.; et al. HDAC4 promotes growth of colon cancer cells via repression of p21. *Mol. Biol. Cell* **2008**, *19*, 4062–4075. [CrossRef]
201. Shen, Y.F.; Wei, A.M.; Kou, Q.; Zhu, Q.Y.; Zhang, L. Histone deacetylase 4 increases progressive epithelial ovarian cancer cells via repression of p21 on fibrillar collagen matrices. *Oncol. Rep.* **2016**, *35*, 948–954. [CrossRef]
202. Spaety, M.E.; Gries, A.; Badie, A.; Venkatasamy, A.; Romain, B.; Orvain, C.; Yanagihara, K.; Okamoto, K.; Jung, A.C.; Mellitzer, G.; et al. HDAC4 Levels Control Sensibility toward Cisplatin in Gastric Cancer via the p53-p73/BIK Pathway. *Cancers* **2019**, *11*, 1747. [CrossRef]
203. Zhang, X.; Qi, Z.; Yin, H.; Yang, G. Interaction between p53 and Ras signaling controls cisplatin resistance via HDAC4- and HIF-1alpha-mediated regulation of apoptosis and autophagy. *Theranostics* **2019**, *9*, 1096–1114. [CrossRef]
204. Ye, M.; Fang, Z.; Gu, H.; Song, R.; Ye, J.; Li, H.; Wu, Z.; Zhou, S.; Li, P.; Cai, X.; et al. Histone deacetylase 5 promotes the migration and invasion of hepatocellular carcinoma via increasing the transcription of hypoxia-inducible factor-1alpha under hypoxia condition. *Tumor Biol.* **2017**, *39*, 1010428317705034. [CrossRef]
205. Zhong, L.; Sun, S.; Yao, S.; Han, X.; Gu, M.; Shi, J. Histone deacetylase 5 promotes the proliferation and invasion of lung cancer cells. *Oncol. Rep.* **2018**, *40*, 2224–2232. [CrossRef]

206. Ma, C.; D'Mello, S.R. Neuroprotection by histone deacetylase-7 (HDAC7) occurs by inhibition of c-Jun expression through a deacetylase-independent mechanism. *J. Biol. Chem.* **2011**, *286*, 4819–4828. [CrossRef]
207. Zhu, C.; Chen, Q.; Xie, Z.; Ai, J.; Tong, L.; Ding, J.; Geng, M. The role of histone deacetylase 7 (HDAC7) in cancer cell proliferation: Regulation on c-Myc. *J. Mol. Med.* **2011**, *89*, 279–289. [CrossRef]
208. Sang, Y.; Sun, L.; Wu, Y.; Yuan, W.; Liu, Y.; Li, S.W. Histone deacetylase 7 inhibits plakoglobin expression to promote lung cancer cell growth and metastasis. *Int. J. Oncol.* **2019**, *54*, 1112–1122. [CrossRef]
209. Cutano, V.; Di Giorgio, E.; Minisini, M.; Picco, R.; Dalla, E.; Brancolini, C. HDAC7-mediated control of tumour microenvironment maintains proliferative and stemness competence of human mammary epithelial cells. *Mol. Oncol.* **2019**, *13*, 1651–1668. [CrossRef]
210. Shinke, G.; Yamada, D.; Eguchi, H.; Iwagami, Y.; Asaoka, T.; Noda, T.; Wada, H.; Kawamoto, K.; Gotoh, K.; Kobayashi, S.; et al. Role of histone deacetylase 1 in distant metastasis of pancreatic ductal cancer. *Cancer Sci.* **2018**, *109*, 2520–2531. [CrossRef]
211. Zeng, L.S.; Yang, X.Z.; Wen, Y.F.; Mail, S.J.; Wang, M.H.; Zhang, M.Y.; Zheng, X.F.; Wang, H.Y. Overexpressed HDAC4 is associated with poor survival and promotes tumor progression in esophageal carcinoma. *Aging* **2016**, *8*, 1236–1249. [CrossRef]
212. Yu, Y.; Cao, F.; Yu, X.; Zhou, P.; Di, Q.; Lei, J.; Tai, Y.; Wu, H.; Li, X.; Wang, X.; et al. The expression of HDAC7 in cancerous gastric tissues is positively associated with distant metastasis and poor patient prognosis. *Clin. Transl. Oncol.* **2017**, *19*, 1045–1054. [CrossRef]
213. Lagger, G.; O'Carroll, D.; Rembold, M.; Khier, H.; Tischler, J.; Weitzer, G.; Schuettengruber, B.; Hauser, C.; Brunmeir, R.; Jenuwein, T.; et al. Essential function of histone deacetylase 1 in proliferation control and CDK inhibitor repression. *EMBO J.* **2002**, *21*, 2672–2681. [CrossRef]
214. Montgomery, R.L.; Davis, C.A.; Potthoff, M.J.; Haberland, M.; Fielitz, J.; Qi, X.; Hill, J.A.; Richardson, J.A.; Olson, E.N. Histone deacetylases 1 and 2 redundantly regulate cardiac morphogenesis, growth, and contractility. *Genes Dev.* **2007**, *21*, 1790–1802. [CrossRef]
215. Trivedi, C.M.; Luo, Y.; Yin, Z.; Zhang, M.; Zhu, W.; Wang, T.; Floss, T.; Goettlicher, M.; Noppinger, P.R.; Wurst, W.; et al. Hdac2 regulates the cardiac hypertrophic response by modulating Gsk3 beta activity. *Nat. Med.* **2007**, *13*, 324–331. [CrossRef]
216. Zhang, Y.; Kwon, S.; Yamaguchi, T.; Cubizolles, F.; Rousseaux, S.; Kneissel, M.; Cao, C.; Li, N.; Cheng, H.L.; Chua, K.; et al. Mice lacking histone deacetylase 6 have hyperacetylated tubulin but are viable and develop normally. *Mol. Cell. Biol.* **2008**, *28*, 1688–1701. [CrossRef]
217. Sun, L.; Telles, E.; Karl, M.; Cheng, F.; Luetteke, N.; Sotomayor, E.M.; Miller, R.H.; Seto, E. Loss of HDAC11 ameliorates clinical symptoms in a multiple sclerosis mouse model. *Life Sci. Alliance* **2018**, *1*, e201800039. [CrossRef]
218. Blander, G.; Guarente, L. The Sir2 family of protein deacetylases. *Annu. Rev. Biochem.* **2004**, *73*, 417–435. [CrossRef]
219. Schwer, B.; Verdin, E. Conserved metabolic regulatory functions of sirtuins. *Cell Metab.* **2008**, *7*, 104–112. [CrossRef]
220. Bordone, L.; Cohen, D.; Robinson, A.; Motta, M.C.; van Veen, E.; Czopik, A.; Steele, A.D.; Crowe, H.; Marmor, S.; Luo, J.; et al. SIRT1 transgenic mice show phenotypes resembling calorie restriction. *Aging Cell* **2007**, *6*, 759–767. [CrossRef]
221. Howitz, K.T.; Bitterman, K.J.; Cohen, H.Y.; Lamming, D.W.; Lavu, S.; Wood, J.G.; Zipkin, R.E.; Chung, P.; Kisielewski, A.; Zhang, L.L.; et al. Small molecule activators of sirtuins extend Saccharomyces cerevisiae lifespan. *Nature* **2003**, *425*, 191–196. [CrossRef] [PubMed]
222. Eckschlager, T.; Plch, J.; Stiborova, M.; Hrabeta, J. Histone Deacetylase Inhibitors as Anticancer Drugs. *Int. J. Mol. Sci.* **2017**, *18*, 1414. [CrossRef] [PubMed]
223. Chen, J.; Li, N.; Liu, B.; Ling, J.; Yang, W.; Pang, X.; Li, T. Pracinostat (SB939), a histone deacetylase inhibitor, suppresses breast cancer metastasis and growth by inactivating the IL-6/STAT3 signalling pathways. *Life Sci.* **2020**, *248*, 117469. [CrossRef] [PubMed]
224. Kusaczuk, M.; Bartoszewicz, M.; Cechowska-Pasko, M. Phenylbutyric Acid: Simple structure—Multiple effects. *Curr. Pharm. Des.* **2015**, *21*, 2147–2166. [CrossRef] [PubMed]
225. Kaletsch, K.; Pinkerneil, M.; Hoffmann, M.J.; Jaguva Vasudevan, A.A.; Wang, C.; Hansen, F.K.; Wiek, C.; Hanenberg, H.; Gertzen, C.; Gohlke, H.; et al. Effects of novel HDAC inhibitors on urothelial carcinoma cells. *Clin. Epigenet.* **2018**, *10*, 100. [CrossRef] [PubMed]
226. Duong, V.; Bret, C.; Altucci, L.; Mai, A.; Duraffourd, C.; Loubersac, J.; Harmand, P.O.; Bonnet, S.; Valente, S.; Maudelonde, T.; et al. Specific activity of class II histone deacetylases in human breast cancer cells. *Mol. Cancer Res.* **2008**, *6*, 1908–1919. [CrossRef] [PubMed]
227. Sawas, A.; Radeski, D.; O'Connor, O.A. Belinostat in patients with refractory or relapsed peripheral T-cell lymphoma: A perspective review. *Ther. Adv. Hematol.* **2015**, *6*, 202–208. [CrossRef]
228. Barbarotta, L.; Hurley, K. Romidepsin for the Treatment of Peripheral T-Cell Lymphoma. *J. Adv. Pract. Oncol.* **2015**, *6*, 22–36.
229. Baertsch, M.A.; Hillengass, J.; Blocka, J.; Schonland, S.; Hegenbart, U.; Goldschmidt, H.; Raab, M.S. Efficacy and tolerability of the histone deacetylase inhibitor panobinostat in clinical practice. *Hematol. Oncol.* **2018**, *36*, 210–216. [CrossRef]
230. Ghodke-Puranik, Y.; Thorn, C.F.; Lamba, J.K.; Leeder, J.S.; Song, W.; Birnbaum, A.K.; Altman, R.B.; Klein, T.E. Valproic acid pathway: Pharmacokinetics and pharmacodynamics. *Pharmacogenet. Genom.* **2013**, *23*, 236–241. [CrossRef]
231. Munster, P.; Marchion, D.; Bicaku, E.; Lacevic, M.; Kim, J.; Centeno, B.; Daud, A.; Neuger, A.; Minton, S.; Sullivan, D. Clinical and biological effects of valproic acid as a histone deacetylase inhibitor on tumor and surrogate tissues: Phase I/II trial of valproic acid and epirubicin/FEC. *Clin. Cancer Res.* **2009**, *15*, 2488–2496. [CrossRef]

232. Lee, P.; Murphy, B.; Miller, R.; Menon, V.; Banik, N.L.; Giglio, P.; Lindhorst, S.M.; Varma, A.K.; Vandergrift, W.A., 3rd; Patel, S.J.; et al. Mechanisms and clinical significance of histone deacetylase inhibitors: Epigenetic glioblastoma therapy. *Anticancer Res.* **2015**, *35*, 615–625.
233. Kim, Y.S.; Cha, H.; Kim, H.J.; Cho, J.M.; Kim, H.R. The Anti-Fibrotic Effects of CG-745, an HDAC Inhibitor, in Bleomycin and PHMG-Induced Mouse Models. *Molecules* **2019**, *24*, 2792. [CrossRef]
234. Wells, C.E.; Bhaskara, S.; Stengel, K.R.; Zhao, Y.; Sirbu, B.; Chagot, B.; Cortez, D.; Khabele, D.; Chazin, W.J.; Cooper, A.; et al. Inhibition of histone deacetylase 3 causes replication stress in cutaneous T cell lymphoma. *PLoS ONE* **2013**, *8*, e68915. [CrossRef]
235. Saito, S.; Zhuang, Y.; Shan, B.; Danchuk, S.; Luo, F.; Korfei, M.; Guenther, A.; Lasky, J.A. Tubastatin ameliorates pulmonary fibrosis by targeting the TGFbeta-PI3K-Akt pathway. *PLoS ONE* **2017**, *12*, e0186615. [CrossRef]
236. Deskin, B.; Yin, Q.; Zhuang, Y.; Saito, S.; Shan, B.; Lasky, J.A. Inhibition of HDAC6 Attenuates Tumor Growth of Non-Small Cell Lung Cancer. *Transl. Oncol.* **2020**, *13*, 135–145. [CrossRef]
237. Balasubramanian, S.; Ramos, J.; Luo, W.; Sirisawad, M.; Verner, E.; Buggy, J.J. A novel histone deacetylase 8 (HDAC8)-specific inhibitor PCI-34051 induces apoptosis in T-cell lymphomas. *Leukemia* **2008**, *22*, 1026–1034. [CrossRef]
238. Pulya, S.; Amin, S.A.; Adhikari, N.; Biswas, S.; Jha, T.; Ghosh, B. HDAC6 as privileged target in drug discovery: A perspective. *Pharmacol. Res.* **2021**, *163*, 105274. [CrossRef]
239. Hu, J.; Jing, H.; Lin, H. Sirtuin inhibitors as anticancer agents. *Future Med. Chem.* **2014**, *6*, 945–966. [CrossRef]
240. Zhou, Z.; Ma, T.; Zhu, Q.; Xu, Y.; Zha, X. Recent advances in inhibitors of sirtuin1/2: An update and perspective. *Future Med. Chem.* **2018**, *10*, 907–934. [CrossRef]
241. Kee, H.J.; Kook, H. Roles and targets of class I and IIa histone deacetylases in cardiac hypertrophy. *J. Biomed. Biotechnol.* **2011**, *2011*, 928326. [CrossRef] [PubMed]
242. Chelladurai, P.; Boucherat, O.; Stenmark, K.; Kracht, M.; Seeger, W.; Bauer, U.M.; Bonnet, S.; Pullamsetti, S.S. Targeting histone acetylation in pulmonary hypertension and right ventricular hypertrophy. *Br. J. Pharmacol.* **2021**, *178*, 54–71. [CrossRef] [PubMed]
243. Williams, S.M.; Golden-Mason, L.; Ferguson, B.S.; Schuetze, K.B.; Cavasin, M.A.; Demos-Davies, K.; Yeager, M.E.; Stenmark, K.R.; McKinsey, T.A. Class I HDACs regulate angiotensin II-dependent cardiac fibrosis via fibroblasts and circulating fibrocytes. *J. Mol. Cell. Cardiol.* **2014**, *67*, 112–125. [CrossRef] [PubMed]
244. Loh, Z.; Fitzsimmons, R.L.; Reid, R.C.; Ramnath, D.; Clouston, A.; Gupta, P.K.; Irvine, K.M.; Powell, E.E.; Schroder, K.; Stow, J.L.; et al. Inhibitors of class I histone deacetylases attenuate thioacetamide-induced liver fibrosis in mice by suppressing hepatic type 2 inflammation. *Br. J. Pharmacol.* **2019**, *176*, 3775–3790. [CrossRef]
245. Xiong, C.; Guan, Y.; Zhou, X.; Liu, L.; Zhuang, M.A.; Zhang, W.; Zhang, Y.; Masucci, M.V.; Bayliss, G.; Zhao, T.C.; et al. Selective inhibition of class IIa histone deacetylases alleviates renal fibrosis. *FASEB J.* **2019**, *33*, 8249–8262. [CrossRef]
246. Jones, D.L.; Haak, A.J.; Caporarello, N.; Choi, K.M.; Ye, Z.; Yan, H.; Varelas, X.; Ordog, T.; Ligresti, G.; Tschumperlin, D.J. TGFbeta-induced fibroblast activation requires persistent and targeted HDAC-mediated gene repression. *J. Cell Sci.* **2019**, *132*, jcs233486. [CrossRef]
247. Coward, W.R.; Watts, K.; Feghali-Bostwick, C.A.; Jenkins, G.; Pang, L. Repression of IP-10 by interactions between histone deacetylation and hypermethylation in idiopathic pulmonary fibrosis. *Mol. Cell. Biol.* **2010**, *30*, 2874–2886. [CrossRef]
248. Sanders, Y.Y.; Tollefsbol, T.O.; Varisco, B.M.; Hagood, J.S. Epigenetic regulation of thy-1 by histone deacetylase inhibitor in rat lung fibroblasts. *Am. J. Respir. Cell Mol. Biol.* **2011**, *45*, 16–23. [CrossRef]
249. Korfei, M.; Stelmaszek, D.; MacKenzie, B.; Skwarna, S.; Chillappagari, S.; Bach, A.C.; Ruppert, C.; Saito, S.; Mahavadi, P.; Klepetko, W.; et al. Comparison of the antifibrotic effects of the pan-histone deacetylase-inhibitor panobinostat versus the IPF-drug pirfenidone in fibroblasts from patients with idiopathic pulmonary fibrosis. *PLoS ONE* **2018**, *13*, e0207915. [CrossRef]
250. Guo, W.; Shan, B.; Klingsberg, R.C.; Qin, X.; Lasky, J.A. Abrogation of TGF-beta1-induced fibroblast-myofibroblast differentiation by histone deacetylase inhibition. *Am. J. Physiol. Lung Cell. Mol. Physiol.* **2009**, *297*, L864–L870. [CrossRef]
251. Ye, Q.; Li, Y.; Jiang, H.; Xiong, J.; Xu, J.; Qin, H.; Liu, B. Prevention of Pulmonary Fibrosis via Trichostatin A (TSA) in Bleomycin Induced Rats. *Sarcoidosis Vasc. Diffus. Lung Dis.* **2014**, *31*, 219–226.
252. Rao, S.S.; Zhang, X.Y.; Shi, M.J.; Xiao, Y.; Zhang, Y.Y.; Wang, Y.Y.; Zhang, C.Z.; Shao, S.J.; Liu, X.M.; Guo, B. Suberoylanilide hydroxamic acid attenuates paraquat-induced pulmonary fibrosis by preventing Smad7 from deacetylation in rats. *J. Thorac. Dis.* **2016**, *8*, 2485–2494. [CrossRef]
253. Glenisson, W.; Castronovo, V.; Waltregny, D. Histone deacetylase 4 is required for TGFbeta1-induced myofibroblastic differentiation. *Biochim. Biophys. Acta* **2007**, *1773*, 1572–1582. [CrossRef]
254. Kabel, A.M.; Omar, M.S.; Elmaaboud, M.A.A. Amelioration of bleomycin-induced lung fibrosis in rats by valproic acid and butyrate: Role of nuclear factor kappa-B, proinflammatory cytokines and oxidative stress. *Int. Immunopharmacol.* **2016**, *39*, 335–342. [CrossRef]
255. Jiang, X.; Fang, G.; Dong, L.; Jin, P.; Ding, L.; Zhang, H.; Fan, J.; Mao, S.; Fan, X.; Gong, Y.; et al. Chemical chaperone 4-phenylbutyric acid alleviates the aggregation of human familial pulmonary fibrosis-related mutant SP-A2 protein in part through effects on GRP78. *Biochim. Biophys. Acta Mol. Basis Dis.* **2018**, *1864*, 3546–3557. [CrossRef]
256. Zhao, H.; Qin, H.Y.; Cao, L.F.; Chen, Y.H.; Tan, Z.X.; Zhang, C.; Xu, D.X. Phenylbutyric acid inhibits epithelial-mesenchymal transition during bleomycin-induced lung fibrosis. *Toxicol. Lett.* **2015**, *232*, 213–220. [CrossRef]
257. Sanders, Y.Y.; Liu, H.; Scruggs, A.M.; Duncan, S.R.; Huang, S.K.; Thannickal, V.J. Epigenetic Regulation of Caveolin-1 Gene Expression in Lung Fibroblasts. *Am. J. Respir. Cell Mol. Biol.* **2017**, *56*, 50–61. [CrossRef]

258. Chen, F.; Gao, Q.; Zhang, L.; Ding, Y.; Wang, H.; Cao, W. Inhibiting HDAC3 (Histone Deacetylase 3) Aberration and the Resultant Nrf2 (Nuclear Factor Erythroid-Derived 2-Related Factor-2) Repression Mitigates Pulmonary Fibrosis. *Hypertension* **2021**, *78*, e15–e25. [CrossRef]
259. Wilborn, J.; Crofford, L.J.; Burdick, M.D.; Kunkel, S.L.; Strieter, R.M.; Peters-Golden, M. Cultured lung fibroblasts isolated from patients with idiopathic pulmonary fibrosis have a diminished capacity to synthesize prostaglandin E2 and to express cyclooxygenase-2. *J. Clin. Investig.* **1995**, *95*, 1861–1868. [CrossRef]
260. Honda, S.; Lewis, Z.A.; Shimada, K.; Fischle, W.; Sack, R.; Selker, E.U. Heterochromatin protein 1 forms distinct complexes to direct histone deacetylation and DNA methylation. *Nat. Struct. Mol. Biol.* **2012**, *19*, 471–477. [CrossRef]
261. O'Shea, J.J.; Kanno, Y.; Chen, X.; Levy, D.E. Cell signaling. Stat acetylation—A key facet of cytokine signaling? *Science* **2005**, *307*, 217–218. [CrossRef]
262. Gupta, M.; Han, J.J.; Stenson, M.; Wellik, L.; Witzig, T.E. Regulation of STAT3 by histone deacetylase-3 in diffuse large B-cell lymphoma: Implications for therapy. *Leukemia* **2012**, *26*, 1356–1364. [CrossRef]
263. Cotto, M.; Cabanillas, F.; Tirado, M.; Garcia, M.V.; Pacheco, E. Epigenetic therapy of lymphoma using histone deacetylase inhibitors. *Clin. Transl. Oncol.* **2010**, *12*, 401–409. [CrossRef]
264. Tang, S.; Cheng, B.; Zhe, N.; Ma, D.; Xu, J.; Li, X.; Guo, Y.; Wu, W.; Wang, J. Histone deacetylase inhibitor BG45-mediated HO-1 expression induces apoptosis of multiple myeloma cells by the JAK2/STAT3 pathway. *Anticancer Drugs* **2018**, *29*, 61–74. [CrossRef]
265. Barter, M.J.; Pybus, L.; Litherland, G.J.; Rowan, A.D.; Clark, I.M.; Edwards, D.R.; Cawston, T.E.; Young, D.A. HDAC-mediated control of ERK- and PI3K-dependent TGF-beta-induced extracellular matrix-regulating genes. *Matrix Biol.* **2010**, *29*, 602–612. [CrossRef]
266. Jaeger, B.; Schupp, J.C.; Plappert, L.; Terwolbeck, O.; Kayser, G.; Engelhard, P.; Adams, T.S.; Zweigerdt, R.; Kempf, H.; Lienenklaus, S.; et al. Airway Basal Cells show a dedifferentiated KRT17^{high} Phenotype and promote Fibrosis in Idiopathic Pulmonary Fibrosis. *bioRxiv* **2020**. [CrossRef]
267. Paroni, G.; Mizzau, M.; Henderson, C.; Del Sal, G.; Schneider, C.; Brancolini, C. Caspase-dependent regulation of histone deacetylase 4 nuclear-cytoplasmic shuttling promotes apoptosis. *Mol. Biol. Cell* **2004**, *15*, 2804–2818. [CrossRef]
268. Scott, F.L.; Fuchs, G.J.; Boyd, S.E.; Denault, J.B.; Hawkins, C.J.; Dequiedt, F.; Salvesen, G.S. Caspase-8 cleaves histone deacetylase 7 and abolishes its transcription repressor function. *J. Biol. Chem.* **2008**, *283*, 19499–19510. [CrossRef]
269. Meja, K.K.; Rajendrasozhan, S.; Adenuga, D.; Biswas, S.K.; Sundar, I.K.; Spooner, G.; Marwick, J.A.; Chakravarty, P.; Fletcher, D.; Whittaker, P.; et al. Curcumin restores corticosteroid function in monocytes exposed to oxidants by maintaining HDAC2. *Am. J. Respir. Cell Mol. Biol.* **2008**, *39*, 312–323. [CrossRef]
270. Osoata, G.O.; Yamamura, S.; Ito, M.; Vuppusetty, C.; Adcock, I.M.; Barnes, P.J.; Ito, K. Nitration of distinct tyrosine residues causes inactivation of histone deacetylase 2. *Biochem. Biophys. Res. Commun.* **2009**, *384*, 366–371. [CrossRef]
271. Min, T.; Bodas, M.; Mazur, S.; Vij, N. Critical role of proteostasis-imbalance in pathogenesis of COPD and severe emphysema. *J. Mol. Med.* **2011**, *89*, 577–593. [CrossRef] [PubMed]
272. Li, M.; Zheng, Y.; Yuan, H.; Liu, Y.; Wen, X. Effects of dynamic changes in histone acetylation and deacetylase activity on pulmonary fibrosis. *Int. Immunopharmacol.* **2017**, *52*, 272–280. [CrossRef] [PubMed]
273. Yuan, H.; Jiao, L.; Yu, N.; Duan, H.; Yu, Y.; Bai, Y. Histone Deacetylase 3-Mediated Inhibition of microRNA-19a-3p Facilitates the Development of Rheumatoid Arthritis-Associated Interstitial Lung Disease. *Front. Physiol.* **2020**, *11*, 549656. [CrossRef] [PubMed]
274. Simonsson, M.; Heldin, C.H.; Ericsson, J.; Gronroos, E. The balance between acetylation and deacetylation controls Smad7 stability. *J. Biol. Chem.* **2005**, *280*, 21797–21803. [CrossRef] [PubMed]
275. Davies, E.R.; Haitchi, H.M.; Thatcher, T.H.; Sime, P.J.; Kottmann, R.M.; Ganesan, A.; Packham, G.; O'Reilly, K.M.; Davies, D.E. Spiruchostatin A inhibits proliferation and differentiation of fibroblasts from patients with pulmonary fibrosis. *Am. J. Respir. Cell Mol. Biol.* **2012**, *46*, 687–694. [CrossRef] [PubMed]
276. Kramer, O.H.; Zhu, P.; Ostendorff, H.P.; Golebiewski, M.; Tiefenbach, J.; Peters, M.A.; Brill, B.; Groner, B.; Bach, I.; Heinzel, T.; et al. The histone deacetylase inhibitor valproic acid selectively induces proteasomal degradation of HDAC2. *EMBO J.* **2003**, *22*, 3411–3420. [CrossRef]
277. Ni, L.; Wang, L.; Yao, C.; Ni, Z.; Liu, F.; Gong, C.; Zhu, X.; Yan, X.; Watowich, S.S.; Lee, D.A.; et al. The histone deacetylase inhibitor valproic acid inhibits NKG2D expression in natural killer cells through suppression of STAT3 and HDAC3. *Sci. Rep.* **2017**, *7*, 45266. [CrossRef]
278. Noguchi, S.; Eitoku, M.; Moriya, S.; Kondo, S.; Kiyosawa, H.; Watanabe, T.; Suganuma, N. Regulation of Gene Expression by Sodium Valproate in Epithelial-to-Mesenchymal Transition. *Lung* **2015**, *193*, 691–700. [CrossRef]
279. Kamio, K.; Azuma, A.; Usuki, J.; Matsuda, K.; Inomata, M.; Nishijima, N.; Itakura, S.; Hayashi, H.; Kashiwada, T.; Kokuho, N.; et al. XPLN is modulated by HDAC inhibitors and negatively regulates SPARC expression by targeting mTORC2 in human lung fibroblasts. *Pulm. Pharmacol. Ther.* **2017**, *44*, 61–69. [CrossRef]
280. Rubio, K.; Singh, I.; Dobersch, S.; Sarvari, P.; Gunther, S.; Cordero, J.; Mehta, A.; Wujak, L.; Cabrera-Fuentes, H.; Chao, C.M.; et al. Inactivation of nuclear histone deacetylases by EP300 disrupts the MiCEE complex in idiopathic pulmonary fibrosis. *Nat. Commun.* **2019**, *10*, 2229. [CrossRef]
281. Petkova, D.K.; Clelland, C.A.; Ronan, J.E.; Lewis, S.; Knox, A.J. Reduced expression of cyclooxygenase (COX) in idiopathic pulmonary fibrosis and sarcoidosis. *Histopathology* **2003**, *43*, 381–386. [CrossRef]

282. Hecker, L.; Logsdon, N.J.; Kurundkar, D.; Kurundkar, A.; Bernard, K.; Hock, T.; Meldrum, E.; Sanders, Y.Y.; Thannickal, V.J. Reversal of persistent fibrosis in aging by targeting Nox4-Nrf2 redox imbalance. *Sci. Transl. Med.* **2014**, *6*, 231ra47. [CrossRef]
283. Waltregny, D.; De Leval, L.; Glenisson, W.; Ly Tran, S.; North, B.J.; Bellahcene, A.; Weidle, U.; Verdin, E.; Castronovo, V. Expression of histone deacetylase 8, a class I histone deacetylase, is restricted to cells showing smooth muscle differentiation in normal human tissues. *Am. J. Pathol.* **2004**, *165*, 553–564. [CrossRef]
284. Waltregny, D.; Glenisson, W.; Tran, S.L.; North, B.J.; Verdin, E.; Colige, A.; Castronovo, V. Histone deacetylase HDAC8 associates with smooth muscle alpha-actin and is essential for smooth muscle cell contractility. *FASEB J.* **2005**, *19*, 966–968. [CrossRef]
285. Borok, Z.; Horie, M.; Flodby, P.; Wang, H.; Liu, Y.; Ganesh, S.; Firth, A.L.; Minoo, P.; Li, C.; Beers, M.F.; et al. Grp78 Loss in Epithelial Progenitors Reveals an Age-linked Role for Endoplasmic Reticulum Stress in Pulmonary Fibrosis. *Am. J. Respir. Crit. Care Med.* **2020**, *201*, 198–211. [CrossRef]
286. Jing, X.; Sun, W.; Yang, X.; Huang, H.; Wang, P.; Luo, Q.; Xia, S.; Fang, C.; Zhang, Q.; Guo, J.; et al. CCAAT/enhancer-binding protein (C/EBP) homologous protein promotes alveolar epithelial cell senescence via the nuclear factor-kappa B pathway in pulmonary fibrosis. *Int. J. Biochem. Cell Biol.* **2021**, *143*, 106142. [CrossRef]
287. Yao, C.; Carraro, G.; Konda, B.; Guan, X.; Mizuno, T.; Chiba, N.; Kostelny, M.; Kurkciyan, A.; David, G.; McQualter, J.L.; et al. Sin3a regulates epithelial progenitor cell fate during lung development. *Development* **2017**, *144*, 2618–2628. [CrossRef]
288. Wang, Y.; Tian, Y.; Morley, M.P.; Lu, M.M.; Demayo, F.J.; Olson, E.N.; Morrisey, E.E. Development and regeneration of Sox2+ endoderm progenitors are regulated by a Hdac1/2-Bmp4/Rb1 regulatory pathway. *Dev. Cell* **2013**, *24*, 345–358. [CrossRef]
289. Wang, Y.; Frank, D.B.; Morley, M.P.; Zhou, S.; Wang, Y.; Lu, M.M.; Lazar, M.A.; Morrisey, E.E. HDAC3-Dependent Epigenetic Pathway Controls Lung Alveolar Epithelial Cell Remodeling and Spreading via miR-17-92 and TGF-beta Signaling Regulation. *Dev. Cell* **2016**, *36*, 303–315. [CrossRef]
290. Guo, W.; Saito, S.; Sanchez, C.G.; Zhuang, Y.; Gongora Rosero, R.E.; Shan, B.; Luo, F.; Lasky, J.A. TGF-beta1 stimulates HDAC4 nucleus-to-cytoplasm translocation and NADPH oxidase 4-derived reactive oxygen species in normal human lung fibroblasts. *Am. J. Physiol. Lung Cell Mol. Physiol.* **2017**, *312*, L936–L944. [CrossRef]
291. Zhang, C.L.; McKinsey, T.A.; Chang, S.; Antos, C.L.; Hill, J.A.; Olson, E.N. Class II histone deacetylases act as signal-responsive repressors of cardiac hypertrophy. *Cell* **2002**, *110*, 479–488. [CrossRef]
292. Davis, F.J.; Gupta, M.; Camoretti-Mercado, B.; Schwartz, R.J.; Gupta, M.P. Calcium/calmodulin-dependent protein kinase activates serum response factor transcription activity by its dissociation from histone deacetylase, HDAC4. Implications in cardiac muscle gene regulation during hypertrophy. *J. Biol. Chem.* **2003**, *278*, 20047–20058. [CrossRef]
293. Backs, J.; Song, K.; Bezprozvannaya, S.; Chang, S.; Olson, E.N. CaM kinase II selectively signals to histone deacetylase 4 during cardiomyocyte hypertrophy. *J. Clin. Investig.* **2006**, *116*, 1853–1864. [CrossRef]
294. Kang, D.H.; Yin, G.N.; Choi, M.J.; Song, K.M.; Ghatak, K.; Minh, N.N.; Kwon, M.H.; Seong, D.H.; Ryu, J.K.; Suh, J.K. Silencing Histone Deacetylase 7 Alleviates Transforming Growth Factor-beta1-Induced Profibrotic Responses in Fibroblasts Derived from Peyronie's Plaque. *World J. Mens Health* **2018**, *36*, 139–146. [CrossRef]
295. Hemmatazad, H.; Rodrigues, H.M.; Maurer, B.; Brentano, F.; Pileckyte, M.; Distler, J.H.; Gay, R.E.; Michel, B.A.; Gay, S.; Huber, L.C.; et al. Histone deacetylase 7, a potential target for the antifibrotic treatment of systemic sclerosis. *Arthritis Rheum.* **2009**, *60*, 1519–1529. [CrossRef]
296. Hua, H.S.; Wen, H.C.; Weng, C.M.; Lee, H.S.; Chen, B.C.; Lin, C.H. Histone deacetylase 7 mediates endothelin-1-induced connective tissue growth factor expression in human lung fibroblasts through p300 and activator protein-1 activation. *J. Biomed. Sci.* **2021**, *28*, 38. [CrossRef]
297. Sarvari, P.; Chelladurai, P.; Korfei, M.; Olson, E.; Gunther, A.; Seeger, W.; Pullamsetti, S.S. The role of histone deacetylase 9 in idiopathic pulmonary fibrosis. *Am. J. Respir. Crit. Care Med.* **2017**, *195*, A2396.
298. Mannaerts, I.; Eysackers, N.; Onyema, O.O.; Van Beneden, K.; Valente, S.; Mai, A.; Odenthal, M.; van Grunsven, L.A. Class II HDAC inhibition hampers hepatic stellate cell activation by induction of microRNA-29. *PLoS ONE* **2013**, *8*, e55786. [CrossRef] [PubMed]
299. Gu, S.; Liu, Y.; Zhu, B.; Ding, K.; Yao, T.P.; Chen, F.; Zhan, L.; Xu, P.; Ehrlich, M.; Liang, T.; et al. Loss of alpha-Tubulin Acetylation Is Associated with TGF-beta-induced Epithelial-Mesenchymal Transition. *J. Biol. Chem.* **2016**, *291*, 5396–5405. [CrossRef] [PubMed]
300. Lam, H.C.; Cloonan, S.M.; Bhashyam, A.R.; Haspel, J.A.; Singh, A.; Sathirapongsasuti, J.F.; Cervo, M.; Yao, H.; Chung, A.L.; Mizumura, K.; et al. Histone deacetylase 6-mediated selective autophagy regulates COPD-associated cilia dysfunction. *J. Clin. Investig.* **2013**, *123*, 5212–5230. [CrossRef] [PubMed]
301. Kathiriya, J.J.; Wang, C.; Zhou, M.; Brumwell, A.; Cassandras, M.; Le Saux, C.J.; Cohen, M.; Alysandratos, K.D.; Wang, B.; Wolters, P.; et al. Human alveolar type 2 epithelium transdifferentiates into metaplastic KRT5(+) basal cells. *Nat. Cell Biol.* **2022**, *24*, 10–23. [CrossRef]
302. Korfei, M.; Schmitt, S.; Ruppert, C.; Henneke, I.; Markart, P.; Loeh, B.; Mahavadi, P.; Wygrecka, M.; Klepetko, W.; Fink, L.; et al. Comparative proteomic analysis of lung tissue from patients with idiopathic pulmonary fibrosis (IPF) and lung transplant donor lungs. *J. Proteome Res.* **2011**, *10*, 2185–2205. [CrossRef]
303. Ganai, S.A. Panobinostat: The Small Molecule Metalloenzyme Inhibitor with Marvelous Anticancer Activity. *Curr. Top. Med. Chem.* **2016**, *16*, 427–434. [CrossRef]
304. Frew, A.J.; Johnstone, R.W.; Bolden, J.E. Enhancing the apoptotic and therapeutic effects of HDAC inhibitors. *Cancer Lett.* **2009**, *280*, 125–133. [CrossRef]

305. Larsson, P.; Alwis, I.; Niego, B.; Sashindranath, M.; Fogelstrand, P.; Wu, M.C.; Glise, L.; Magnusson, M.; Daglas, M.; Bergh, N.; et al. Valproic acid selectively increases vascular endothelial tissue-type plasminogen activator production and reduces thrombus formation in the mouse. *J. Thromb. Haemost.* **2016**, *14*, 2496–2508. [CrossRef]
306. Saluveer, O.; Larsson, P.; Ridderstrale, W.; Hrafnkelsdottir, T.J.; Jern, S.; Bergh, N. Profibrinolytic effect of the epigenetic modifier valproic acid in man. *PLoS ONE* **2014**, *9*, e107582. [CrossRef]
307. Larsson, P.; Ulfhammer, E.; Magnusson, M.; Bergh, N.; Lunke, S.; El-Osta, A.; Medcalf, R.L.; Svensson, P.A.; Karlsson, L.; Jern, S. Role of histone acetylation in the stimulatory effect of valproic acid on vascular endothelial tissue-type plasminogen activator expression. *PLoS ONE* **2012**, *7*, e31573. [CrossRef]
308. Svennerholm, K.; Haney, M.; Biber, B.; Ulfhammer, E.; Saluveer, O.; Larsson, P.; Omerovic, E.; Jern, S.; Bergh, N. Histone deacetylase inhibition enhances tissue plasminogen activator release capacity in atherosclerotic man. *PLoS ONE* **2015**, *10*, e0121196.
309. Jiang, P.; Gil de Rubio, R.; Hrycaj, S.M.; Gurczynski, S.J.; Riemondy, K.A.; Moore, B.B.; Omary, M.B.; Ridge, K.M.; Zemans, R.L. Ineffectual Type 2-to-Type 1 Alveolar Epithelial Cell Differentiation in Idiopathic Pulmonary Fibrosis: Persistence of the KRT8(hi) Transitional State. *Am. J. Respir. Crit. Care Med.* **2020**, *201*, 1443–1447. [CrossRef]
310. Strunz, M.; Simon, L.M.; Ansari, M.; Kathiriya, J.J.; Angelidis, I.; Mayr, C.H.; Tsidiridis, G.; Lange, M.; Mattner, L.F.; Yee, M.; et al. Alveolar regeneration through a Krt8+ transitional stem cell state that persists in human lung fibrosis. *Nat. Commun.* **2020**, *11*, 3559. [CrossRef]
311. Pang, M.; Kothapally, J.; Mao, H.; Tolbert, E.; Ponnusamy, M.; Chin, Y.E.; Zhuang, S. Inhibition of histone deacetylase activity attenuates renal fibroblast activation and interstitial fibrosis in obstructive nephropathy. *Am. J. Physiol. Ren. Physiol.* **2009**, *297*, F996–F1005. [CrossRef] [PubMed]
312. Singh, A.; Patel, P.; Jageshwar; Patel, V.K.; Jain, D.K.; Kamal, M.; Rajak, H. The Safety, Efficacy and Therapeutic Potential of Histone Deacetylase Inhibitors with Special Reference to Panobinostat in Gastrointestinal Tumors: A Review of Preclinical and Clinical Studies. *Curr. Cancer Drug Targets* **2018**, *18*, 720–736. [CrossRef] [PubMed]
313. Wawruszak, A.; Borkiewicz, L.; Okon, E.; Kukula-Koch, W.; Afshan, S.; Halasa, M. Vorinostat (SAHA) and Breast Cancer: An Overview. *Cancers* **2021**, *13*, 4700. [CrossRef]
314. Claveria-Cabello, A.; Colyn, L.; Arechederra, M.; Urman, J.M.; Berasain, C.; Avila, M.A.; Fernandez-Barrena, M.G. Epigenetics in Liver Fibrosis: Could HDACs be a Therapeutic Target? *Cells* **2020**, *9*, 2321. [CrossRef] [PubMed]
315. Bajbouj, K.; Al-Ali, A.; Ramakrishnan, R.K.; Saber-Ayad, M.; Hamid, Q. Histone Modification in NSCLC: Molecular Mechanisms and Therapeutic Targets. *Int. J. Mol. Sci.* **2021**, *22*, 11701. [CrossRef]
316. Hervouet, E. The Promising Role of New Generation HDACis in Anti-Cancer Therapies. *EBioMedicine* **2018**, *32*, 6–7. [CrossRef]
317. Weichert, W.; Roske, A.; Niesporek, S.; Noske, A.; Buckendahl, A.C.; Dietel, M.; Gekeler, V.; Boehm, M.; Beckers, T.; Denkert, C. Class I histone deacetylase expression has independent prognostic impact in human colorectal cancer: Specific role of class I histone deacetylases in vitro and in vivo. *Clin. Cancer Res.* **2008**, *14*, 1669–1677. [CrossRef]
318. Khabele, D. The therapeutic potential of class I selective histone deacetylase inhibitors in ovarian cancer. *Front. Oncol.* **2014**, *4*, 111. [CrossRef]
319. King, T.E., Jr.; Schwarz, M.I.; Brown, K.; Tooze, J.A.; Colby, T.V.; Waldron, J.A., Jr.; Flint, A.; Thurlbeck, W.; Cherniack, R.M. Idiopathic pulmonary fibrosis: Relationship between histopathologic features and mortality. *Am. J. Respir. Crit. Care Med.* **2001**, *164*, 1025–1032. [CrossRef]

Article

Pulmonary Fibroelastotic Remodelling Revisited

Peter Braubach [1,2,*], Christopher Werlein [1,2], Stijn E. Verleden [3,4,5], Isabell Maerzke [1], Jens Gottlieb [2,6], Gregor Warnecke [2,7], Sabine Dettmer [2,8], Florian Laenger [1,2] and Danny Jonigk [1,2]

1. Institute for Pathology, Hannover Medical School, 30625 Hannover, Germany; Werlein.Christopher@mh-hannover.de (C.W.); maerzke.isabell@mh-hannover.de (I.M.); laenger.florian@mh-hannover.de (F.L.); jonigk.danny@mh-hannover.de (D.J.)
2. German Center for Lung Research (DZL), Biomedical Research in Endstage and Obstructive Lung Disease Hannover (BREATH), 30625 Hannover, Germany; gottlieb.jens@mh-hannover.de (J.G.); Warnecke.Gregor@mh-hannover.de (G.W.); dettmer.sabine@mh-hannover.de (S.D.)
3. Department of ASTARC, University of Antwerp, 2610 Wilrijk, Belgium; Stijn.Verleden@uantwerpen.be
4. Respiratory Division, University Hospital Antwerp, 2650 Edegem, Belgium
5. Division of Thoracic and Vasculature Surgery, University Hospital Antwerp, 2650 Edegem, Belgium
6. Department of Respiratory Medicine, Hannover Medical School, 30625 Hannover, Germany
7. Department of Cardiothoracic and Transplant and Vascular Surgery, Hannover Medical School, 30625 Hannover, Germany
8. Department of Radiology, Hannover Medical School, 30625 Hannover, Germany
* Correspondence: Braubach.Peter@mh-hannover.de

Abstract: Pulmonary fibroelastotic remodelling occurs within a broad spectrum of diseases with vastly divergent outcomes. So far, no comprehensive terminology has been established to adequately address and distinguish histomorphological and clinical entities. We aimed to describe the range of fibroelastotic changes and define stringent histological criteria. Furthermore, we wanted to clarify the corresponding terminology in order to distinguish clinically relevant variants of pulmonary fibroelastotic remodelling. We revisited pulmonary specimens with fibroelastotic remodelling sampled during the last ten years at a large European lung transplant centre. Consensus-based definitions of specific variants of fibroelastotic changes were developed on the basis of well-defined cases and applied. Systematic evaluation was performed in a steps-wise algorithm, first identifying the fulcrum of the respective lesions, and then assessing the morphological changes, their distribution and the features of the adjacent parenchyma. We defined typical alveolar fibro-elastosis as collagenous effacement of the alveolar spaces with accompanying hyper-elastosis of the remodelled and paucicellular alveolar walls, independent of the underlying disease in 45 cases. Clinically, this pattern could be seen in (idiopathic) pleuroparenchymal fibro-elastosis, interstitial lung disease with concomitant alveolar fibro-elastosis, following hematopoietic stem cell and lung transplantation, autoimmune disease, radio-/chemotherapy, and pulmonary apical caps. Novel in-transit and activity stages of fibroelastotic remodelling were identified. For the first time, we present a comprehensive definition of fibroelastotic remodelling, its anatomic distribution, and clinical associations, thereby providing a basis for stringent patient stratification and prediction of outcome.

Keywords: interstitial fibrosis; lung; alveolar fibroelastosis

1. Introduction

Fibroelastotic remodelling (FER) is a common morphological injury pattern occurring in a number of different clinical settings [1–3]. Within the broad scope of FER, distinct patterns with slightly diverging histopathological features and clinical phenotypes are recognized. A rare entity of interstitial lung disease (ILD) with a predominant pattern of FER, Pleuroparenchymal fibro-elastosis (PPFE), was first implemented by Frankel et al. in 2004 [4] and was officially recognized by the American Thoracic Society in 2013 [5]. PPFE often occurs idiopathically without a known trigger (iPPFE), but there are also cases of secondary PPFE linked to autoimmune disorders (AID). Moreover, PPFE-like patterns of FER have also been observed following radio- and/or chemotherapy [6] as well as after lung (LTX) and hematopoietic stem cell transplantation (HSCT) [7–11]. All these manifestations share a rather poor prognosis and similar histological features—a fibrous obliteration of the alveolar airspaces associated with preservation and hyper-elastosis of the embedded alveolar septa [6,12]. This histologic pattern of remodelling has been addressed by a variety of terms, including airway-cantered fibro-elastosis [13], intra-alveolar fibrosis with elastosis [14] or (intra)alveolar fibro-elastosis (IAFE, AFE) [15,16]. Moreover, it has also been recognized that the so-called "pulmonary apical caps" (PAC) of the upper lobes share strikingly similar histologic features with PPFE, but usually remain asymptomatic and are often discovered incidentally in resection or autopsy specimens [17]. A comprehensive review of the clinical manifestations of FER and the associated clinical settings is given by Chua et al. (2019) [18] which also attempts to separate clinical and pathological terminology; however, no clearly applicable minimum requirements for the histopathological diagnosis of AFE have been defined thus far. This lack of clear separation and of clinical features and nomenclature on the one hand and morphological terminology, on the other hand hampers the scientific and clinical dialogue. For instance, the clinical term PPFE is still used widely in current studies to describe the histologic pattern of FER [3,19]. In this study, we have reviewed cases with well-defined AFE pattern from the archive of Europe's largest lung-transplant centre and systematically analysed the histological features and distribution of the FER in order to i. define stringent histological criteria, ii. clarify the corresponding terminology and iii. to distinguish relevant variants of FER.

2. Materials and Methods

We identified pulmonary specimens with FER in the archives of the Institute of Pathology at Hannover Medical School, sampled within the last ten years. To avoid conflicting terms we used stringent definitions for clinical and histological nomenclature (see Table 1).

For histologic evaluation, sections with approximately 1 μm thickness were cut from the formalin-fixed and paraffin-embedded archival tissue blocks and stained with haematoxylin and eosin (HE), periodic acid-Schiff (PAS) and elastic van Gieson (EvG) stains.

Table 1. Terminology on fibroelastotic remodelling.

Term	Description
Fibroelastotic remodelling (FER)	Unspecific term describing matrix predominant structural changes in lung parenchyma with loss of original tissue replaced by collagenous and elastic fibers.
Alveolar fibroelastosis (AFE)	Specific histological pattern of FER characterized by collagenous effacement of the alveolar spaces with accompanying hyperelastosis of the remodelled and paucicellular alveolar walls.
Idiopathic pleuroparenchymal fibroelastosis (iPPFE)	A form of interstitial lung disease (ILD) characterized by typical clinical and radiological presentation and of unknown cause. Histologically predominant AFE pattern in subpleural, paraseptal and parabronchial distribution.
PPFE-like disease	FER, with clinical presentation similar to PPFE, AFE histology and known underlying disease/lung injury. Specifically PPFE secondary to autoimmune disease (AID), - alloimmune triggers (Chronic lung allograft dysfunction after lung transplantation, pulmonary fibrosis after hematopoetic stem cell transplantation) and radio-/chemotherapy etc.
ILD with concomitant AFE	Interstitial lung disease of any other type (e.g., usual interstitial pneumonia, nonspecific interstitial pneumonia) with AFE as a minor component.
Pulmonary apical cap (PAC)	Localized FER of the upper lobe with AFE histology and benign clinical course.

To avoid conflicting terms we stringently use definitions for clinical and histological nomenclature.

To define a basis for systematic evaluation, 14 PPFE and PPFE-like as well as 12 PAC cases were systematically reviewed to develop a reference catalogue of morphological features. Subsequently, all included cases included were systematically evaluated and the observed morphological features methodically catalogued.

We defined typical AFE as i. collagenous effacement of the alveolar spaces with ii. accompanying hyperelastosis of the remodelled and paucicellular alveolar walls characterized by fourfold thickening of the elastic layer when compared with normal alveoli and iii. at least 4 connected alveoli showing these changes.

The systematic evaluation was performed by two trained pulmonary pathologists (P.B. and C.W. or I.M.) in four steps on a dual-observer transmitted light microscope (Olympus BX43) equipped with 2×–40× objective lenses. First, areas of typical AFE were identified, their size (in n alveoli) estimated and the morphological features within the typical AFE regions assessed. In steps two and three, morphological features directly adjacent to the typical AFE and their respective distribution in the anatomical compartments of the lung were evaluated. Finally, the cases were re-evaluated for pathological changes in the lung but not in direct spatial association with the AFE. The consensus of both observers was recorded for future analysis. In case of disagreement cases were discussed with two consulting pulmonary pathologists (D.J. and F.L.). The study was in accordance with the regulation of the ethics committee of the Hannover Medical School (ethics vote no. 2050−2013).

The last available in vivo CT before resection was assessed by a single trained thoracic radiologist to assess if radiologic changes were completely conclusive with the histological changes, were partly conclusive or inconclusive.

3. Results

We evaluated a total of 45 cases. In detail, the PPFE collective consisted of 31 cases. Of these, 6 were iPPFE and 25 had PPFE-like pulmonary fibrosis due to other causes: with underlying AID ($n = 2$), after radio-/chemotherapy ($n = 2$), chronic allograft dysfunction (CLAD) after LTX ($n = 12$) and following HSCT ($n = 7$). Two cases had AFE pattern as a minor companion pattern in other ILD.

The PAC collective consisted of samples from a total of 14 patients; of these, 12 were incidental PAC (surgery due to unrelated indications) and 2 patients had undergone primary resection due to an unclear pulmonary apical mass.

The patients were between 9 and 61 years old (See Table 2). Detailed patient information and the diagnoses of our collective are shown in Supplementary Table S1.

Table 2. Patient collective.

Group		n	Age (Range)	Ratio m/f
	PAC	14	57.3 (23–77)	5/9
	iPPFE	6	52 (24–61)	3/3
PPFE-like disease	CLAD	12	45 (23–59)	4/8
	HSCT	7	24.6 (9–57)	5/2
	AID	2	44.5 (44–45)	1/1
	RCTX	2	55 (52–58)	0/2
	ILD	2	48 (47–49)	0/2

Characteristics of patient population in the investigated groups of patients with pulmonary apical caps (PAC), idiopathic pleuropulmonary fibroelastosis (iPPFE) and PPFE-like disease comprising of chronic lung allograft dysfunction (CLAD) after lung transplantation, pulmonary fibrosis after hematopoetic stem cell transplantation (HSCT), linked to autoimmune disease (AID) or radio-/chemotherapy (RCTX) and interstitial lung disease (ILD) with concomitant alveolar fibroelastosis pattern. The number of cases analysed (n), the age of the patient in years (mean and range) at the time of surgical intervention and the ratio of males (m) to females (f).

After a review of representative AFE cases, we could identify different patterns within typical AFE and a range of common changes in direct proximity to the AFE lesions (Table 3).

Table 3. Histological patterns.

Pattern	Description
Fibroelastic interstitial expansion	Expanded alveolar septa with increased interstitial elastic and collagen fibres—often but not always—with emphysematous changes.
Normal lung parenchyma	AFE lesions can show a direct and abrupt transition to morphologically (mostly) non-remodelled lung parenchyma.
Incomplete alveolar fibrosis	Distinct hyperelastosis of the alveolar septa, similar to typical AFE. However the fibrous obliteration of the alveolar lumen is incomplete and small remnant spaces, lined by cuboidal or flat epithelium remain.
Pulmonary arterial sclerosis	Expansion of media and intima of pre-capillary pulmonary arteries.
Pleural fibrosis	Fibrotic expansion of the visceral pleura, usually with only scant cellularity.
Emphysema	Loss of alveolar septa with irreversible widening of the airspaces.
Bronchiolitis obliterans	Fibrous obliteration of small pre-terminal airways
Fibroelastotic scar	Irregularly distributed elastic and collagenous fibers without preservation of the original alveolar outlines.
Macrophage aggregates	Dominant aggregates of intraalveolar macrophages, filling upt the airspaces completely, comparable to those seen in the desquamative interstitial pneumonia (DIP) pattern.
Cholesterol granulomas	Aggregates of multinucleated macrophages with slit-like impressions of crystalline material.
Nonspecific interstitial pneumonia (NSIP)	Widening of alveolar septa. To qualify as NSIP vs. fibroelastic interstitial expansion (see above), the remodelling was required to extend uniformly throughout the lung without a gradient towards the areas of typical AFE.
Organizing pneumonia (OP), acute fibrinous organizing pneumonia (AFOP)	Aggregates of intraalveolar connective tissue (OP) or intermixed fibrin and connective tissue (AFOP) with variable, often prominent infiltration by inflammatory cells.
Myogenic metaplasia	Scattered strands of smooth muscle fibers, not associated with a bronchus or a blood vessel.
Architectural distortion	Complete loss of alveolar architecture with cystic airspace remodelling and metaplastic epithelium, as seen in usual interstitial pneumonia (UIP) pattern of lung fibrosis.

Patterns in direct spatial association with alveolar fibroelastosis (AFE) lesions were systematically evaluated in all cases.

Within areas of typical AFE, the pattern of intra-alveolar fibrosis/fibrotic obliteration was classified as coarse fibrillary if broad hyalinised bundles of collagenous fibres (usually ~2 μm in diameter) were present and as fine fibrillary if delicate, mostly curled fibres were demonstrable. The presence of anthracophages and lymphoid aggregates was noted as well as an increase in cellularity with diffuse infiltration of lymphocytes or the presence of an increased number of mesenchymal cells such as (myo) fibroblasts in the obliterated alveolar lumen (see Figure 1).

In the majority of cases (67%) both coarse and fine fibrillary fibrosis could be detected, in the other cases either only fine fibrillary or only coarse fibrillary fibrosis (20% and 13% respectively) were detectable. Features found regularly in areas of AFE were aggregates of lymphatic cells (73%), often at the leading edge of the remodelling process (see Table 4). These appear well circumscribed, organized in an organoid manner, sometimes contain specialized vessels with the appearance of highly endothelialised venules (HEV) and can be distinguished from a diffuse infiltration of the AFE lesion by lymphatic cells which can be observed in approximately 30–40% of cases. Macrophages containing phagocytosed anthracotic pigment can be detected in 53% of total cases and appear less frequently in patients of the HSCT group (14%). Typical fibroblastic foci (FF) could be detected in 11% of cases. Overall, the areas of AFE showed similar morphological characteristics in all investigated groups. PAC showed overall less cellular mesenchymal (0%) and lymphatic (7%) infiltration when compared to the PPFE and PPFE-like cases (45% and 45% respectively).

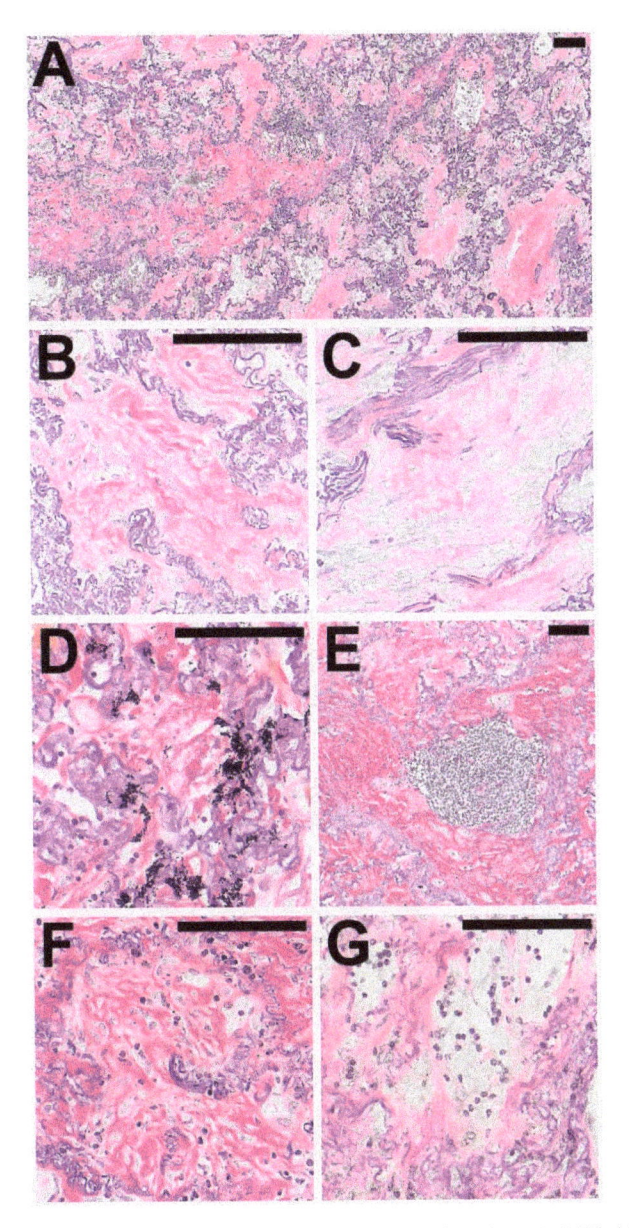

Figure 1. Typical histological patterns of alveolar fibroelastosis (AFE). (**A**) Typical AFE is characterized by a complete obliteration of the alveolar lumen with collagenous material with formation of either coarse (**B**) or fine (**C**) fibrils. In some cases, aggregates of macrophages containing anthracotic pigment can be observed (**D**). Lymphoid aggregates are a common finding in or at the border of AFE lesions (**E**). Increased cellularity with presence of mesenchymal cells (**F**) or lymphocytes (**G**) can be observed in the fibrotic areas to a variable degree. All images are elastic van Gieson stainings. Scale bars are 100 µm each.

We observed and catalogued several morphological patterns in direct spatial association with regions of typical AFE. Besides structurally intact lung parenchyma, various forms of FER with either fibro-elastic expansion of alveolar septa, incomplete alveolar fibrosis, or irregularly distributed collagenous and elastic fibers could be observed (See Figure 2 and Table 3 for a comprehensive list of catalogued features).

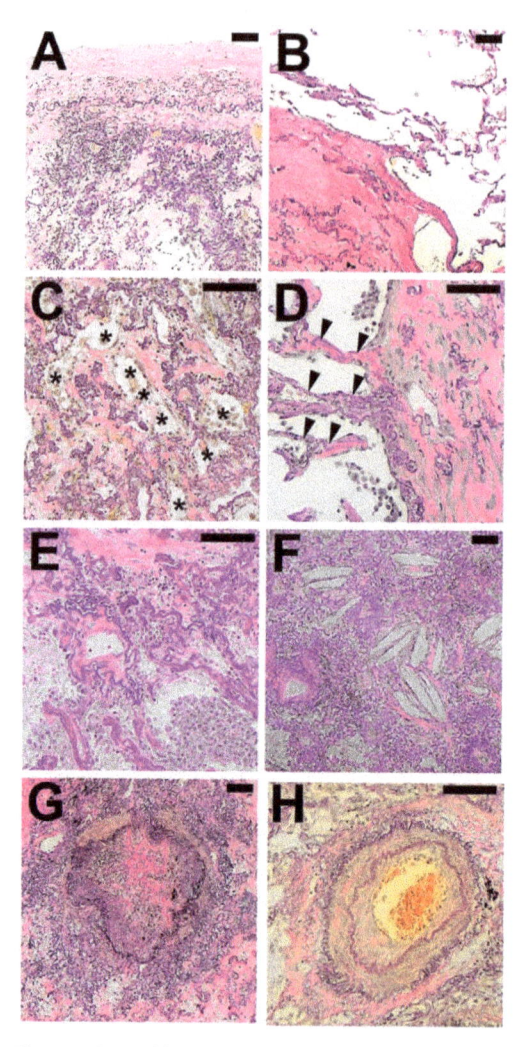

Figure 2. Typical histological patterns in special association with alveolar fibroelastosis (AFE). A set of typical features regularly found in spatial association with AFE: (**A**) Pronounced fibrosis of the visceral pleura. (**B**) Emphysema with an irreversible loss of alveolar septa. (**C**) Elastosis of the alveolar wall with incomplete alveolar fibrosis of the alveolar lumen with residual airspaces lined by cuboidal epithelium (*). (**D**) Fibroelastic interstitial expansion of the alveolar septa adjacent to the AFE lesion. (**E**) Aggregates of intraalveolar macrophages. (**F**) Cholesterol granulomas with multinucleated giant cells with clefts of cholesterol crystals. (**G**) Bronchiolitis obliterans with fibrous obliteration of small airways and (**H**) sclerosis of pulmonary arteries with hypertrophy of the media and intimal hyperplasia. Images are elastic van Gieson stains. Scale bars are 100 μm each.

In the majority of cases (93%) fibroelastic expansion of alveolar septa could be observed at the border of typical AFE besides a direct and abrupt transition to structurally intact alveolar parenchyma (91%). In 84% of cases, areas of incomplete fibroelastosis could be detected. Frequently, pleural fibrosis could be observed adjacent to typical AFE (79%).

Patterns spatially associated with AFE were mostly similar in all cases examined, with the exception of obliterative airway remodelling (bronchiolitis obliterans; BO), which was observed in all cases of CLAD after LTX, and fibrotic pulmonary remodelling following HSCT. BO was also present in half of the PPFE cases but not present in APC.

The compartmental anatomical distribution of the delimitable changes was categorized as subpleural, parabronchial, para-arterial and paraseptal, when AFE was found in association with the respective anatomical structures. Areas of AFE in the parenchyma not associated with the anatomical structures lined out above were classified as "centrolobular" (see Figure 3).

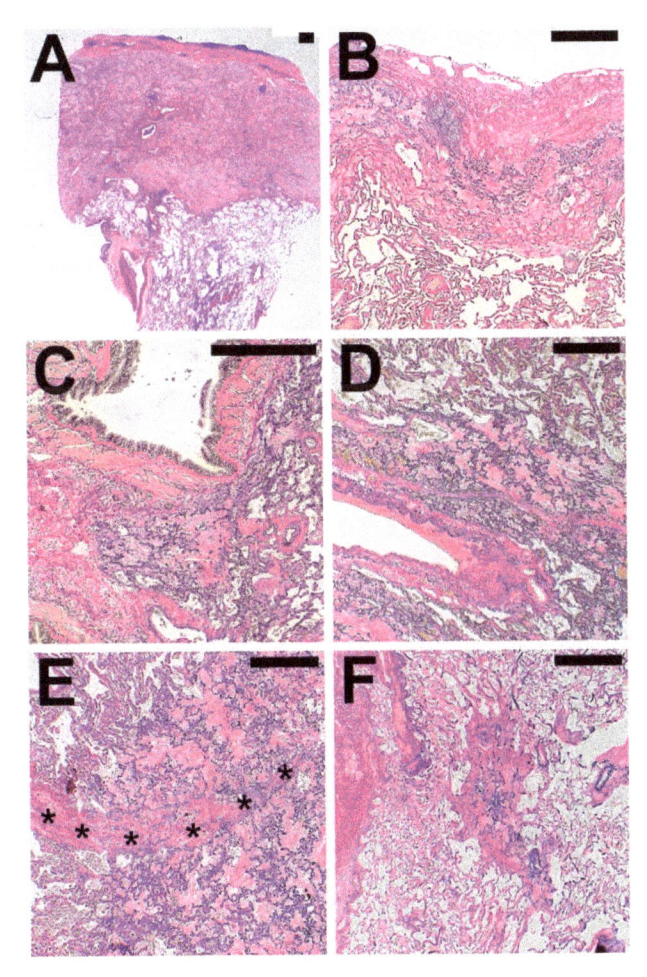

Figure 3. Compartmental distribution of alveolar fibroelastosis (AFE). AFE is commonly found in the subpleural parenchyma (**A**,**B**), in parabronchial (**C**) and paravascular (**D**) distribution and along interlobular septa (*, **E**). When not in association with these structures, we classified the localization as centrolobular (**F**). Images are haematoxylin and eosin (**A**) and elastic van Gieson (**B**–**F**) stains. Scale bars are 500 µm each.

Table 4. Histological characteristics of alveolar fibroelastosis, its surroundings and compartmental distribution.

	Pattern	PAC	CLAD	HSCT	ILD	PPFE	All	PPFE & PPFE-Like
	n =	14	12	7	2	10	45	31
Characteristics of AFE	Fine fibrillary	100	58	57	100	90	80	71
	Coarse fibrillary	71	92	86	100	100	87	94
	Lymphatic aggregates	50	75	67	100	78	67	76
	Mesenchymal cell rich	0	50	43	50	40	31	45
	Lymphocyte rich	7	50	57	0	40	33	45
	Anthracophages	86	58	14	100	60	62	52
	Fibroblast foci	0	0	0	50	30	9	13
Spatially associated patterns	Fibroelastic interstitial expansion	93	83	100	100	100	93	94
	Normal parenchyma	100	92	71	100	90	91	87
	Incomplete alveolar fibrosis	86	75	86	100	90	84	84
	Pulmonal arterial sclerosis	64	92	71	100	90	80	87
	Pleural fibrosis	79	91	100	50	57	79	79
	Emphysema	93	83	43	50	40	69	58
	Bronchiolitis obliterans	0	92	71	0	40	44	65
	Fibroelastotic scar	21	33	14	50	50	31	35
	Macrophage aggregates	21	0	57	50	20	22	23
	Cholesterol granuloma	0	25	33	0	22	16	24
	Nonspecific interstitial pneumonia	0	0	43	0	10	9	13
	Organizing pneumonia	0	8	0	50	0	4	6
	Myogenic metaplasia	7	0	0	50	10	7	6
	Architectural distortion	0	0	0	50	10	5	7
Compartmental distribution	Subpleural	100	91	100	100	90	95	93
	Paraarterial	14	100	100	100	90	71	97
	Paraseptal	8	100	83	100	67	60	85
	Parabronchial	7	50	86	100	90	53	74
	Centrolobular	0	25	14	50	30	18	26

A total of 45 cases were systematically evaluated to assess the characteristics of typical alveolar fibroelastosis (AFE) lesions, the patterns in direct spatial association with the AFE lesion and their compartmental distribution. The cases consisted of so called "pulmonary apical caps" (PAC), chronic lung allograft dysfunction (CLAD) after lung transplantation, pulmonary fibrosis after hematopoetic stem cell transplantation (HSCT), interstitial lung disease (ILD) of other patterns with concomitant AFE and pleuroparenchymal fibroelastosis (PPFE)—either idiopathic or secondary due to autoimmune disease or radio/chemotherapy. Values are given in percentage of positive cases per group, in all 45 investigated in cases and pooled PPFE and PPFE-like cases.

In PAC, the AFE pattern was always found in direct spatial association with the visceral pleura (in not-PAC cases in 93%) and only extended to other compartments in a minority of cases. In contrast to PAC, PPFE and PPFE-like disease showed AFE affection of the para-arterial (97%), paraseptal (85%) and parabronchial (74%) compartments.

Other typical histologic features of ILD such as architectural distortion, myogenic metaplasia or an NSIP pattern are rarely found in direct association with AFE lesions, even if present within the same lung.

Further radiological information was available in 38 (84%) patients. Of these 38 CT scans, 26 (68%) confirmed a main pattern of alveolar fibro-elastosis, in 10 (26%) patients this was a minor pattern and in 2 (5%) remaining patients, there was no radiologic evidence for AFE (see Figure 4 for representative images)

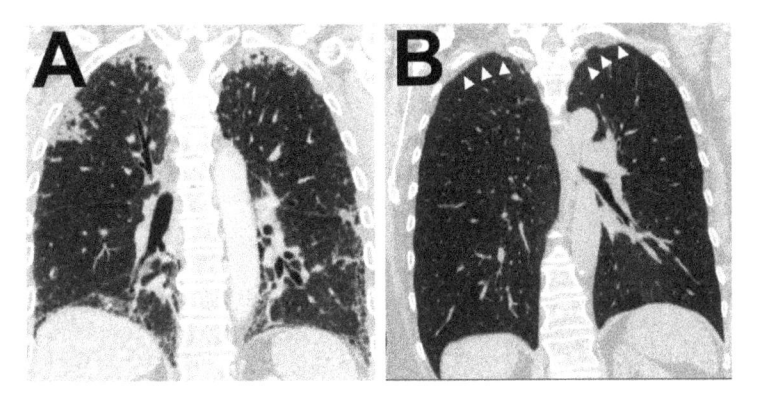

Figure 4. Radiological correlate of AFE Illustration of the two typical radiological patterns accompanying a histologic AFE diagnosis. (**A**). Radiological PPFE pattern with typical (sub)pleural distribution of fibrosis. (**B**) Apical cap.

4. Discussion

FER is has been considered a rather unspecific process in a multitude of diseases for over a century, until Frankel defined FER as the morphological component of a specific form of ILD termed iPPFE. However, some of the patients investigated for their study had received chemotherapy [4] and in the following years we and others identified AFE pattern as sequelae of—amongst other injuries—radiotherapy, LTX and HSCT and also concomitant with other ILD.

In their initial study, Frankel and colleagues used a rather descriptive approach and classified histological features of PPFE without establishing formal criteria. Kusagaya et al. went on to develop criteria, which were then adopted and refined by Thüsen and colleagues in 2013. These not only include intra-alveolar fibrosis and septal elastosis but also comprise a subpleural distribution in the upper lobes with concomitant pleural fibrosis.Therefore, a clear separation of the clinical and histological entities in FER is still lacking and authors often utilize "PPFE" to describe clinical, radiological and histological presentations indiscriminately [3,19]. In addition, authors consistently point out that due to the striking differences in prognosis, PPFE and PAC have to be distinguished, even though i. the histologic patterns of both are very similar and ii. both affect the upper pulmonary compartment and iii. both differ only in some aspects of spatial distribution [16]. Depending on clinical context, manifestations of AFE areassociated with different clinical outcomes (see Figure 5).

PAC are regarded as typically benign lesions in contrast to PPFE with a mean survival time of approximately 24 months [18]. Survival in patients with ILD and concomitant PPFE varies considerably depending on the cohort reported either following the disease trajectory of the underlying ILD or of iPPFE [20,21].

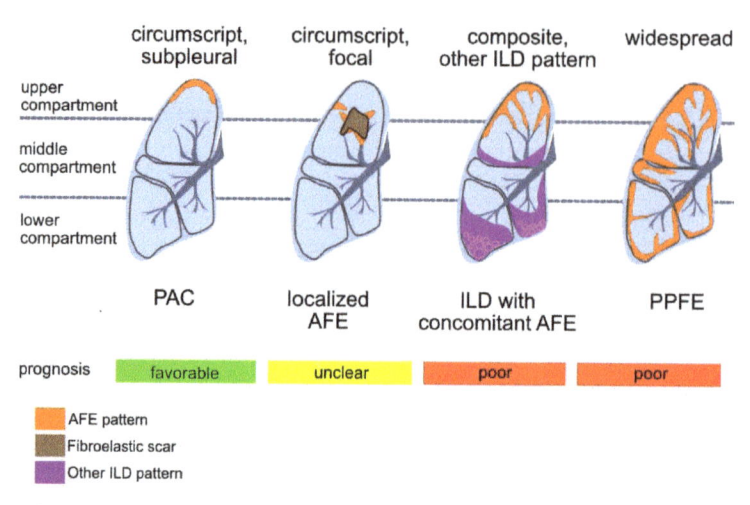

Figure 5. Patterns of compartmental distribution of alveolar fibroelastosis (AFE): AFE is a pattern defined by the typical fibrous obliteration of the alveolar airspace with hyper-elastosis of the preserved alveolar structure. Similar histologic patterns can be observed in a variety of diseases which are distinguishable by a characteristic distribution of the AFE pattern. When AFE is found circumscript in the subpleural parenchyma of the upper lobe without any other indication of interstitial lung disease (ILD), a prognostic favourable pulmonal apical cap (PAC) is the most likely diagnosis. Further, circumscript focal AFE can be found e.g., after radiotherapy and around (unspecific) scars of the lung parenchyma. When found in association with other ILD patterns (e.g., usual interstitial pneumonia, UIP) the prognosis of the patient may be worse than when concomitant AFE is not found. AFE as dominant pattern with subpleural, parabronchial and paraseptal distribution and accentuation in the upper compartments of the lung is indicative of pleuroparenchymal fibroelastosis (PPFE), a rare ILD with poor prognosis.

To separate the clinical from the histological presentation, the term AFE was coined, describing the typical histological pattern of collagenous effacement of the alveolar spaces with accompanying hyperelastosis of the remodelled alveolar walls [15,16]. In our present study, we provide a systematic review of cases with AFE pattern histology to comprehensively document the features, distribution and pulmonary surroundings of AFE. To this end, we have employed a pattern-based approach, assessing AFE indiscriminately of its respective manifestation.

4.1. Features in AFE

The AFE-defining features of intra-alveolar fibrosis and septal elastosis were present in all patient groups. However, we noticed a difference in the cellular composition with an increase of lymphatic and mesenchymal cells embedded in the AFE of approximately half PPFE and PPFE-like cases, a feature we could not observe in PAC. This might point towards different states of activity within AFE lesions. Further studies are required to determine if cellularity can be used as prognostic marker. The low cellularity of AFE lesions in ILD cases with concomitant AFE is likely due to the low number of cases included in this study and typical lymphocytic inflammation could be observed in fibrotic (non-AFE) remodelled parenchyma (see Supplemental Figure S1).

Anthracophages, however, were frequently encountered in PAC, PPFE and PPFE-like cases, especially in older patients, pointing towards entrapment of otherwise innocent bystanders in the fibrotic process, unlike in other ILD, where exposure to small particles is known to be a causative agent.

The presence of FF in AFE has been pointed out in several studies. Frankel et al. reported them to be rare (4). Kusagaya et al. [22] described them as appearing in "small numbers" and Von der Thüsen et al. finally as "at most in small numbers" [23]. In our study, FF can be observed in 13% of cases. Increased detection of FF in other studies could be explained by a systematic bias of the respective authors in what they consider to qualify as FF. Unlike in UIP, groups of (myo) fibroblasts observed in AFE do not readily form classical FF with perpendicularly aligned (myo) fibroblasts, embedded in an immature, myxoid extracellular matrix and accompanied by hyperplastic type 2 pneumocytes. The presence of fully formed, typical FF should, therefore, prompt the pathologist to consider AFE concomitant to another ILD.

4.2. Features Surrounding AFE

Incomplete AFE is very common in close spatial proximity to AFE lesions and should possibly be interpreted as an equivalent to typical AFE in the context of the clinical setting. So far it is unclear whether incomplete AFE represents an incomplete transitional state or a premature consolidation. Emphysematous and even inconspicuous alveolar parenchyma can be often observed in direct proximity to AFE lesions, which typically expand with a "pushing border" aspect into the adjacent lung. Pleural fibrosis is common and can easily be recognized. However, it is present in only about 79% of cases and should not be considered as a mandatory criterion for establishing the diagnosis.

Pulmonary arterial sclerosis is common in AFE lesions or in their close proximity both in patients with PPFE, PPFE-like disease and PAC. Some authors have suggested pulmonary arteriolosclerosis and the resulting ventilation-perfusion disparity as a trigger of AFE-type fibrosis [24].

BO is commonly found in close proximity to AFE lesions in CLAD and following HSCT, where it has long been recognized as a defining feature of the disease. In the context of PPFE-like disease, our recent study on fibrotic airway remodelling points towards shared pathways in BO and AFE development [15].

AFOP and intraalveolar macrophage aggregates can be observed in some cases. These features have been proposed to represent a transitory step in the formation of AFE [15]. The rather infrequent detection in our cohort may be explained by a temporal bias with the majority of cases being end-stage lung disease, in which AFE lesions have already consolidated. This is in agreement with a report by Von der Thüsen et al. which described AFOP in 38% of their explanted lungs following redo transplantation [23].

4.3. Compartmental Distribution of AFE

In our study, AFE pattern fibrosis was most commonly found in the subpleural compartment, compatible with current literature [14]. However, when excluding PAC from the analysis, AFE pattern fibrosis is also found para-arterial and para-septal in 80% of patients and para-bronchial in two-thirds of cases. This indicates that these compartments are also commonly affected in PPFE (and PPFE-like) ILD, which has a significant impact on patient survival when compared to PAC. These findings are relevant as they indicate that AFE found in other than subpleural compartments should not preclude the diagnosis of PPFE or PPFE-like disease. Moreover, the subpleural parenchyma can only be accessed by open, but not by conventional transbronchial lung biopsy. However, relevant AFE can be detected in a sufficiently large transbronchial cryobiopsy specimen [13] because fibroelastic changes extend along bronchovascular bundles and interlobular septae. Nonetheless, data regarding the sensitivity of transbronchial biopsies for diagnosing AFE is currently not available for larger patient collectives.

5. Conclusions

i. Cardinal features of AFE are collagenous effacement of the alveolar spaces with accompanying hyperelastosis of remodelled alveolar walls and ii. pleural fibrosis does not represent a condition sine qua non for the diagnosis. iii. Incomplete AFE has to be considered an equivalent lesion to typical AFE, provided an appropriate clinical setting. iv. FF are not a typical feature of AFE and should raise suspicion of a concomitant lung injury pattern, such as UIP. AFE is commonly distributed along the visceral pleura, the bronchovascular bundles and the paraseptal parenchyma, and compartmental involvement can give an indication towards the identification of the underlying disease. vi. The previously proposed, step-wise progression model of AFE from initial fibrinous exudation, over macrophage-rich, insufficient resolution to fully developed AFE has possibly to be complemented by active and inactive AFE, according to the intra-alveolar cellularity in the remodelled alveolar spaces.

Outlook

The exact definition of what makes up AFE is important, not only to help to identify the underlying diseases and therefore specific treatment options, but also to stratify patients and predict their individual outcome. Moreover, the systematic application of exact histological criteria is needed as a basis for all morpho-molecular studies in order to gain further insights into the mechanisms of pulmonary FER.

Supplementary Materials: The following are available online at https://www.mdpi.com/article/10.3390/cells10061362/s1, Figure S1: ILD with concomitant alveolar fibroelastosis, Table S1: Detailed patient information.

Author Contributions: P.B. and D.J. conceptualized the Study. P.B., C.W. and I.M. systematically assessed histology cases. P.B., C.W., I.M., S.E.V., F.L. and D.J. reviewed the histology scoring. S.D. reviewed radiological images. J.G. and G.W. treated the patients. All authors gave critical feedback on the manuscript. All authors have read and agreed to the published version of the manuscript.

Funding: Sonderforschungsbereich, "SFB" 738 (Projekt B9) of the German Research Foundation to Danny Jonigk. The grants of the European Research Council (ERC); European Consolidator Grant, XHale to Danny Jonigk (ref. no. 771883).

Institutional Review Board Statement: The study was approved by the local ethics committee. See materials and methods.

Informed Consent Statement: Patients provided informed consent for scientific investigation.

Data Availability Statement: Datasets are freely available upon request.

Acknowledgments: The authors thank Regina Engelhardt, Annette Mueller Brechlin and Christina Petzold for their excellent technical support and Harshit Shah and Mark Kühnel for editing the manuscript.

Conflicts of Interest: The authors declare no conflict of interest.

References

1. Parra, E.R.; Kairalla, R.A.; De Carvalho, C.R.R.; Capelozzi, V.L. Abnormal deposition of collagen/elastic vascular fibres and prognostic significance in idiopathic interstitial pneumonias. *Thorax* **2007**, *62*, 428–437. [CrossRef] [PubMed]
2. Wynn, T.A.; Ramalingam, T.R. Mechanisms of fibrosis: Therapeutic translation for fibrotic disease. *Nat. Med. Nat. Publ. Group* **2012**, *18*, 1028–1040. [CrossRef] [PubMed]
3. Rosenbaum, J.N.; Butt, Y.M.; Johnson, K.A.; Meyer, K.; Batra, K.; Kanne, J.P.; Torrealba, J.R. Pleuroparenchymal fibroelastosis: A pattern of chronic lung injury. *Hum. Pathol.* **2015**, *46*, 137–146. [CrossRef] [PubMed]
4. Frankel, S.K.; Cool, C.D.; Lynch, D.A.; Brown, K.K. Idiopathic Pleuroparenchymal Fibroelastosis. *Chest* **2004**, *126*, 2007–2013. [CrossRef] [PubMed]
5. Travis, W.D.; Costabel, U.; Hansell, D.M.; King, T.E.; Lynch, D.A.; Nicholson, A.G.; Ryerson, C.J.; Ryu, J.H.; Selman, M.; Wells, A.U.; et al. An Official American Thoracic Society/European Respiratory Society Statement: Update of the International Multidisciplinary Classification of the Idiopathic Interstitial Pneumonias. *Am. J. Respir. Crit. Care Med.* **2013**, *188*, 733–748. [CrossRef] [PubMed]
6. Khiroya, R.; Macaluso, C.; Montero, M.A.; Wells, A.U.; Chua, F.; Kokosi, M.; Devaraj, A.; Rice, A.; Renzoni, E.A.; Nicholson, A.G. Pleuroparenchymal Fibroelastosis Between Histologic Parameters and Survival. *Am. J. Surg. Pathol.* **2017**, *41*, 1683–1689. [CrossRef] [PubMed]
7. Ofek, E.; Sato, M.; Saito, T.; Wagnetz, U.; Roberts, H.C.; Chaparro, C.; Waddell, T.K.; Singer, L.G.; Hutcheon, M.A.; Keshavjee, S.; et al. Restrictive allograft syndrome post lung transplantation is characterized by pleuroparenchymal fibroelastosis. *Mod. Pathol. Nat. Publ. Group* **2013**, *26*, 350–356. [CrossRef] [PubMed]
8. Fujikura, Y.; Kanoh, S.; Kouzaki, Y.; Hara, Y.; Matsubara, O.; Kawana, A. Pleuroparenchymal Fibroelastosis as a Series of Airway Complications Associated with Chronic Graft-versus-host Disease following Allogeneic Bone Marrow Transplantation. *Intern. Med.* **2014**, *53*, 43–46. [CrossRef] [PubMed]

9. Okimoto, T.; Tsubata, Y.; Hamaguchi, M.; Sutani, A.; Hamaguchi, S.; Isobe, T. Pleuroparenchymal fibroelastosis after haematopoietic stem cell transplantation without graft-versus-host disease findings. *Respirol. Case Rep.* **2018**, *6*, e00298. [CrossRef] [PubMed]
10. Greer, M.; Riise, G.C.; Hansson, L.; Perch, M.; Hämmäinen, P.; Roux, A.; Hirschi, S.; Lhuillier, E.; Reynaud-Gaubert, M.; Philit, F.; et al. Dichotomy in pulmonary graft-versus-host disease evident among allogeneic stem-cell transplant recipients undergoing lung transplantation. *Eur. Respir. J.* **2016**, *48*, 1807–1810. [CrossRef] [PubMed]
11. Ishii, T.; Bandoh, S.; Kanaji, N.; Tadokoro, A.; Watanabe, N.; Imataki, O.; Dobashi, H.; Kushida, Y.; Haba, R.; Yokomise, H. Air-leak Syndrome by Pleuroparenchymal Fibroelastosis after Bone Marrow Transplantation. *Intern. Med.* **2016**, *55*, 105–111. [CrossRef]
12. Watanabe, K. Pleuroparenchymal Fibroelastosis: Its Clinical Characteristics. *Curr. Respir. Med. Rev.* **2013**, *9*, 229–237. [CrossRef] [PubMed]
13. Kronborg-White, S.; Ravaglia, C.; Dubini, A.; Piciucchi, S.; Tomassetti, S.; Bendstrup, E.; Poletti, V. Cryobiopsies are diagnostic in Pleuroparenchymal and Airway-centered Fibroelastosis. *Respir. Res.* **2018**, *19*, 1–7. [CrossRef] [PubMed]
14. Cheng, S.K.H.; Chuah, K.L. Pleuroparenchymal fibroelastosis of the lung: A review. *Arch. Pathol. Lab. Med.* **2016**, *140*, 849–853. [CrossRef] [PubMed]
15. Jonigk, D.; Rath, B.; Borchert, P.; Braubach, P.; Maegel, L.; Izykowski, N.; Warnecke, G.; Sommer, W.; Kreipe, H.; Blach, R.; et al. Comparative analysis of morphological and molecular motifs in bronchiolitis obliterans and alveolar fibroelastosis after lung and stem cell transplantation. *J. Pathol. Clin. Res.* **2016**, *3*, 17–28. [CrossRef] [PubMed]
16. Reddy, T.L.; Tominaga, M.; Hansell, D.M.; Von Der Thusen, J.; Rassl, D.; Parfrey, H.; Guy, S.; Twentyman, O.; Rice, A.; Maher, T.M.; et al. Pleuroparenchymal fibroelastosis: A spectrum of histopathological and imaging phenotypes. *Eur. Respir. J.* **2012**, *40*, 377–385. [CrossRef] [PubMed]
17. Lagstein, A. Pulmonary apical cap-what's old is new again. *Arch. Pathol. Lab. Med.* **2015**, *139*, 1258–1262. [CrossRef] [PubMed]
18. Chua, F.; Desai, S.R.; Nicholson, A.G.; Renzoni, E.; Rice, A.; Wells, A.U. Pleuroparenchymal Fibroelastosis. A Review of Clinical, Radiological, and Pathological Characteristics. *Ann. Ats* **2019**, *16*, 1351–1359. [CrossRef] [PubMed]
19. Kinoshita, Y.; Watanabe, K.; Ishii, H.; Kushima, H.; Hamasaki, M.; Fujita, M.; Nabeshima, K. Pleuroparenchymal fibroelastosis as a histological background of autoimmune diseases. *Virchows Arch.* **2018**, *474*, 97–104. [CrossRef] [PubMed]
20. Oda, T.; Ogura, T.; Kiatamura, H.; Hagiware, E.; Baba, T.; Enomoto, Y.; Iwasawa, T.; Okudela, K.; Takemura, T.; Sakai, F.; et al. Distinct Characteristics of Pleuroparenchymal Fibroelastosis With Usual Interstitial Pneumonia Compared with Idiopathic Pulmonary Fibrosis. *Chest* **2014**, *146*, 1248–1255. [CrossRef] [PubMed]
21. Tanizawa, K.; Handa, T.; Kubo, T.; Chen-Yoshikawa, T.F.; Aoyama, A.; Motoyama, H.; Hijiya, K.; Yoshizawa, T.; Oshima, Y.; Ikezoe, K.; et al. Clinical significance of radiological pleuroparenchymal fibroelastosis pattern in interstitial lung disease patients registered for lung transplantation: A retrospective cohort study. *Respir. Res.* **2018**, *19*, 162. [CrossRef] [PubMed]
22. Kusagaya, H.; Nakamura, Y.; Kono, M.; Kaida, Y.; Kuroishi, S.; Enomoto, N.; Fujisawa, T.; Koshimizu, N.; Yokomura, K.; Inui, N.; et al. Idiopathic pleuroparenchymal fibroelastosis: Consideration of a clinicopathological entity in a series of Japanese patients. *BMC Pulm Med.* **2012**, *5*, 72. [CrossRef] [PubMed]
23. Von der Thüsen, J.H. Pleuroparenchymal Fibroelastosis: Its Pathological Characteristics. *Curr. Respir. Med. Rev.* **2013**, *9*, 238–247. [CrossRef] [PubMed]
24. Zhang, S.; Xie, W.; Wang, Z.; Tian, Y.; Da, J.; Zhai, Z. Pleuroparenchymal fibroelastosis secondary to autologous hematopoietic stem cell transplantation: A case report. *Exp. Ther. Med.* **2019**, *17*, 2557–2560. [CrossRef] [PubMed]